HERBAL REMEDIES

Herbal Remedies

A Quick and Easy Guide to Common Disorders and Their Herbal Treatments

Asa Hershoff, N.D.
Andrea Rotelli, N.D.

Avery
a member of
Penguin Putnam Inc.
New York

Every effort has been made to ensure that the information contained in this book is complete and accurate. However, neither the publisher nor the author is engaged in rendering professional advice or services to the individual reader. The ideas, procedures, and suggestions contained in this book are not intended as a substitute for consulting with your health practitioner. All matters regarding health require supervision by a health professional. Neither the author nor the publisher shall be liable or responsible for any loss, injury, or damage allegedly arising from any information or suggestion in this book.

a member of
Penguin Group (USA) Inc.
375 Hudson Street
New York, NY 10014
www.penguin.com

Published simultaneously in Canada

Library of Congress Cataloging-in-Publication Data

Hershoff, Asa, date.
Herbal remedies : a quick and easy guide to common disorders and their herbal treatments / Asa Hershoff, Andrea Rotelli.
p. cm
Includes bibliographical references and index.
ISBN 0-89529-949-6
1. Herbs—Therapeutic use. I. Rotelli, Andrea. II. Title.

RM666.H33 H476 2001 00-066508
615'.321—dc21

Printed in the United States of America
10 9 8 7 6

This book is printed on acid-free paper. ♾

Book design by Asa Hershoff

To Our Mothers
Carol and Henrietta

Contents

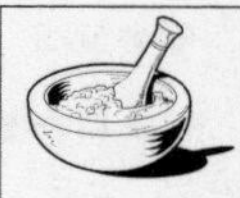

1. How to Use Herbs

2. Body Systems

3. A-Z Herbal Prescriber

4. Herbal Sources, Dosage & Safety

5. Herbal Resources

PREFACE

Herbal medicine has gone from fringe to mainstream. It has changed from the exclusive realm of zealous health seekers in natural food stores to mainstream consumers in supermarkets and drugstores everywhere. Everyone is jumping on the herb bandwagon. Yet though there are many herbal texts on the market, this book is a pioneering effort. It is the answer to a problem arising in my own clinical practice of 26 years, and while lecturing and teaching natural medicine around the world to both doctors and the general public alike. I simply have been unable to find or to recommend a quick and easy guide to the effective use of herbs for a variety of conditions.

Most herb books require an intense study of each plant, and information about the treatment of a specific condition is scanty at best. With no models to follow, this book took thousands of hours of painstaking work on the part of Dr. Rotelli and myself to put together all the pieces of information scattered in hundreds of books, articles and research. What we created, I believe, is the most accurate, useful and user-friendly herb book available. The information here is as current and accurate as possible, yet avoids unnecessary jargon or pharmacological terminology, making it suitable for both professionals and lay people.

I designed and laid out the book similarly to my previous work, *Homeopathic Remedies* (Avery 1999), as it provided an extremely easy-to-use and accessible format. Almost a hundred of my own line drawings are included, so that the whole book is visually appealing and readable. Each condition has a two-page format—since I personally dislike having to turn pages to find information!

Today, in discussing herbs, one can err on two sides. Some authors ignore thousands of years of clinical herbal experience, feeling that even one poorly designed piece of modern research is superior to traditional knowledge. The German Commission E, so highly touted in herbal circles, falls into this category. On the other hand, exaggerated claims or unfounded statements are equally misleading about the strengths and limitations of herbal medicine. We hope that this book takes a middle path. It comes from practicing naturopathic physicians, not researchers, writers or herbal spokespeople. Our own tradition stretches back to the very roots of the ancient healing arts, and it is our commitment to follow this path with integrity and diligence. We love and respect plants deeply and feel fortunate to be able to apply this knowledge to help others in a world that is so badly in need of healing.

Asa Hershoff & Andrea Rotelli

New York

USING THIS BOOK

Part 1. How to Use Herbs

The first part of this book contains basic information about herbal medicines necessary for prescribing for oneself or for treating others.

- Herbal principles provide a framework for understanding and using herbs. These ideas are not mere theory, but objective principles and accurate perceptions of how biological healing works, i.e., how the body heals itself and how herbs enable this process.
- These ideas and observations are based on the experience of millions of healing practitioners and their patients across time and space.
- While they are a reliable guide to the intelligent use of herbs, these concepts are not complex, esoteric or obscure. Quite the contrary, they are simple and almost self-evident, as any truth should be.

Part 2. Body Systems

- The body has separate and distinct systems of organs and tissues. Though powerfully interrelated, each system performs unique and highly specialized functions in the organism, and each has its own needs.
- The traditional studies of anatomy, physiology, disease and treatment have all been done according to body systems, such as the digestive, respiratory, nervous and immune systems.
- The Body Systems section, beginning on page 51, follows this same classification, but also includes a number of "condition categories" such as Infections, Trauma, and Detoxification.
- This section can serve as a visual summary and rapid reference for locating a health problem and its herbal solution.
- For each system, there is a general discussion, followed by a description of the conditions detailed in this book in Part 3.
- A diagram of the system (or condition category) is included, showing the specific illnesses discussed in this book and their corresponding herbs. A page number is shown under each of these conditions, leading you to a full discussion of the illness in the A-Z Herbal Prescriber.

There is a further advantage to Body Systems. An individual often does not fit neatly into any one single disease category, and because of this, a large percentage of chronic conditions are never properly diagnosed. Looking at body systems helps get around this problem. Any named condition or disease should be interpreted in the broadest possible sense. For example, the herbs listed under Memory Loss apply to problems as simple as poor performance in school or business to Alzheimer's disease.

BODY SYSTEMS

NERVOUS SYSTEM

The System

The intricate system of nerves that interweaves throughout the body provides constant surveillance and regulation of many thousands of body functions on a moment-to-moment and long-term basis.

BRAIN
- The brain handles incoming sensory and outgoing motor commands.
- A hierarchy of developmental layers regulates automatic acts, such as breathing, and complex pathways for thought and feeling.

SPINAL NERVES
- The spinal cord transmits signals from the periphery to the brain and vice versa, or travels directly in a reflex arc from sense organ to muscle.
- Sensory nerves transmit sensations like pain and heat to the brain.
- The motor nerves transmit impulses from the brain to muscles for conscious movement, but are also the medium for spasms or cramps.

AUTONOMIC SYSTEM
- The autonomic nervous system regulates all the "unconscious" systems of the body, such as breathing, circulation, digestion and elimination.
- It has two opposing systems: the sympathetic and parasympathetic.
- The sympathetic or "fight or flight" system shuts down digestion and prepares for action, increasing blood pressure and adrenal activity.
- The parasympathetic system promotes digestion, relaxes muscles and improves metabolism, reducing blood flow to the periphery.
- Imbalances between these two systems are part of many disease syndromes, including asthma, colitis, anxiety and stress disorders.

Herbal Approaches

HEADACHE
- Herbal treatment can provide non-toxic pain relief for tension or migraine headache and reduce the frequency and intensity of attacks
- They help address related toxic, circulatory or hormonal imbalances.

INSOMNIA
- Herbs are a gentle and non-addictive treatment for inducing sleep.
- With time, nervine plants can help underlying stress patterns.

MEMORY LOSS
- Herbs can improve brain circulation and metabolism in the aged.
- They also help with overall mental performance and concentration.

PAIN/NEURALGIA
- Herbal medicines have direct sedative and analgesic properties.
- They also help with related inflammation, muscle spasm and anxiety.

54

The System

A brief overview of the anatomy and function of each body system and its component parts are given. This conveys an understanding of its relation to health and disease.

Icon

The icon shown here also appears in each condition within the Herbal Prescriber that is related to that body system. These conditions are also listed below.

Herbal Approaches

Here a summary is given of the value and usefulness of herbal treatment for each condition that will be dealt with in the A-Z Herbal Prescriber.

Body System

The usual name for the system heads the page. Condition categories such as Detoxification and Trauma are included.

Conditions

The most common problems in this body system—those detailed in the A-Z Herbal Prescriber section—head the top of each herb list.

Herbal Medicines

A summarized list of the herbs that will be discussed in detail in the Prescriber section is given here.

Page Reference

The listed page takes you to a detailed look at the condition in the A-Z Herbal Prescriber.

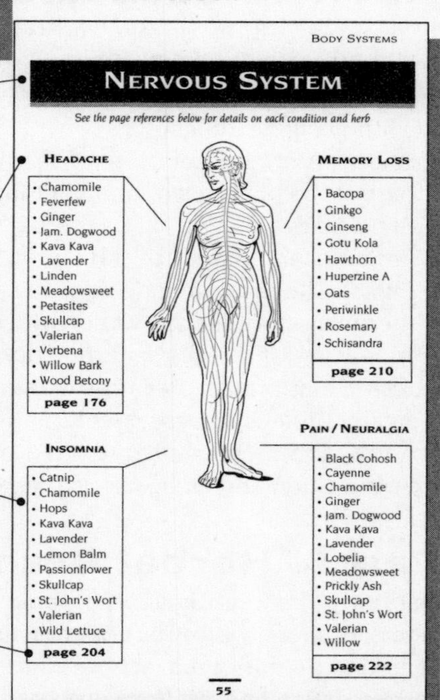

BODY SYSTEMS

NERVOUS SYSTEM

See the page references below for details on each condition and herb

HEADACHE
- Chamomile
- Feverfew
- Ginger
- Jam. Dogwood
- Kava Kava
- Lavender
- Linden
- Meadowsweet
- Petasites
- Skullcap
- Valerian
- Verbena
- Willow Bark
- Wood Betony

page 176

MEMORY LOSS
- Bacopa
- Ginkgo
- Ginseng
- Gotu Kola
- Hawthorn
- Huperzine A
- Oats
- Periwinkle
- Rosemary
- Schisandra

page 210

INSOMNIA
- Catnip
- Chamomile
- Hops
- Kava Kava
- Lavender
- Lemon Balm
- Passionflower
- Skullcap
- St. John's Wort
- Valerian
- Wild Lettuce

page 204

PAIN / NEURALGIA
- Black Cohosh
- Cayenne
- Chamomile
- Ginger
- Jam. Dogwood
- Kava Kava
- Lavender
- Lobelia
- Meadowsweet
- Prickly Ash
- Skullcap
- St. John's Wort
- Valerian
- Willow

page 222

55

Part 3. A-Z Herbal Prescriber

Apart from looking in the Body Systems section, the easiest way to find the condition or illness that concerns you is through the main section of the book, the A-Z Herbal Prescriber. This alphabetical list of conditions allows one to quickly see what herbal medicines can do for a variety of common problems like fibromyalgia, headache, ADD and so on.

- The condition pages in the Prescriber list the ten to fifteen most important herbs used for each problem, disease or symptom complex.
- Herbs are listed by their commonly used name, followed by their Latin name. Sometimes an additional common name is listed as well.
- The effects of each herb *for that condition* are described, making for easy selection. More information about that herb for other conditions can be found by checking the herb's listing in the index.
- The Herbal Reading List also contains recommended books (with three asterisks***) for learning more about individual herbs.
- Cross-references are provided at the end of each condition page so that one can look up a closely related or contributing problem.
- An icon in the margin of each page indicates the body system involved, which helps in both finding the right condition and cross-referencing it to similar problems.

Part 4. Herbal Sources, Dosage & Safety

To avoid repetition, dosage and safety information is not given for each herb in the A-Z Herbal Prescriber. Instead, this data is grouped in a separate section, where the herbs are listed alphabetically. Each herb has the following headings:

- *Sources*: A brief description of the herb is given, which may include the part of the plant used, the plant family, its history and effects.
- *Standardization*: For those herbs that have been standardized, the amounts and names of standardized ingredients are shown.
- *Dosage*: The recommended dosage for capsules, tinctures or other commonly available forms are provided. Note that this information varies widely and thus following directions on the bottle is useful.
- *Safety*: Important precautions and safety notes are described here. Again, there is disagreement on the relative safety and toxicity of some herbs, and we have tried to strike a reasonable balance between excessive caution and overzealous prescribing.

Part 5. Herbal Resources & Index

Naturally, the index is another rapid way to find cross-references to specific conditions, herbs (by common names) or herbal effects. A brief guide to herbal practitioners, schools and products is included, in addition to an Herbal Reading List that serves as an excellent resource for herbal books.

A-Z HERBAL PRESCRIBER

HERBAL REMEDIES

ADD / ADHD

Select the herbs that are most suitable for your condition.

Kava Kava

The Herbal Approach

Attention deficit disorder and hyperactivity are the epidemic of our age, but current treatment is woefully inadequate. While our society wages an ongoing "war on drugs," millions of small children are hooked on "speed" in the form of Ritalin and amphetamines. Apart from serious and permanent side effects, these do not remotely address underlying causes, and can in no way be regarded as a cure. Diagnoses such as learning disability, hyperactivity, poor impulse control, etc., are usually attributed to a brain chemistry imbalance. A better term might be "toxic brain syndrome," since the overriding factor is a constant bombardment of the child's nervous system with pesticides, mercury, lead, food additives, artificial sweeteners, vaccines, antibiotics and allergenic foods. Each one of these factors has been shown to significantly and profoundly impact developing brain cells, and combine together with devastating effect.

A full-scale assault on these problems requires a homeopathic, herbal and nutritional program to undo the developmental and biological damage caused by chronic exposure to toxins. Herbs have the short term gain of relaxing and calming, while improving brain function and neurotransmitter production. In the long run, nervine and adaptogenic plants can protect, detoxify and heal the nervous system—all without the significant toxicity or side effects of drugs. See also ▪ Anxiety ▪ Fatigue ▪ Insomnia ▪ Depression ▪ Memory ▪ Stress.

Bacopa**—Brahmi/Bacopa monnieri
- Calming and sedative. Improves anxiety; important for hyperactivity.
- Improves intellectual capacity, acuity, clarity of thought, concentration.
- Improves memory, especially in the elderly; shortens learning time.

California Poppy***—Eschscholtzia californica
- A gentle sedative that relieves psychological and emotional disturbances in kids. Soothes and balances an overactive nervous system.
- Reduces anxiety and tension in overactive states, decreases spasms.
- Effective for difficulty in falling asleep or frequent, regular waking.

Catnip*—Nepeta cataria
- Relieves anxiety, restlessness, tension, stress and hyperactivity.
- A mild relaxant that promotes restful sleep. Helps diarrhea, headache, colic or stomach ache due to stress. Balances mood swings or hysteria.

92

Condition

Each condition is displayed in the header. They should be interpreted broadly, i.e., herbs for attention deficit disorder also help anyone with concentration, attention or learning problems.

The Herbal Approach

After a brief introduction to the condition and some of its causes, from a holistic viewpoint, the herbal approach to its treatment and cure is discussed.

Cross-References

Other conditions discussed in the book are cross-referenced for a broader range of useful herbs.

PSYCHOLOGICAL STATES

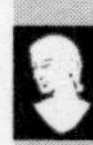

Ginkgo**—Ginkgo biloba
- Improves focus, memory, cognition, knowledge retention, perception.
- Increases neurotransmitters, boosts the brain's ability to use oxygen.
- Increases circulation to brain; High in nutritive antioxidants that protects the brain and nervous system from damage by various toxins.

Grape Seed Extract***—Vitis vinifera
- Contains bioflavonoids with the most potent antioxidant effects known.
- Able to cross the blood brain barrier and directly protect the brain against a wide variety of toxins and damaging free radicals.
- Improves brain blood flow, strengthens brain capillaries.

Hops**—Humulus lupulus
- Indicated for nervous tension, excitability, restlessness and irritability.
- Excellent for insomnia, taken orally or as a hops and lavender pillow.
- Calms and improves the mood, but should be avoided in depression.
- Strengthens and stimulates digestion, relieves intestinal discomfort.

Kava Kava**—Piper methysticum
- Valuable in attention deficit disorder; relieves anxiety without any cognitive or mental impairment. Reduces insomnia, tension and stress.
- Produces a sense of tranquility and softens angry or violent feelings.
- Significantly improves mood, tension level and sleep patterns.

Lemon Balm**—Melissa officinalis
- A gentle, safe and calming children's herb for depression and anxiety.
- Relaxes the nervous system; eases agitation while soothing digestion.

Oats***—Avena sativa
- Nervous system tonic and nutritive; for mental stress, nervousness, overwork, exhaustion, weakness. Improves mental concentration, focus.
- Eases stress, tension, depression, insomnia—but improves clarity.
- Excellent for transitioning and weaning off neurological medications.

Skullcap**—Scutellaria laterifolia
- Helps anxiety, restlessness, crying spells, irritability and nervousness.
- A useful daytime sedative, with no mental impairment or drowsiness.
- Nervine action relieves frequent headaches, relaxes muscular spasms.

St. John's Wort***—Hypericum perforatum
- An herb of choice for attention deficit or hyperactive children.
- Calms an agitated nervous system, yet safe for long term usage.
- Regulates mood and attention, relieves feelings of sadness, apathy, low self-esteem, isolation, anger, guilt, shame. Good for nervous exhaustion.

Valerian***—Valeriana officinalis
- Relaxing and sedating, reduces restlessness, nervousness, improves sleep; should be taken for 2-4 weeks to improve mood and sleep.
- Shows improvements in learning skills, with less aggressive behavior.

93

Individual Herbs

Herbs are arranged alphabetically by their common name, followed by their Latin name. Then indications are given for the use of each herb in treating the condition at hand.

Grading System

Each herb name is followed by one to three asterisks (*), to convey its relative usefulness for treating the condition.

Icon

A visual key indicates the body system involved and provides a cross-referenced index to related conditions in the book.

Part 1

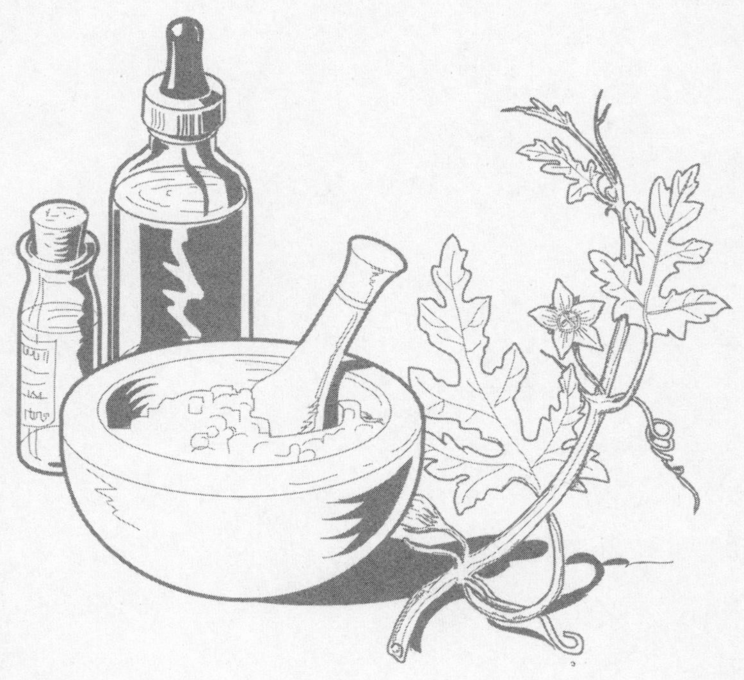

How to Use Herbs

THE WORLD OF PLANTS

It is difficult to truly appreciate the immense role that plants play in our lives. All forms of food and even the air we breathe are by-products of plant life. Plants provide fuel, clothing, lumber, furniture, paints and resins, perfumes, colorants, cosmetics, spices—a seemingly endless flow of essential and practical tools for everyday living. Apart from the material ways that plants support us, they also provide the background for endless recreation and enjoyment. Human ingenuity has found further ways to enhance our homes and cities with parks, landscaping and ornamental gardens. Plants continually refresh us with their beauty and inspiration. In their deepest aspect, they reconnect us with our spiritual core and our sense of the pervasive intelligence and wholeness of nature.

A special aspect of our relationship to plants are the healing herbs. Disease and infirmity are an intrinsic part of existence, and the search for efficient and effective ways to deal with these problems has occupied a large amount of humanity's time and effort. The most readily available and successful medicines have proved to be, since time immemorial, the herbs, grasses, trees, fungi and living plants that surround us. The ancient beginnings of herbal medicine are a matter of speculation. The modern perspective is that primitive peoples, by observing animals and through trial and error, eventually came to understand the medicinal use of plants over the centuries and millennia. The other view, held by most traditional societies, is that plant knowledge came through divine inspiration or revelation—a gift from God or the gods. The answer likely lies between these two extremes. Humans have far more intuition and sensitivity than we moderns realize, and "primitive" people were much more discriminating and inventive than we give them credit for being. Whatever the real story is, the systematic use of plants and the expertise to use them has developed among people everywhere.

Yet after several thousand years as an integral part of our lives, plant medicines were suddenly submerged by the scientific and economic phenomena of the pharmaceutical revolution of the 20th century. Today they have gained a new focus—like a long lost friend who has come home to take his rightful place in the community. Still, plant medicines are different things to different people. Some see herbs as glorified drugs, repositories of biochemistry and active ingredients. Others see them as part of the natural, user-friendly, traditional way to improve health, prevent disease and promote longevity. Others see these plants as living energies, carrying intrinsic healing vibrations and having deep spiritual impact. All of these are true. All are individual paradigms, a spectrum of meanings perfectly embraced by the living tapestry of the plant world.

THE GIFT OF HERBS

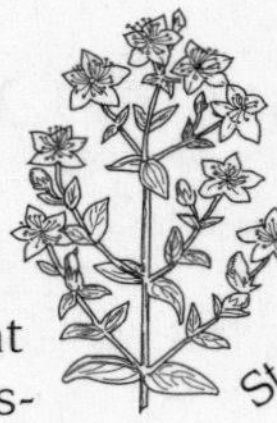

St. John's Wort

With the rush to embrace holistic medicine, it is useful to begin by looking at the unique qualities that make herbs so attractive and desirable. Each characteristic sets apart the world's oldest, most widespread form of medicine.

Natural

In spite of its overuse and hype, here the word "natural" has a genuine meaning. Having evolved over millions of years with plants as our main foodstuff, our human physiology and biochemistry have a natural affinity and compatibility with medicinal herbs. Far from being primitive or basic, herbs used in their whole, natural state are far more complex and advanced than the synthetic, laboratory-created drugs that mimic them.

Effective

Herbs have proved themselves effective in treating every conceivable type of health problem in tens of millions of patients. In fact, herbs are still the main system of health care for 80% of the world's population. While the current standard of double-blind scientific studies is useful, it takes second place to the centuries of consistent action and clinical results observed by healing practitioners in every culture and time period.

Holistic

No one part of the person can be sick without the involvement of the whole. Even catching a simple cold implies a temporary weakness in the spleen, thymus, respiratory tract, etc. Conversely, any sick organ will affect the entire person; i.e. intestinal dysbiosis causes toxic build-up in the liver and kidney, weakening immunity. These relationships are the basis of combination herbal formulas, designed to influence total health.

Synergistic

Because of their complex nature, herbs affect multiple organ systems and functions. For example, a plant may be an all-in-one antioxidant, immune stimulant, anti-inflammatory, anti-spasmodic and pain reliever! This kind of remarkable synergism is exemplified in *meadowsweet*. Its "active ingredient," aspirin, is the single leading cause of stomach hemorrhage and ulceration, yet the *whole herb* is a soothing antacid and digestive tonic.

Safe

There are food plants, medicinal plants and poisonous plants. Yet, relative to drugs, herbs have an extremely high benefits-to-risk ratio. This is evidenced by the fact that fatalities from medicinal herbs are almost unheard of—as opposed to at least 100,000 deaths annually from medical drugs. Thus a recent news item described a woman who attempted suicide by taking a *bottleful* of valerian pills—resulting in a restful sleep!

Herbs should always (yes, always) be considered before taking more drastic, toxic or risky synthetic medicines, which are acceptable last resorts.

Consistent

Medical drugs are basically experimental—most have had only limited human trials when they are put on the market. This is why over 3,000 drugs are taken off the shelves annually, due to previously unknown side effects or toxicity. Plants, on the other hand, have a track record that often goes back thousands of years. While science continues to deepen our understanding of herbal action, we can currently rely on their long-established record of safety and effectiveness.

Non-Suppressive

Even when effective for short-term gains, most mainstream treatments simply thwart or block our normal immune and neurological responses. The long-term effect of this suppression and interference is to weaken and damage the body's defense mechanisms, causing deeper problems later on. This is seen, for example, in several studies where each bout of antibiotics increased the susceptibility to both otitis and tonsillitis.

Family-Based Medicine

Herbs are a relatively gentle medicine, making them ideal for children, the aged and for those in long-term treatment. They are valuable anytime there is very real concern about the toxicity and side effects of short- and long-term drug use. Also, a great many plants are perfectly suited for self-care and for treating one's family and friends.

Multiple Choice

In traditional systems around the globe, there are many herbal choices for seemingly identical conditions. The subtle yet unique differences in the nature and qualities of each herb allow one to fine-tune the prescription. Through knowledge, or trial and error, one can find the most compatible plant. And if a particular herb begins to be less effective over time, there are always alternatives.

Cost Effective

Herbal medicines are not always cheap, but are far, far less expensive than medical drugs. Their greatest savings, however, comes in their ability to prevent chronic disease, whose cost in medical expenses, lost work and emotional strain is beyond estimate.

Environmental

Last, but not least, herbs are a truly environmentally friendly form of medicine. Using organically grown, naturally processed herbs, the land, sea and air are not further despoiled. It is imperative to use herbs that are minimally processed and which avoid the use of solvents or toxic chemicals. Herbs need to be true to their own unique heritage, quite separate and distinct from the petrochemical industry.

The Scope of Herbs

Individuals experience herbs in a variety of ways. Some may find the colorful bottles lined up in health food stores a curiosity. Others may try out ginkgo for memory, based on a recent cover story of a national magazine. Still others may see echinacea, goldenseal and milk thistle as a way of life and a true alternative to more toxic pharmaceuticals. The scope of herbal treatment includes all this and much more. From refreshing teas, to home care, to professional treatment of serious disease by an herbal expert, herbs have a range of capabilities as broad as humanity itself. They also work on many integrated levels, simultaneously, as described below. Here we need only hint at the vast usefulness of herbs. Note that if illness is of a serious nature, professional/medical diagnosis and treatment is highly advisable. Yet here too, for optimal benefit, the first line of treatment tried should be non-invasive herbal medicines.

Acute Conditions

Generally we think of acute problems as being relatively superficial and of short duration. By definition, if such a condition does not resolve within a few days or a week, it is redefined as subacute or chronic.

- Herbal medicines are extremely effective and quick-acting for acute infections, inflammations, bleeding, injuries or temporary stresses.
- Rather than just acting on symptoms, herbs simultaneously promote tissue repair and prevent long-term consequences of illness.

Chronic Disease

Chronic diseases are those that linger on and, if left unchecked, progressively worsen. Arising insidiously, they result in increasing debility, interfering with organic functions and begin to permanently damage tissues.

- Herbal treatment can *slow* the progress of most chronic diseases.
- In less-advanced cases, they can *stop* further disease progression.
- The optimal goal is complete *reversal* of the condition, and this can happen, even in cases labeled "incurable" by mainstream medicine.
- Where cure is not possible, herbs can often alleviate symptoms.
- Herbs are extremely valuable in hospice work and in aiding the dying.

Prevention

Prevention has a number of meanings, and herbs fulfill them all.

- When contagious diseases abound, herbs can bolster the immune system, so that one's statistical chance of getting sick no longer applies.
- Long-term use definitely helps prevent chronic, degenerative disease.
- The antioxidant and anti-cancer effects of numerous herbs is well established, from *garlic* and *green tea*, to *reishi* and *ginseng*.

Thus both judicious self-care and professional herbal treatment has the potential to eradicate the tendency to chronic diseases before it begins.

Physical Ailments

As the main form of medicine in all times and places, herbs have been used to treat literally every physical symptom or condition. In fact most herbs have a very definite affinity to specific organs or tissues. Herbs can be used to treat *acute conditions* like allergies and back pain, as well as *chronic conditions* such as psoriasis, arthritis and arteriosclerosis. Beyond this, herbs can be used as an excellent form of disease prevention.

Psychological Conditions

Herbs are nature's tranquilizers and are amply suited to depression, anxiety and hyperactivity. Many recent studies have shown how herbs like *St. John's wort* and *kava* work as effectively as medical tranquilizers and anti-anxiety drugs, without their risks or addictive tendencies. Herbs combine well with psychotherapy because they often sharpen cognition, rather than dulling the emotional life like psychotropic drugs.

Anti-aging

Along with appropriate vitamins and nutrients, herbs play a huge role in the important area of anti-aging. There are dozens of herbs with special rejuvenating properties and a long tradition of promoting longevity. There is simply no other known form of therapy that has the ability to prevent the potential ravages of aging quite as well. With antioxidant protection, improved circulation, enhanced immunity and increased neurological function, a reversal of age-related degeneration is a realizable goal.

Geriatrics

The most over-medicated segment of society, the aging population is also the group with the highest rate of side effects and mortality from prescribed drugs. Herbal medicines can be a gentle healing alternative to harsh drugs. Dozens of conditions typical of the elderly, including heart disease, are very responsive to herbal medicine. Their remarkable ability to reestablish vitality, appetite, sexual function and zest for life makes them the treatment of choice for the elderly.

Universality

Not only are there plant medicines for every conceivable problem, there are almost no conditions where adaptogens, nervines and tonics cannot improve vitality and help ease a variety of physical and mental suffering. Many herbs are gentle and safe enough for long-term use or when there is already a weakened state that cannot tolerate heroic measures.

Immune Strengthening

Immunity has now been recognized as a cornerstone of our health. The old principles of Hippocrates, nature cure and traditional medical systems have been vindicated—it is the body's defense system that is the real key to longevity and freedom from infection and chronic illness. Herbs possess unique abilities to augment and maintain immune health.

Herbal Paradigms

Daisy

While herbal healing encompasses a wide range of systems and practices, there are common threads and understandings that hold true over time and place. Herbs are more than a natural form of medical drugs. Simply substituting an herbal medicine for a pharmaceutical drug will certainly work, but does not do it justice. In fact, herbal medicine is part of a different *paradigm* than the current medical system. This means that its way of viewing, understanding and working with health, disease and cure are radically different, and the expected outcome is also radically different. Like most truths, the concepts of healing are so simple and straightforward that they easily go unperceived. Some of the basic principles of the herbal paradigm known since the time of Hippocrates are outlined below.

Health

- The organism possesses a remarkable and profound ability to self-correct, adapt, change and heal, and is constantly engaged in this.
- The healthy body and mind function as an integrated whole, not as fragmented elements, which is more characteristic of disease.
- Health is not just an absence of symptoms, but a dynamic, energetic and vibrant state, in which one can access all their deepest strengths.
- From this healthy state, one can respond effectively to environmental stress, toxins or infection, quickly adapting or returning to normal.

Disease

- From a logical standpoint, disease is not an independent, self-existing entity that attacks. We are not "struck" by cancer or any other disease.
- Diseases have definite causes, such as a virus, an injury or a toxin.
- Disease *symptoms* themselves are the reactions of the individual, body and mind, to the causes and stresses it is trying to deal with.
- These reactions are intelligent and adaptive. They are attempts at self-cure, even if they are not successful or are uncomfortable.
- By suppressing symptoms, one is thwarting the body's attempts at cure, while the underlying causes go unchecked.

Cure

- Symptoms are guideposts to cure, to how the body wants to be helped.
- Cure thus means removal of causes, eradicating both the obvious and, as much as possible, basic underlying factors that create disease.
- Curing should proceed in the gentlest way possible, using methods that are in harmony with the working of the human organism.
- Cure means changing basic tendencies and predispositions, so that its highest goal becomes prevention of both acute and chronic disease.

Vitalism

Intelligent Life

Vitalism is part of the herbal paradigm, a view of nature that is holistic, ecological and integrative. These ancient, yet very contemporary concepts, include the following ideas and understandings:

- Life in all its forms is rich, complex and highly organized. It adapts, responds and creates, showing continual intelligence and ingenuity.
- That same intelligence also coordinates every aspect of our physical life: digesting, breathing, clearing of toxins and healing of tissues.
- The appreciation and respect for life as intelligent, rather than mechanical, is what dramatically differentiates traditional and holistic health care from contemporary medical thinking and drug therapy.

Universal Understanding

These principles have been universally recognized and rediscovered throughout all times and cultures, and integrated into the worldview of these diverse peoples and regions.

- Biological intelligence, known variously as chi, prana, dynamis, pneuma and vital or life force, is the cornerstone of Chinese medicine, Ayurveda, homeopathy, Hippocratean medicine and other systems.
- The organizing life force pervades the individual and is at one's core.
- We now recognize that the immune, nervous and hormonal systems are key components of this biological intelligence.
- While it exerts its control through these response systems and directs their activity, it is not identical to them.
- Psychoneuroimmunology demonstrates that these systems function as a unified whole and also interface with our emotions and thoughts.
- Other, subtler energy systems, are also part of biological intelligence.
- The chakra system of Ayurveda and meridian system of Chinese medicine are advanced systems that utilize the pathways of the life force.

Response to Disease

In practical terms, the above understandings reframe the way health and disease are approached, and the way treatment is applied.

- All disease starts with, and affects, biological intelligence/the life force.
- In acute disease, the biological intelligence responds dramatically, using intense means to push disease away from the center.
- In chronic disease, it tries to compensate and prevent deeper entrenchment of the process of deterioration.
- Biological intelligence has clear priorities to protect the most vital organs and functions, as discussed at the end of this section.
- Once again, disease symptoms become guides to cure, not merely nuisances to be removed without regard for their underlying meaning.

THE 5 STEPS OF HEALING

The body does not heal in a haphazard, accidental way, but according to a deep biological intelligence. Thus, a true healing art is based on principles that mirror the body's own processes and its inherent healing tendencies. These principles are the sum of centuries of astute human observation, insight and experience. Thus, even though this book is a handbook for self care and for treating specific illnesses with specific groups of herbs, it should be kept in mind that total healing requires an overall strategy. It is not about a single effective herb, but an attempt to first understand, and then to help, the way our minds and bodies cure themselves. There are many ways to formulate the principles of healing. Here, we discuss all herbal effects as falling into five categories of action. These stages often follow one another, but can proceed simultaneously.

1. Symptom Relief

What drives most of us to seek a health practitioner is relief from some kind of pain, discomfort or lack of freedom on a physical or psychological level. All systems of medicine are involved with alleviating these symptoms, in order to restore ease and functionality to the person. No less than mainstream medicine, herbal and other natural therapies can be extremely effective in allaying symptoms of both acute and chronic

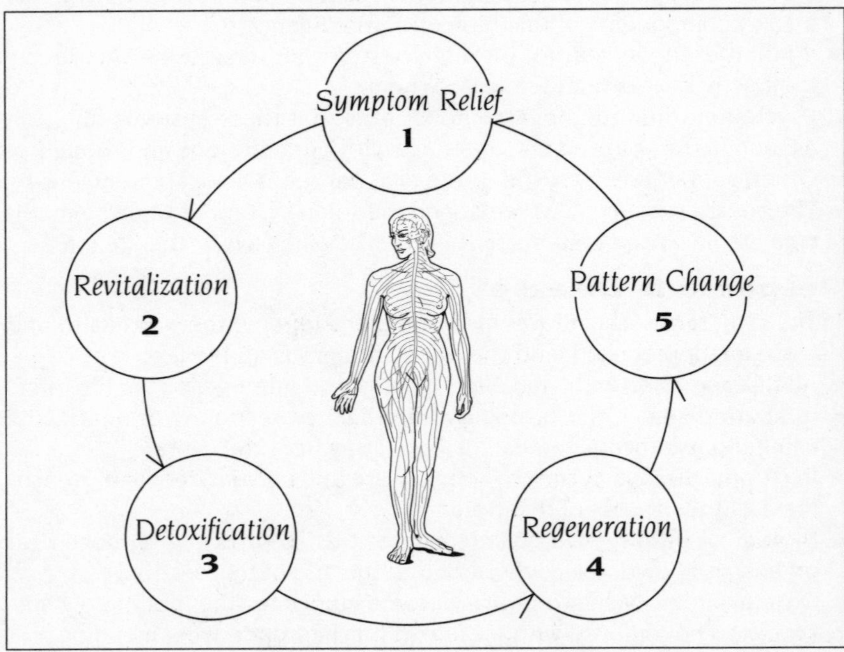

suffering that debilitates and weakens the individual. But while this is the mainstay of regular medicine, herbal treatment also seeks to unravel deeper causes and promotes lasting changes in one's level of health.

2. Revitalization

Revitalization of the organism is a crucial part of healing and a unique capability of herbal medicines. Unknown in mainstream medicine, it is also easily overlooked in the field of natural healing. When individuals are weakened by illness, they become reduced in vitality and internal resources. Nutrients, antioxidants, amino acids and all kinds of gross and subtle elements are depleted. Any attempt at promoting and stimulating healing should take into account how well the person can respond to healing measures. Adaptogenic and tonic herbs are well suited to building up an exhausted system. All future treatments should be adjusted to the tempo and level of the organism's vital strength.

3. Detoxification

Detoxification is a cornerstone of every great system of healing. Free radicals and damaging toxins play a major role in the creation of illness. This includes external toxins (viruses, fungi, heavy metals, chemicals) and internal accumulations of the body's own by-products. These wastes slowly and inexorably weaken the organism on all levels, generating both chronic disease states and acute illness—the body's attempts to throw off these wastes. Clearing debris from cells, tissues and organs relieves the body of a tremendous burden. And before tissues can be regenerated or healed, these impediments must be removed through detoxifying techniques. Otherwise, it is like pouring fine wine into vinegar!

4. Regeneration

Once vitality is enhanced and detoxification is proceeding adequately, herbs can be used to help regenerate damaged, weakened and devitalized tissue. The extent of this repair depends on the nature, duration and location of illness. But many plants are *cell proliferants*, promoting the creation of new cells in tissues that can regenerate, such as the skin, liver and white blood cells, or replacing worn-out components of irreplaceable cells, such as those found in the heart and nerves.

5. Pattern Change

When the body has regained its strength, cleansed at a deep level, and repaired weak and damaged areas, healing is almost complete. Yet there is a crucial next step. Pattern change simply means changing the underlying patterns, predisposition and forces that contribute to ill health or that will cause a relapse back to a weakened state. External changes include changing damaging lifestyle habits, diet and activities. Internal change is possible as we slowly change or even eradicate our deep susceptibilities and tendencies toward disease. Long expert treatment with plants gives evidence that this profound level of healing is possible.

GLOBAL HERBS

Ancient Roots

To really understand herbs, it is necessary to delve, even briefly, into their history, for the history of herbs is the history of humankind, interweaving with daily life as far back as we can peer into prehistory. The use of healing plants is rooted in the hunting and gathering societies wandering over the globe some 50,000 years ago. The cultivation and use of herbs had further development with the beginnings of agriculture, when barley, wheat, rice and corn became staple crops of agricultural societies 5,000 to 10,000 years ago. Yet in all the diverse cultures, places, climates and environments that formed a backdrop for the human drama, healing plants played a crucial role in the life of people. Indigenous herbs were known and valued, and as travel across land and sea became more common, the herbal treasures of distant regions were sought out. The global trade in herbs and spices reached a crescendo in the great silk routes from Asia to Europe and subsequent sea routes to the Americas and Far East. This exchange has continued up until today. Coffee from Africa, tea from Asia, tobacco from South America: global culture has continually enriched itself with "plants that changed the world." Apart from foods, spices and stimulants, dedicated plant explorers also brought back herbal medicines from far flung regions: *curare* from South America, *rauwolfia* from India, *strophanthus* from Africa. These items have found lasting and important places in the world of healing plants.

Integrated Traditions

Today we are at another crossroads. A few years ago, for example, the rich herbal heritage of Ayurveda was almost unknown outside its native India. Now dozens of these irreplaceable herbal medicines are used side by side with Asian *ginseng*, American *goldenseal*, European *elderberry*, South American *cat's claw* and Australian *tea tree oil*. Every year, new herbs come to prominence. Some are neglected herbs from our own Western tradition, with new, scientifically verified uses, such as St. *John's wort* or *saw palmetto*. Others are more esoteric, but quickly become stars on the herbal horizon—like *kava* or *reishi* mushrooms. The result of all this cross-cultural exchange, discovery and research is a rich melting pot of both time-tested and innovative herbal medicines. While this provides an unprecedented wealth of herbs to cure our ails, it also brings some confusion. The choices may seem too vast and overlapping. In the next pages, an overview of the components of this global herb marketplace will be provided. From this, we can gain a deeper understanding of the origin, traditions and relationship of the many herbs available today.

European Herbs

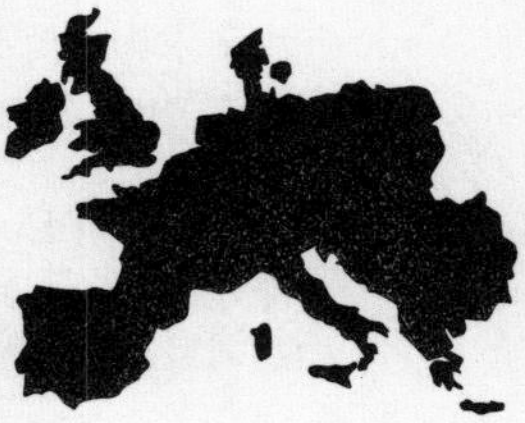

The Roots of Phytotherapy

The European tradition forms the basis for the practice of herbal medicine in the Western world today. The history of this tradition has its roots in both the sophisticated systems that developed in Greece and Rome, as well as the folk traditions that existed throughout the numerous tribes and ethnic groups scattered across Europe. This interweaving tapestry over time and space can be only briefly traced here.

Greece and Rome

The history of European herbalism always begins with the Roman Galen in the first century A.D. Taking his information from Hippocrates and Aristotle, he instituted the theory of the four humors. This system in turn was based on more ancient ideas coming from Chinese and Indian systems of thought and medicine. Illness was seen to arise from imbalances in the four elements: earth, water, air and fire (corresponding to black bile, phlegm, yellow bile and blood). While these ideas may seem quaint, they do relate to definite physiological tendencies and biological functions (such as fire relating to inflammation) and represent a workable and effective healing system. As far as healing substances, the classic Greek works of Dioscorides and Pliny from the first century B.C. held sway, and their observation and comments on hundreds of herbs still influence herbal use today. With the fall of the Roman empire, much of this knowledge was lost—temporarily.

Medieval Traditions

During the dark ages, invading "barbarians" destroyed centers of learning as well as texts and scholars who had been carrying on the traditions of science and healing. Fortunately Galen and all the other classic authors had been translated into Arabic. By the 9th century, Avicenna was the world's most renowned physician, and both his Middle Eastern teachings and the classical texts were translated back into Latin again. It was the monastic centers of Europe that kept the tradition of medicine, and even writing, alive. Galen again held sway for 400 years.

Folk Traditions

Until the 15th century, all writings had to be transcribed by hand, limiting both knowledge and literacy. With the invention of the printing press, folk medicine in every country and every language, not just Latin, became available as published books, and a growing population was able to use them. For the first time, not only physicians, but lay herbalists were able to communicate and further popularize herbal knowledge. A mixture of folk medicine, classic Dioscorides and personal experience, these herbal texts were immensely popular. John Gerard's book was a landmark in 1597, and was the prominent English-language text on the subject for centuries. It is still in print 400 years later. Culpeper, flourishing in the 1600s, may be the world's most well-known herbalist, and his books are still very readable—and available—today.

The Schism in Healing Thought

A split began to develop in how healing was practiced during the "age of rationalism." Educated doctors and institutions began to use imported herbs almost exclusively, and sought ways to make them more concentrated and heroic in their effects. It was the heyday of bloodletting, and the main treatment was calomel (mercury). Herbs were combined with a variety of minerals and chemical solvents to create a more "medicinal" concoction. By the late 1800s, herbs began to be looked upon as mere folklore or at best as poor substitutes for the chemicalized medicine of the day. As Europe's commercial and scholarly powers were consolidated, laws were enacted in many countries to prevent lay people, and even doctors, from using herbal medicine. Homeopathy emerged during this time as well, partly in reaction to what would surely be termed barbaric medicine today—leeches, opium, arsenic, strychnine and a witches brew of "rational" medicine. Meanwhile, it took Lister sixty years to convince his medical brethren to wash their hands before doing surgery!

Modern Phytomedicine

Britain was the only country that had a system of lay herbal medicine. It is only in the last twenty-five years that rational phytotherapy or herbal medicine has once again been allowed to come into its own. In France, for example, every pharmacy proudly advertises the sale of three kinds of medicine: allopathy (medical drugs), homeopathy and phytotherapy (herbal medicine). Today European phytomedicine represents an advanced and integrated approach to herbal medicine. In this model, each herb is considered as a drug entity, in sharp contrast to pharmacological medicine. There is no attempt to isolate and use a single "active ingredient" at the expense of the whole plant.

At the same time, numerous European governments have taken an active role in integrating traditional herbal knowledge and science. The landmark German Commission E in Germany recently completed their examination of several hundred plants, comparing their historical and clinical uses with current scientific evidence of their effectiveness. Though this important study was extremely conservative in their findings and recommendations, it is a model of the kind of interchange that is taking place in Europe between pharmacological and herbal medicine.

North American herbs

Brave New World

Instead of finding a new (and cheaper) trade route to Eastern spices and medicinals, early explorers to North American shores discovered a whole "New World" of plant substances. Native Americans already had well-established and intricate medical systems, with herbs at the center of curative activity. When European settlers arrived, they carried with them both herbs and the knowledge of their uses from their own countries of origin. However, out of necessity and opportunity, they soon became aware of the wealth of very different and effective healing plants in their new home. This created an explosion in the number of plants that were available to European countries. New foods, such as potatoes, tomatoes, corn and squashes, would soon change the face of European culture. New World medicines were in great demand. Plants like *American ginseng* were overharvested almost to extinction. Scores of new plant medicines emerged: *cascara, senna, slippery elm* and *witch hazel*. Women's medicine was enriched by *true unicorn root, trillium* and *blue cohosh*. Powerful new antiseptic plants came into vogue, including *goldenseal, echinacea* and *wild indigo*.

European Influences

The merging of North American and European herbs was natural. The climates of these continents made it easy to transplant species onto one's native soil and the similarity of temperate species brought a familiarity with them. Several schools of healing rose up in North America, based on integrating local herbs into medical practice. The Thompsonian school was a lay movement that had a simple theory and small group of medicines that were considered panaceas. Meanwhile, a considerable number of regular physicians joined the rank of the Eclectics, integrating the best of European and Native American herbal formulas and single remedies. Homeopathy also began to flourish, with its intense use of plant medicines in small doses. All of these schools became eclipsed for a variety of reasons, but especially because of the emerging pharmaceutical industry, headed by America's most powerful, influential families.

The Naturopathic Profession

Integrating the Nature Cure of Europe with the holistic practices of the day (including homeopathy, botanical medicine and hydrotherapy), the naturopathic profession was born just as the modern system of medicine was being consolidated by pharmaceutical interests. As a monopolized system of patented, synthetic drugs took over, herbal medicine was overshadowed. Until recent times, naturopathic physicians were the prime carriers of the torch of European and North American herbal practice.

CHINESE HERBS

The Way of TCM

The first known herbal records date back over 4,500 years to the famous Yellow Emporer's Classic. This system has remained almost unchanged today. Traditional Chinese Medicine (TCM) involves a complex philosophy and cosmology of yin and yang. Herbs are not prescribed based on the principles of anatomy and physiology that are familiar to Western medicine. A person's symptoms and signs expressed in their tongue, pulse and urine can show imbalances in the basic five elements that constitute matter. Medicines are then prescribed to balance qualities of heat, cold, moisture and dryness.

East Meets West

Chinese medicine left its stamp on Japan and Korea, but also began to migrate westward many centuries ago, giving us the *peach* and *lemon*, and specific drugs like *opium* and *ginseng*. Today the detailed system of Chinese medicine has become hugely popular in the West, largely due to the use of acupuncture. Meanwhile, in China, TCM and Western pharmacological medicine now coexist on an equal basis. Similarly, traditional Chinese doctors have migrated West, while Western doctors have travelled far to bring back, and put into practice, these ancient healing arts.

In with the New

Chinese herbs, however, have found their way into the European style of single herb prescribing. While *ginseng* and *dong quai* have been integrated into mainstream herbalism for decades, powerful new additions have arrived in recent years. These include *schisandra*, *codonopsis*, *baical skullcap*, *ephedra* and immune-boosting *astragalus*. Medicinal mushrooms are another unique contribution, including *reishi*, *maitake* and *shiitake*: all immune stimulating and life-enhancing fungi. With a passionate interest in longevity herbs, TCM promotes adaptogen plants like *fo-ti* that have far-reaching effects, enhancing both the duration and the quality of life.

Further Integration and Research

Textbooks abound detailing the healing virtues of more than 5,000 Chinese plants. At the same time, China and other countries around the world have invested significant resources to scientifically validate the action of traditional herbs. A significant difference in the use of herbs in TCM is that they are almost exclusively used in complex formulas, taken as a tea or boiled together—and anything but pleasant to taste. Naturally, many of these are used in the West in the form of easy-to-take capsules or alcoholic tinctures. It is only a matter of time until more of them become known, validated and made available to an eager world.

South American herbs

Amazonian Treasures

The South American continent is a veritable treasure-trove of herbal medicines, containing as much as 50% of all plant species. The rich tapestry of plant life in the equatorial jungles of the Amazon River basin are more familiar to us nowadays because of media coverage of rain forest destruction in these areas. However, beyond the jungles of this vast continent, there is a much wider range of plant groups, inhabiting mountains, grasslands, forests, semi-deserts, moist coastal regions and Mediterranean-like climates. Many herbs in these areas have been used for healing since prehistory.

Everyday Herbs

These herbs are not restricted to indigenous tribes or the descendants of the ancient Incas. Large open air markets sell hundreds of locally grown herbs to the populace of largely Spanish descent who, much like their European brethren, treat herbs as a natural part of daily life. And though transplanted European herbs have become mixed with native species since the 1700s, the rich tradition of the "curendaro," or indigenous healers, continues. Also, because of the strong European roots in the Latin culture, the medical profession has been more open to treating herbs as an integral part of mainstream practice. To test the validity of age-old herbal cures, several research centers and hospital-based facilities, as well as major drug companies and private foundations, continue investigations into these important South American resources.

Gifts of the Americas

Already the continent has contributed many plants that are now consumed in vast quantities the world over. Tomatoes, potatoes, tobacco, chili peppers and bell peppers—all came from circumscribed areas of the western Andes in the 1600s. Corn, yams, papayas, pineapples, avocados and many types of squashes and melons are South American natives. Important drugs include *curare*, *quinine* (the main cure for malaria for 300 years), *wild yam* (the source of commercial of estrogen) and *ipecac* (used in every emergency ward). The region also contributes mightily to our list of stimulants and herb-based drugs, including coffee, chocolate and cocaine—one of the two main ingredients of the original Coca-Cola. Other South American herbs in common use today include *sarsaparilla* (once Europe's greatest herbal import), *guaiacum* (a former syphilis cure), *cat's claw*, *lapacho* and *suma* (Brazilian ginseng). Brazil alone has twice the number of native plant species as North America, and forty times that of England! This vast, largely unexplored region is sure to provide some of the most exciting herbal discoveries of the new century.

INDIAN HERBS

Ancient Origins

Ayurveda is the most recent healing system to find its way into the melting pot of global herbalism. The ancient tradition of the subcontinent of India has its roots in the mythic past and is known to have been practiced over 5,000 years ago. Ancient Ayurvedic texts codified the system in 1500 B.C., which today uses some 600 herbs. In India this effective medical system treats millions who rely solely on physicians trained in Ayurvedic colleges, and Ayurvedic products are available in every pharmacy.

East Meets West

With the development of spice routes between Asia and Europe, exotic condiments and herbs found their way into European marketplaces and pharmacy shelves. Thus, numerous native Indian plants have been integrated into Western herbalism for centuries, including *garlic*, *licorice*, *black pepper*, *sandalwood* and *cinnamomum*. Potent pharmaceutical plants, such as *rauwolfia*, source of the cardiac drug reserpine, were also gleaned from the wealth of traditional Ayurvedic healing plants. Known for millennia in India, but never before seen in America and Europe, a new crop of healing plants have come on the scene. These include *curcumin*, *arjuna*, *boswellia*, *holy basil*, *guggul* and *ashwaganda*. It is now difficult to imagine being without these unique herbs, which have found instant popularity.

The Ayurvedic System

The traditional context of these herbs—the system of Ayurvedic medicine—has also found adherents. However, the influence of Ayurveda is already an old one. The system of five elements, pulse diagnosis and pharmacology contained within Ayurveda formed the basis of systems that later developed in the Middle East and Tibet. The tradition pervaded the medicine of Greece and Europe, this impact continuing until the modern era. Influences were mutual however, and both Middle Eastern and Greco-Roman systems still exist in present-day India. While Islamic conquests, British rule and modern pharmacology have all presented challenges to the survival of Ayurveda, over the last sixty years it has found a renewed vitality and dynamism, gaining global popularity.

Future of Indian Herbalism

Millions of acres in India are turned over to the growing of medicinal herbs. Today three systems exist side by side—medical, ayurvedic and homeopathic—demonstrating a level of integration and coexistence that we still aspire to in the West. From this vast medicinal heritage, we can look forward to the yearly integration of new herbs into everyday use.

African Herbs

Out of Africa

Africa has a greater variety of herbal traditions than any other continent. With its vast ecology of deserts, arid woodlands and scrub, rain forests, grasslands and moist coastal regions, it has always had a rich diversity of plant life. The ancient trade routes provided an interchange between Indian, Arabian and African herbal knowledge for three millennium. At the same time, many isolated tribal herbal systems and folk medicines have continued as they were in ancient times. In the north, Egypt boasts the world's oldest medical text, the Ebers papyrus, a 3,500-year-old document describing over 700 herbs. Many of these plants are still revered today, including *opium* (e.g., codeine, morphine), *aloe* and *gentian*. Egyptian medical teachings relied heavily on detoxification and intestinal health, and this formed the basis of the later Greek, Roman and Middle Eastern systems of medicine. This profoundly influenced the entire Western herbal tradition, right up to recent times.

African Contributions

From Africa we have obtained many foods, including *okra* and *kola nut*, high in caffeine and the original basis of Coca-Cola. But nothing can compare to the impact of *coffee*, one of the most important items of global food trade. Medicinal herbs native to the African continent have also become essential to global herbalism. *Senna* entered Western herbalism and medicine in the ninth century and has been an important herb for constipation in American and European pharmacopoeia ever since. Other African plants that have been known for at least a hundred years include *calabar bean* (physostigma), used as a pupil dilator; *castor bean* (*Ricinus communis*), source of the famous castor oil; *strophanthus*, a powerful cardiac drug; and *buchu*, an important kidney tonic. *Myrrh*, so vital to Middle Eastern herbalism, is native to southern Africa.

Modern Imports

However, neither the advent of Western medicine nor historical suppression of native traditions by colonizing nations have diminished herbal use. Today 70 to 80% of the population still depends on the literally thousands of native herbs for their primary health care, with some thirty traditional healers to every medical doctor. Herbs new to the West have appeared in recent years, with gratifying results. Examples include *devil's claw*, for arthritis and inflammation, *yohimbe*, a potent aphrodisiac and *pygeum*, an important prostate herb. Part of a long folk tradition, many African herbs are the focus of intensive research and integration into mainstream medical practices.

MIDDLE EASTERN HERBS

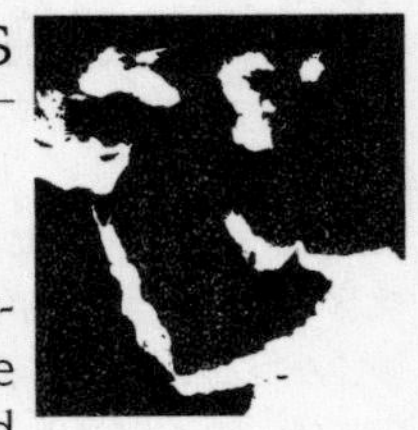

Islamic Civilization

While Europe was plunged into the Dark Ages in the seventh century, the heritage of Greek and Roman medicine and the ancient works of Dioscorides, Galen, Pliny and Hippocrates were all lost. Meanwhile, the rising Islam culture began collecting and translating all the medical and scientific texts of the ancient world. By 800 A.D., and for 600 years, Arabian physicians, using herbal medicines, were the most advanced in the civilized world. With further conquests, their influence reached back to Egypt, where it made a permanent impression on North African medicine. Likewise, innovations in medical education, licensing, surgery, ideas of contagion and quarantine, and pharmaceutical compounding would return to reform and revitalize European medicine.

Herbal Additions

The teachings of Avicenna, as well as other Middle Eastern botanists and physicians, formed the basis of European herbal practice. At the crossroads of the silk routes linking East and West, Arabian physicians were able to start with the 500 plants mentioned in classic Greek texts and integrate herbs and healing concepts of Persia, Arabia, Egypt, India and even Asia. The effects of hundreds of herbs were carefully observed and their clinical effectiveness evaluated. Both single herbs and effective formulas were utilized. By 1000 A.D., Avicenna was Islam's greatest doctor, and his texts became standards for the eventual rebirth of European medicine in Solerno, Italy, and Montpelier, France. Hundreds of herbs thus found their way into European medical practice, including *cardamon, cumin, nutmeg, saffron, cloves, tamarind, senna, musk, camphor* and more.

Hebraic and Nomadic Traditions

Paralleling this were the traditions and practices passed along in the 6,000-year-old Jewish tradition. *Sesame, dates, olives, acacia* and other desert plants formed an integrated system, and this knowledge was exchanged with Persian and Arabic doctors. In remote and inhospitable areas, local folk systems—such as that of the nomadic Bedouin—have remained unchanged for millennia, using both local herbs and those that were naturalized a millennia before. The encroachment of modern civilization and Western medical drugs has displaced these systems in many areas. Yet with the resurgence of interest in botanical medicine, many herbs from this continent have caught the attention of ethnobotanists and herbal practitioners. Recently, several books have appeared on plants of the bible, such as *aloe* and *myrrh*. This tradition, which spans more than two millennia, still has much to offer to a world turning back to herbs.

Contemporary Herbs

The Modern Scene

The renewed growth of herbal medicine around the world has been exponential. Currently, sales of herbs are increasing at a remarkable rate of 25 to 30% per year, with sales topping $9 billion. This represents as many as 50% of the population that are now using herbs. Physicians and other health professionals are scrambling to catch up with herbal knowledge, while those who have long been in this field are finding a new, expanded audience. There are now a huge number of herbal companies, growing every day. And the commercial success of herbs has spurred unprecedented scientific investigation into the herbal world. Both well-known and newly rediscovered herbs are being examined to determine their biochemical profiles and healing ingredients. In the global herbal melting pot, herbs from every region and tradition are available.

The Double-Edged Sword

There are up and down sides to the herbal renaissance. Some advantages and disadvantages are listed below here to show the dynamic forces that are at work in the new, emerging face of botanical medicine.

- The quality of herbs has become more variable. With more players in the herbal industry, there are those whose motives are profit, not health.
- With current standards and understandings, some impeccable companies have been able to produce even more effective and valuable products and to compare their value to less desirable competitors.
- The investigation into the chemical nature of plants has tended to "medicalize" them. Active ingredients are considered to be more effective, "real" drugs, while traditional herbs are derided as folk medicine.
- Far greater numbers of people are being exposed to herbs and can make up their own minds about the advantages of natural medicines.
- Popular herbs, like *goldenseal*, have been severely overharvested, so that it is no longer advisable to gather wild plants.
- The age-old controversies between holistic and materialistic medicine have re-emerged with an intensity. Are herbs part of a larger paradigm that encompasses ideas like individualized treatment, detoxification and herbal energetics? Or are they just another form of drug, more trendy and less toxic, yet second class compared to pharmaceutical inventions and their dangerous power?

Time will tell where the trends will take us during the current herbal resurgence. One thing is certain: Herbal popularity will continue to grow at an ever faster rate. The deciding factor will be how educated the public becomes about herbs and herbal healing in all its vast and profound aspects.

PLANT CONSTITUENTS

Herbs contain hundreds, if not thousands, of chemical ingredients, many of which have yet to be discovered! Even for plants like *ginger*, which has over 500 known constituents, the final number, what they all do and how they interact, are light years beyond our current knowledge. Thus, thinking that information about this or that ingredient means we really understand a healing herb in its depth and complexity is scientific narrow-mindedness. However, if seen in its proper context and perspective, facts about plant ingredients are extremely useful. They are another piece of the puzzle in classifying medicinal herbs, explaining traditional uses and discovering new healing capabilities.

Below are some important components of botanical medicines, with examples. Remember that according to the models of Ayurveda, Chinese medicine, European and American shamanism, homeopathy, flower essences, as well as cutting-edge physics, plants also embody healing energies and properties that go far beyond their chemical constituents.

Alkaloids: Nitrogen-containing alkaloids have intense physiological effects. Some are highly narcotic or mind-altering, while others are extremely deadly. However, among the dozen or so groups of very different alkaloid types, many work to heal different organs and tissues and are among the most powerful of plant medicines. Examples include *celandine* (opium family), *goldenseal* and *cayenne* (in the nightshade family). However, caffeine and nicotine are the most well-known alkaloids.

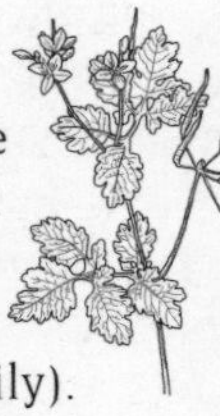

Celandine

Anthroquinones: These substances are well known in pharmacology as the active ingredients in various stimulating laxatives. They act by causing a mild "irritation" or stimulation to the intestinal walls to produce a liquid evacuation, usually within twelve hours. Anthroquinone-containing laxatives include *buckthorn*, *senna*, *cascara*, *rhubarb* and *aloe*.

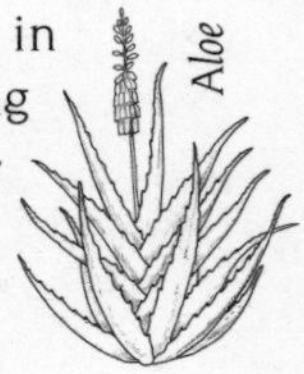

Aloe

Antioxidants: One of the most important developments in nutritional and herbal medicine is the recognition of the role antioxidants play in health and disease. Some must be gotten from food, while others can be manufactured by the body. An excess of toxins in relation to inadequate antioxidants means increased free radical damage to the tissues. The result is a Pandora's box of chronic degenerative diseases and accelerated aging. A great number of herbs are powerful antioxidants, acting both globally and locally. Examples are *ginkgo*, *milk thistle* and *bilberry*.

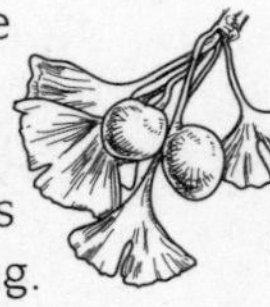

Ginkgo

Bitters: Bitter-tasting herbs stimulate a variety of digestive enzymes and stomach acid. This improves the breakdown and absorption of nutrients, aiding recovery from various debilitating conditions. In spite of their similar taste, the chemical makeup of bitters is quite diverse. Accordingly, they also have other varying effects, which may include antibiotic properties. Traditional bitter appetite stimulants and stomach tonics include *artichoke, gentian, dandelion, hops, horehound*, and the most bitter, *wormwood*.

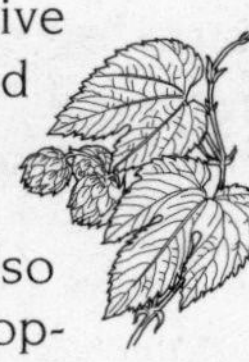

Hops

Cardiac Glucosides: As the name implies, these compounds have a direct impact on the heart, increasing the efficiency of its contraction and output. They are usually diuretic and thus also lower blood pressure. Plants with cardiac glucosides as a main component include *foxglove* (i.e. digitalis), *lily of the valley, pheasant's eye* and *strophanthus*. All of these are restricted, in varying degrees, to medical use because of their intense action, tissue accumulation and potential toxicity.

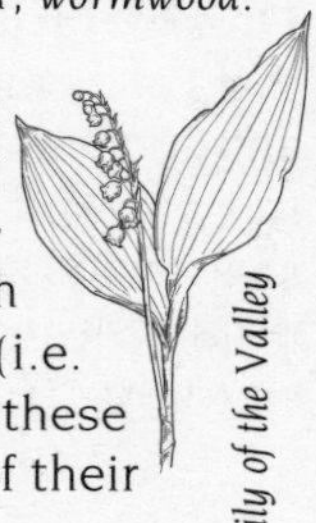

Lily of the Valley

Coumarins: Coumarins are the substances responsible for the smell of newly mown hay. They are also anti-inflammatory, blood-thinning agents and the basis of the medical anti-clotting drug Coumadin. The furocoumarins cause photosensitivity, increasing potential sunburning or tanning. This includes the whole parsley family. Other coumarin-containing herbs include *licorice, arnica, hawthorn* and *chamomile*.

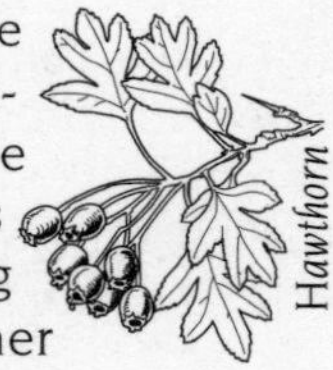

Hawthorn

Flavonoids: Also known as bioflavonoids, these substances are widely dispersed throughout the plant kingdom. They are particularly rich in the colored skin and barks of plants and fruits, and possess many healing properties. With powerful antioxidant, antihistamine, anti-allergy and anti-inflammatory properties, they strengthen connective and elastic tissue in the body. This is particularly important for blood vessels. Specialized kinds of bioflavonoids, proanthocyanidins, are found richly in *grape seed* and *bilberry*. *Green tea* contains the important anti-cancer EGCG bioflavonoids, which are lost in regular *black tea*.

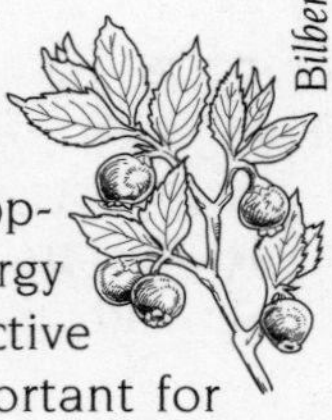

Bilberry

Minerals: As with vitamins, the mineral content and dosage of plant medicines is often not high enough to make up for deficiencies. There are cases, though, where the mix of hard-to-find trace elements, nutraceuticals and absorption factors make herbs invaluable for improving the metabolism of minerals within the body. *Alfalfa* and *nettles* have high amounts of absorbable iron. *Horsetail* provides silica, and *dandelion* is a source of bioavailable potassium.

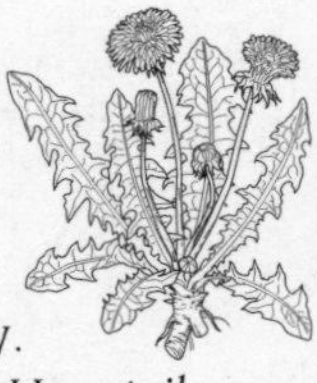

Dandelion

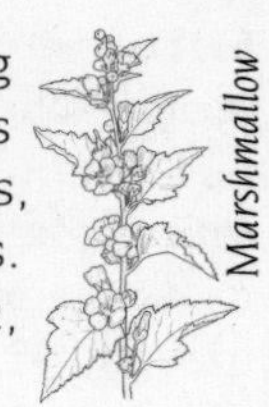

Mucilages: Mucilages are sugars that are water-loving (hydrophilic), so that they swell and form gelatinous masses when ingested. Mimicking the body's own mucus secretions, mucilage-containing herbs are often soothing demulcents. Examples of highly mucilaginous plants include *slippery elm*, *marshmallow*, *coltsfoot*, *plantain*, *linden* and *psyllium seeds*.

Phenols: Phenols are a broad category of plant chemicals that can combine in various ways to form flavonoids, tannins and coumarins. These chemicals are generally anti-inflammatory and anti-microbial. Good examples of phenols are salicylic acid (i.e. aspirin) as found in *meadowsweet*, *willow* and *wintergreen* and thymol, the antiseptic found in *thyme*, *arnica* and *wormwood*. Externally, phenols can be irritating to the skin.

Phytoestrogens: This group of flavonoids includes both isoflavones and lignans. There are high amounts in *soy*, *carrots*, *parsley*, *legumes* and *flaxseed*, though the herb *red clover* is highest in all four known isoflavones, while *soy* has only two. These substances are precursors for the body's own production of hormones, and protect it from estrogen-mimicking carcinogens, such as pesticides, DDT and PCBs.

Plant Acids: Organic acids appear broadly in the plant world, especially in fruits (i.e. malic acid in apples and citric acid in oranges). Both chain and ring acids are found in various medicines. With a wide range of actions, some plant acids, such as *cranberries*, are used for their antiseptic action, while others, like *nettles* (formic acid), help dissolve toxins. Plants containing oxalic acid, like *spinach*, can predispose one to kidney stones.

Pyrrolizidine Alkaloids: This type of alkaloid has been shown to undergo changes in the body, transforming it into toxic compounds. With excess or prolonged use, they can damage the lungs, increase cancer risk and eventually cause liver damage. Plants containing toxic pyrrolizidine alkaloids include *borage*, *gravel root*, *butterbur*, *lungwort* (Pulmonaria), *comfrey*, *coltsfoot* and *golden ragwort* (Senecio). However, limited dosages of these valuable plants is possible for short periods without danger.

Saponins: Saponins are plant constituents that produce a lather when mixed with water. Apart from this similarity, there are two important groups of saponins. The *triterpenoid* saponins have expectorant effects and may also stimulate and improve digestion. Acting as anti-inflammatories as well, they include *mullein* and *figwort*. *Steroidal* saponins can be used by the body to produce its own cortisol, estrogen, DHEA and other hormones. Prime examples are *licorice* and *ginseng*.

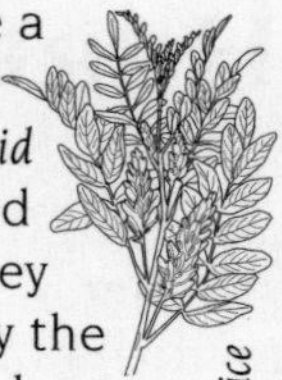

Licorice

Tannins: Tannins are highly astringent compounds, drying excess secretions and strong enough to coagulate protein. Found throughout the plant world, they act as deterrents to animals, insects and microorganisms. Highly concentrated in the bark, leaves or galls of trees, tannins are still used today in curing leather. Medicinally, they are used to heal discharges or diarrhea, and tone, tighten and heal tissues. Examples are many, but include *oak*, *geranium*, and *witch hazel*—and black tea!

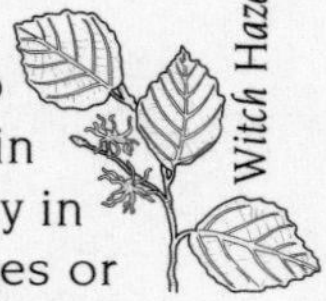

Witch Hazel

Vitamins: All plants contain varying amounts of vitamins. But herbs are generally not consumed in large enough quantities to make up for dietary deficiencies or to have them work like nutritional supplements, therapeutically. However, the unique blend of vitamins and their relationship to hundreds of other substances play a crucial role in a plant's overall effects—and effectiveness. Vitamins C, E and bioflavonoids, for example, are antioxidants for the plant itself, acting as preservatives that keep other chemical components from being degraded or destroyed.

Volatile Oils: Volatile oils are aromatic, easily evaporating substances that impart the familiar odor and flavor to many plants, including *mint*, *ginger* and *garlic*. Extracted from plants by steam distillation, essential oils form the basis of both aromatherapy and perfumery, as well as specific herbal medicines. Though they have a wide possible range of action, most are highly antiseptic, anti-inflammatory, stimulate digestion and are medicinal when excreted on the breath, in the urine and through body secretions. As extracts, they are highly concentrated and their internal use can be extremely dangerous. Examples of plants high in volatile oils are *tea tree*, *chamomile*, *juniper* and *curcumin*.

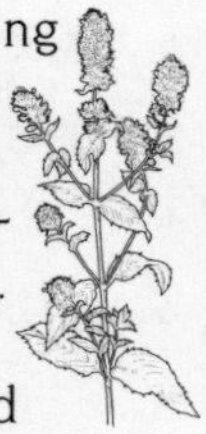

Peppermint

HERBAL ACTIONS

As mentioned earlier, using herbal medicines is not just substituting a natural plant for a similar drug, but involves a different approach to promoting health and correcting imbalances. The traditional way in which herbs have been prescribed in the European tradition for over 500 years is based on body function or physiology. This is an excellent approach, since it allows one to individualize, and to prescribe herbs more for the individual person than the disease. Rather, herbs are applied to correct functional imbalances that underlie those illnesses. Indeed, another name for holistic medicine in much of Europe and America today is functional medicine. This implies getting at causes, instead of symptomatically treating all diseases in the same superficial way.

The terms that follow are based on centuries of careful clinical use, observation and evaluation. There are well over one hundred such terms that have been used to describe the different actions of herbs on the human body and mind. Here we have simplified these sometimes confusing terms and put them into major categories, according to body system as follows:

- General Effects
- Antibiotic Effects
- Nervous System Effects
- Cardiovascular Effects
- Digestive Effects
- Respiratory Effects
- Urinary Effects
- Musculoskeletal Effects
- Female Effects
- Skin Effects

Note that effects on the immune system are included in the general category. Though knowing these terms is not essential to use or even prescribe herbs, they can greatly enrich our understanding. They make it easier to navigate through the rich diversity of healing herbs, and especially to understand why certain herbs are used together or in specific formulas.

GENERAL EFFECTS

There are herbs that have specific effects on a special organ or tissue, while others have universal applications. Below are listed herbal actions that have this kind of system-wide effect. These same plants can also be put in formulas with organ-specific herbs for more focused effect.

Adaptogens: Though the term is a new one, this is a very important class of herbs. Similar to tonics, they have the ability to either increase or decrease body functions, according to its need. They are renowned for their ability to help the body adapt to stress, improve performance and fend off or recuperate from illness. Many also have specific anti-aging effects. An example is *ashwaganda*. See the topics ■ Anti-aging ■ Fatigue ■ Sports Fitness ■ Stress.

Anti-inflammatories: Inflammation is one of the primary defense systems of the body and part of a majority of disease syndromes. Thus anti-inflammatory drugs are a mainstay of medical practice, using either steroids (cortisone), or non-steroidal anti-inflammatories (NSAIDS), like aspirin. However, herbs work in far more complex and comprehensive ways to block inflammation, as many studies have shown. They produce better clinical effects with much fewer side effects. A typical example is *meadowsweet*. See the topic ■ Inflammation.

Anti-mutagens: Anti-cancer agents work in a variety of ways, but many prevent the development of cancer by interfering with the ability of a substance to induce cellular changes. Carcinogens that have the ability to cause genetic mutations can be neutralized by agents high in bioflavonoids, sulphur-containing molecules and a variety of immune-boosting agents. Examples are *garlic* and *ginger*. See the topic ■ Cancer.

Antioxidants: Though the term is a relatively new one, antioxidant herbs have always been valued for their broad healing action. Antioxidants strike at one of the major causes of disease and aging—free radical damage. They prevent destruction to collagen or protein in the body and thus have a profound effect on protecting small blood vessels and enhancing circulation. Examples are *hawthorne* and *bilberry*. See the topics ■ Anti-aging ■ Arteriosclerosis.

Astringents: Astringents are drying agents that reduce the body's secretions and have the ability to coagulate and precipitate proteins. They reduce mucus, have antiseptic capabilities and help all kinds of congestion. Their deeper effect is to tone and tighten tissues that have become weakened and lack tone. They can be applied to almost any system in the body. Powerful astringents include *oak* and *geranium*. Others can be found under many topics, including ■ Hayfever/Allergy.

Demulcents: Demulcents contain mucilage that soothes, coats and softens mucus membranes. They can also be applied to skin. Apart from alleviating symptoms, they reduce inflammation and irritation and provide a protective coating, allowing tissues to heal. There are numerous demulcents that are useful anywhere there are lining membranes, including the mouth, intestines, bronchi, urinary tract and throat. *Licorice* and *slippery elm* are examples of excellent demulcents. These herbs appear in a variety of topics, including ■ Cough ■ Stomach Conditions.

Detoxifiers: A crucial aspect of healing is the clearing of accumulated debris from organs, tissues, lymphatics and cells. Traditionally, these types of herbs are known as *alteratives* or *blood purifiers*. They act by various and different physiological means, but the sum effect is deep tissue cleansing. This can alleviate underlying causes of both acute and chronic diseases, ranging from infections to cancer. There are many detoxifiers mentioned in this book, such as *red clover*, *phytolacca* and *cleavers*. See the topics ■ Acne/Abscess ■ Cancer ■ Detoxification ■ Infection.

Immune Stimulants: A large number of herbs have the ability to affect the immune system. With its far-reaching effect on every possible illness and susceptibility, immune stimulation is useful in a wide range of infections, inflammations and acute and chronic illnesses. Often too, the immune system becomes weakened or suppressed. There are short-term stimulants, like *echinacea*, and those that build the system up progressively, such as *astragalus*. See ■ Fatigue ■ Immune Weakness ■ Stress.

Stimulants: As the name implies, stimulants increases activity of the body's systems and overall nervous excitation. They act directly through the nervous system, or increase circulation, hormonal function or excretion of toxins. They are ideal for sluggish functions, but as activators, they can be overused or abused. See the topic ■ Fatigue.

Tonics: Tonics are among the most important categories of herbs and may be specific to the heart, nerves or liver. While other herbs cause a specific action in one direction, either stimulating or sedating, tonics go both ways. They help balance the organism and act as nurturing, restorative and strengthening factors. *Oats* and *astragalus* are typical tonics. See the topics ■ Anti-aging ■ Fatigue ■ Stress.

ANTIBIOTIC EFFECTS

Antibiotics: Antiseptic or antimicrobial herbs inhibit the growth or disrupt the life cycle of microorganisms. Yet these are not true "anti" (against) biotics (life). Many also have powerful effects on underlying immunity and resistance to microorganisms. They have the advantage of never becoming ineffective due to the development of resistant strains of microbes. And while all antibiotic drugs damage the liver, kidney, immune and nervous systems to some extent, herbal antibiotics promote the health of these organs. Studies show that each bout of antibiotics predisposes one to more frequent infections, especially in the case of otitis, colds and the like. If such drugs are used, herbs still play a role in repair and recuperation, with immune-promoting, detoxifying and tonic herbs.

ANTIBACTERIAL: Plants such as *myrrh*, *oregano*, *garlic*, *peppermint*, *eucalyptus* and *goldenseal* have proven effects on a very wide variety of bacteria, including E. coli, staph, strep. See the topics ■ Acne/Abscess ■ Infection.

ANTIVIRAL: Many herbs slow or halt the replication of invading viruses. Such herbs include *echinacea*, *St. John's wort*, and *olive leaf*. See the topics ■ HIV/AIDS ■ Infection ■ Colds & Flu.

ANTIFUNGAL: These herbs treat infections such as candida, and include herbal medicines like *grapefruit seed extract*, *tea tree oil* and *pau d'arco*. See the topic ■ Candida/Yeast.

ANTIPARASITIC: This class of herbs can eliminate the various kinds of larger organisms that invade the human organism. This includes amoebic infections (dysentery, vaginitis, mouth ulcers) as well as pinworms, roundworms and tapeworms. Some are gentle and safe, such as *garlic*, *pumpkin seeds* and *pomegranate*. In all cases, follow-up herbs are needed to strengthen the digestive system, liver and immune system. See the topics ■ Immune System ■ Parasites.

Febrifuges & Diaphoretics: Febrifuges are herbs that help to reduce fever. Closely related are diaphoretics, which induce sweating to assist the body's cooling process. However, fever is an important part of the body's defense system, reducing or stopping the production of bacteria or viruses. Both febrifuge and diaphoretic herbs do not suppress these natural reactions, but help eliminate toxins and enhance immunity. Most also have antimicrobial action, including *elderflower*, *ginger*, *catnip*, *boneset* and *yarrow*. See the topic ■ Colds & Flu.

Nervous System effects

Nervines: Synonymous with nerve tonics, nervines restore and rebalance the nervous system. They may be stimulating or relaxing, but ultimately nourish and strengthen the brain and nerves. *Oats*, *bacopa* and *gotu kola* are good examples, while *ginseng* and other adaptogens are also nerve tonics. See ■ Fatigue ■ Memory Loss ■ Stress.

Stimulants: This class of herbs is extremely well known to coffee and tea lovers everywhere. If the stimulus is strong enough, such plants are called excitants. Stimulants are best for short-term effects, to be followed by restorative nervines. Stimulants include *kola*, *oats* and *ephedra*. See the topics ■ Fatigue ■ Overweight.

Relaxants: Tranquilizing plants have a wide range of activity. *Relaxants* have a mild action. *Sedatives* take things one step further, calming the nervous system and reducing body functions. At the end of the spectrum, *narcotic* plants cause numbness, decreased awareness and stupor. Relaxant herbs include *valerian* and *skullcap*. See ■ Anxiety ■ Insomnia ■ Stress.

Soporifics: Soporific herbs induce a state of drowsiness and eventually sleep. *Hypnotics* act more strongly to induce a state of profound sleep. Most well-known sleep herbs are soporifics, including *passion flower*, *hops* and *wild lettuce*. See ■ Anxiety ■ Insomnia ■ Stress.

Antispasmodics: Also known as spasmolytic herbs, these plants relax muscles, both in internal organs such as the lungs and bronchi, as well as large and small external muscle masses. Such plants are true muscle relaxants and include herbs such as *black haw*, *black cohosh* and *wild yam*. See the topics ■ Anxiety ■ Colic/Cramps ■ Dysmenorrhea ■ Stress.

Sympathetic Stimulants: The sympathetic nervous system is behind our fight-or-flight reactions. It is also important in managing the body's adaptation to long-term stress. Stimulating the nerves combats fatigue, dilates the bronchi and enhances alertness and performance. Examples include *licorice* and *lobelia*. See ■ Asthma ■ Fatigue ■ Stress.

Parasympathetic Stimulants: Responsible for relaxing the automatic functions of the body, the parasympathetic nervous system promotes digestion, deep breathing and eases the sphincter muscles. Many relaxants, noted above, also tone the parasympathetic nerves.

Cardiovascular Effects

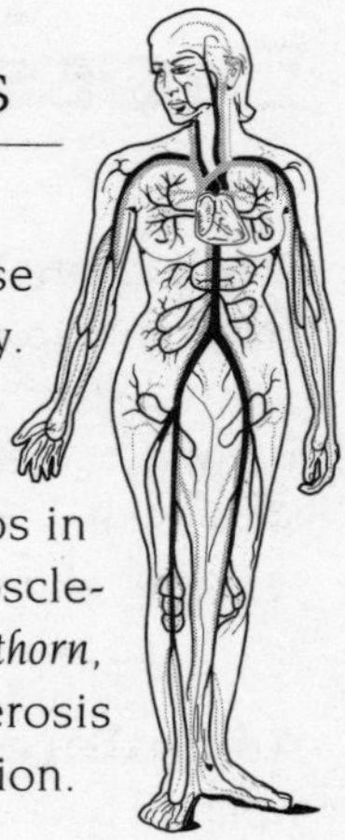

Cardiac Tonics: Also known as cardiotonics, these plants improve the functioning of the heart in a global way. They increase the force and volume of blood pumped, improve the supply of nutrients and oxygen to the heart muscle and regulate its rhythm. Additionally, many herbs in this group work on the blood vessels, influencing arteriosclerosis and high blood pressure. Cardiac tonics include *hawthorn, lily of the valley* and *motherwort*. See the topics ■ Arteriosclerosis ■ Heart Conditions ■ High Blood Pressure ■ Veins/Circulation.

Circulatory Stimulants: Herbs like *cayenne* increase blood flow in general or to specific areas, increasing the flow of oxygen and nutrients and carrying away metabolic wastes. *Ginkgo* has this effect on flow to the brain, extremities and even the gonads. See ■ Veins/Circulation.

Hemostatics: Also called styptics, herbs possessing this effect are able to stop or decrease bleeding. This may act through assisting the body's own clotting mechanisms, decreasing local blood flow or having an astringent effect on small capillaries and veins. Herbs such as *yarrow, witch hazel* and *shepherd's purse* are rightly famous for their historical use in times of war and peace. See the topics ■ Bleeding ■ Injury/Wounds.

Hypotensives: Hypertensive medicines raise blood pressure, while hypotensives (also called anti-hypertensives), do the opposite. Acting through a variety of mechanisms, they affect the nervous system, adrenals and the coats of the arteries themselves. Under the High Blood Pressure topic, typical hypotensive agents include *garlic, olive leaf* and *valerian*.

Vasoconstrictors: Herbs that narrow blood vessels and decrease blood flow are important in conditions such as bleeding or acute allergic reactions. Many vasoconstrictors are also astringents, this dual action being particularly useful for shrinking dilated or swollen blood vessels. Vasoconstrictors include *ephedra, butcher's broom* and *horse chestnut*. See the topics ■ Bleeding ■ Hemorrhoids ■ Veins/Circulation.

Vasodilators: Vasodilators are herbs that relax and widen blood vessels, thus increasing blood flow. They are important in high blood pressure, arteriosclerosis and specifically coronary heart disease. Examples include *hawthorn, siberian ginseng, coleus* and *ginkgo*. See the topics ■ Arteriosclerosis ■ Heart Conditions ■ Veins/Circulation.

Digestive Effects

Digestive Tonics: There are wide number of plants that improve digestion, increasing function in the whole digestive tract. Appetite is increased, gastrointestinal fluids and secretions promoted, and the assimilation of nutrients is improved. Chinese medicine lays great store in these "spleen" herbs that include *ginger, ginseng, licorice* and *peppermint*. All the topics listed below include digestive tonics.

Antimicrobials: While the large intestine has over 400 types of bacteria and fungi, the stomach and small intestine should be free of these organisms. For parasites, see the earlier Antibiotic Effects. Effective antibiotic herbs include *grapefruit seed* and *goldenseal*. See the topics ▪ Diarrhea ▪ Parasites ▪ Stomach Conditions.

Antispasmodics: As in other areas of the body, antispasmodic herbs act to reduce cramps. With indigestion, nausea, diarrhea or other upsets, they can reduce pain and muscle spasm. They also offer safe and gentle relief for infantile colic. Excellent antispasmodics include *chamomile* and *cramp bark*. See the topics ▪ Colic/Cramps ▪ Diarrhea ▪ Nausea.

Astringents: Astringents are important for drying up excess secretions, as well as toning up and tightening weakened tissues. They are used in ulcers, gastroenteritis, diarrhea, dysbiosis and for overall rehabilitation of the digestive tract. *Geranium, oak* and *raspberry* are good examples. See the topics ▪ Stomach Conditions ▪ Diarrhea ▪ Colitis/IBS.

Bitters: Bitters stimulate the digestive tract, increasing appetite, stomach acids, enzymes and mucus secretions. They are most effective when their bitterness can be tasted (i.e. in liquid form) and are the basis of many traditional European "bitters." Important plants in this group include *gentian, goldenseal* and *centaury*. See the topic ▪ Stomach Conditions.

Carminatives: Carminatives relieve belching, flatus and bloating, working on both the stomach and intestines. Often they work by reducing inflammation and underlying bacterial toxicity in the intestinal tract. Important carminatives include *chamomile, caraway* and *ginger*. See the topics ▪ Gas/Bloating ▪ Colitis/IBS ▪ Stomach Conditions.

Demulcents: Digestive demulcents soothe and promote healing of inflamed and irritated gastrointestinal linings and are useful in gastritis, colitis and diarrhea. They provide a protective barrier, and some, like *psyllium*, are also laxatives. Other digestive demulcents include *comfrey* and *marshmallow*. See the topics ■ Colitis/IBS ■ Diarrhea ■ Stomach Conditions.

Emetics: Emetic plants induce vomiting. Some traditional systems, including Native American, relied heavily on this kind of heroic treatment for digestive and liver detoxification. There is little place in today's herbal practice for emetics, though emergency medicine values *ipecac* for inducing vomiting after ingestion of non-caustic poisons or drug overdose.

Laxatives: Laxative herbs increase the passage of wastes through the small and large intestines. A*perient* indicates a mild laxative, *purgative* refers to a more powerful action and *cathartic* is a strongly irritant laxative. Laxatives include *cascara*, *senna* and *buckthorn*. For more detail, see herbs listed under the topics ■ Constipation ■ Gas/Bloating ■ Colitis/IBS.

Sialagogues: Sialagogues are closely related to bitters, stimulating the flow of secretions within saliva. This promotes starch-splitting enzymes in the mouth to aid digestion, but also has a detoxifying effect for use in congested or inflamed mouth conditions. Apart from bitters, other herbs with sialagogue effects include *ginger*, *cayenne* and *licorice*.

Stomachics: Stomachic is a broad term for stomach tonics. They increase the digestive activity of the stomach and may have additional anti-inflammatory and carminative effects. Bitters are a class of stomachic, but other herbs, like *peppermint*, promote digestion in their own, less obvious ways. See the topics ■ Nausea ■ Stomach Conditions.

Hepatics: Hepatics are liver tonics, improving the many functions of that organ and fostering regeneration of liver tissue. Since the liver is involved with literally every phase of body chemistry and detoxification, hepatics also figure prominently in many combination formulas. Many are *hepatoprotective*, protecting the liver from damage by various toxic substances. Most also have a *lipotropic* effect, stimulating the metabolism and breakdown of fats, an important therapy for weight loss and lowering cholesterol. Important hepatics include *celandine*, *fringe tree*, *dandelion* and *milk thistle*. See the topics ■ Gall Bladder ■ Liver Conditions.

Cholegogues: These hepatics stimulate the flow of bile from the liver or gallbladder into the intestine and help the gall bladder to contract. Closely related are *choleretics*, which stimulate the production of bile in the liver. Bile flow helps in the digestion of fats and reduces the incidence of gallstones. Many hepatics are cholegogues, the best of them being *artichoke* and *curcumin*. See ■ Gall Bladder ■ Liver Conditions.

RESPIRATORY EFFECTS

Antimicrobials: The nose, sinus, throat, bronchi and lungs are the most frequent sites of contagious illness. Important antibacterial, antiviral and antifungal respiratory herbs include *garlic*, *echinacea* and *goldenseal*. Additionally, herbs with volatile oils, like *peppermint* have antiseptic effects when exhaled. See the topics ■ Cold & Flu ■ Cough ■ Infection ■ Sore Throat.

Astringents: Drying and toning weak tissues, respiratory astringents are useful for excess mucus condition of the nose, throat or lungs. Thus they are valuable in almost every acute and chronic respiratory condition. Effective respiratory astringents include *myrrh*, *eyebright* and *elderflower*. See ■ Asthma ■ Cold & Flu ■ Cough ■ Sinusitis.

Demulcents: Respiratory demulcents are essential for soothing and healing irritated, dry linings of the throat and bronchi. They also add a protective barrier against further infection or free radical damage. *Licorice* and *marshmallow* are some of our most effective respiratory demulcents. See the topics ■ Cough ■ Hayfever ■ Sore Throat.

Expectorants: Expectorants soften and liquefy hard, dry phlegm and help expel wastes and mucus from the respiratory tract. These are used for moist coughs, asthma and emphysema, but also help clear mucus from post-nasal drip or sinus congestion. Examples include *elecampane*, *mullein* and *fennel*. See the topics ■ Asthma ■ Cough ■ Hayfever ■ Sinusitis.

Antispasmodics: Some herbs are true cough suppressants, acting on the brain and decreasing irritation in nerve endings. Others help calm muscle spasms of the bronchi and diaphragm, sharing this effect with many nervines or relaxants. *Antitussives* are an offshoot of antispasmodics, the Latin word simply meaning "against coughs." Respiratory antispasmodics include *lobelia*, *coltsfoot* and *wild cherry*. See ■ Asthma ■ Cough.

Pectorals: Though now a little-used term, pectorals are basically lung tonics that have a specific affinity for the bronchi and respiratory passages. They are used to correct illness, but also to strengthen the structures of the thoracic cavity. The lungs are an important detoxification pathway, and these herbs ably help it in this function. *Comfrey* (available in a pyrrolizidine-free form) is rightly famous as a healing pectoral herb, along with many other cough herbs. See ■ Asthma ■ Cough.

URINARY EFFECTS

Diuretics: Like their drug counterparts, diuretic herbs increase the flow of urine, useful for clearing infections and inflammations from the urinary tract. However, unlike their medical analogues, herbs like *dandelion* and *cornsilk* do not induce potassium loss because of their high content of that mineral. Diuretics are also useful in other conditions, including heart disease, high blood pressure, obesity, PMS and menopause. *Goldenrod*, *horsetail* and other effective diuretics are listed under the topics ■ Bladder Infections ■ Kidney Conditions.

Urinary Antiseptics: Many antimicrobial herbs have the ability to disinfect the urinary tract. This includes *buchu*, *uva ursi* and *juniper*. Most work through a direct antibiotic effect, while *cranberry* acts by making it impossible for bacteria to adhere to the sides of the bladder. See the topics ■ Bladder Infection ■ Candida ■ Infection ■ Kidney Conditions.

Urinary Astringents: As elsewhere in the body, astringents are useful to help strengthen, tighten and heal mucus membrane linings. This is important after infection or when there is a chronic "catarrh" or mucus condition of the bladder or urethra. Effective herbs in this category include *goldenseal*, *bearberry* (Berberis) and *horsetail*. See topics above.

Urinary Demulcents: When there is infection or inflammation of the urethra or bladder, demulcents need to be combined with diuretics or antiseptics. Demulcent herbs offer both healing and protection against damage to the membrane linings of these tissues. Important urinary demulcents include *althea*, *couchgrass* and *licorice*. See topics above.

Antilithics: This group of herbs has the ability to prevent the formation of calculi or stones. They are also traditionally used to dissolve kidney stones, where possible. This action goes beyond their diuretic action, as they change the acid/base balance of the urine and work by, as yet, poorly understood mechanisms. Such herbs include *hydrangea*, *gravel root*, *parsley root* and *pellitory*. See the topic ■ Kidney Conditions.

Kidney Tonics: Herbs that tone and heal the kidney are also used as part of overall detoxification programs. While they do usually have diuretic or antiseptic properties, they also help regenerate and optimize kidney tissue, which is largely made up of tiny arteries and tubules. See the topics ■ Arteriosclerosis ■ Detoxification ■ Kidney Conditions.

MUSCULOSKELETAL EFFECTS

Analgesics: Pain-relieving herbs, like *meadowsweet* and *chamomile* provide safe and effective action, while also providing anti-inflammatory, anti-spasmodic effects, often addressing the underlying causes for pain. See the topics ■ Arthritis ■ Fibromyalgia ■ Headache ■ Pain/Neuralgia.

Anti-inflammatories: Most musculoskeletal conditions involve inflammation of joint, muscle, ligament or connective tissue. Often working as well as anti-inflammatory drugs, major herbs in this category include *curcumin* and *boswellia*. See the topics ■ Arthritis ■ Fibromyalgia ■ Inflammation ■ Injury/Wounds.

Antispasmodics: All of the spasm-reducing herbs are important for treating both the causes and effects of various musculoskeletal problems. See the topics ■ Colic/Cramps ■ Fibromyalgia ■ Pain/Neuralgia.

FEMALE EFFECTS

Uterine Tonics: Uterine tonics increase the muscular tone of uterine tissues and have been used traditionally for uterine displacements, prolapse, miscarriage, dysmenorrhea and infertility. B*lue cohosh* and *true unicorn root* are well-known uterine tonics. See ■ Dysmenorrhea ■ Miscarriage.

Estrogenics: Many traditional herbs that are used to promote normal menses and relieve symptoms of menopause are now known to contain isoflavones and other chemicals that the body turns into progesterone or estrogen. Closely related are *emmenagogues* that stimulates menses, while balancing the female hormones. See the topics ■ Amenorrhea ■ Infertility ■ Menopause.

Antispasmodics: Relieving spasms is important in painful periods, PMS, excess bleeding or threatened miscarriage. These herbs work by relaxing nerves and muscle fibers, and by neutralizing inflammatory substances like prostaglandins and cytokines. See ■ Dysmenorrhea.

Oxytoxics: Opposite to antispasmodics, herbs like *black cohosh* can stimulate the uterus to contract. These herbs are primarily, and importantly, used as traditional medicines for labor. See the topic ■ Childbirth.

SKIN EFFECTS

Antiseptics: Numerous herbs have antibacterial, antiviral and antifungal activity for various kinds of skin infections. This includes boils, abscesses, pimples and infected wounds, as well as ringworm and nail fungi. Among the best of these are *tea tree oil, calendula* and *goldenseal*. See the topics ▪ Acne/Abscess ▪ Infection ▪ Skin Conditions.

Astringents: For any kind of "moist" condition, astringents dry up secretions and discharges and tone up the skin. They are useful in weeping eczemas, as well as bleeding and bruising. Good skin astringents include *witch hazel* and *plantain*. See ▪ Injury/Wounds ▪ Skin Conditions.

Emollients: Herbal emollients soften the skin when it is chaffed, dry or scaly. Whether due to harsh weather or more serious skin diseases, like psoriasis or eczema, they lubricate and nourish the skin, relieving itching, flaking and discomfort. They also form a basic ingredient in the majority of cosmetics. Examples include *slippery elm* and *olive oil*.

Rubefacients: Herbs with a rubefacient effect stimulate blood flow to the skin. This relieves congestion locally, dispelling heat and bringing needed nutrients and oxygen to the area. Such effects are valuable for various skin ailments, circulatory disorders, as pain relief and to accelerate healing of wounds. The most famous rubefacient is *cayenne*. See the topics ▪ Inflammation ▪ Injury/Wounds ▪ Skin Conditions ▪ Veins/Circulation.

Styptics: Styptics are locally applied herbs that stops blood loss from cuts or wounds. They also arrest bleeding from the mucus membranes and fine venous networks of the nose, ear, anus, rectum or vagina. Often astringent as well, they include herbs like *St. John's wort, horse chestnut, witch hazel* and *green tea*. See the topics ▪ Bleeding ▪ Hemorrhoids ▪ Injury/Wounds ▪ Veins/Circulation.

Vulneraries: Vulneraries have the ability to promote wound healing, something no medical drug has duplicated. Such herbs improve tissue repair and often prevent or minimize scarring. They often combine anti-inflammatory and antimicrobial effects and can be styptics as well. Examples are *calendula, heal all* and *burdock*. See the topics ▪ Inflammation ▪ Injury/Wounds.

HERBAL SOURCES

With herbs commonly available in capsules, dropper bottles and tea bags, we are usually unaware of which part of the plant goes into the making of these products. The plant kingdom is vast and diverse, with both deadly poisons and common foods. The medicinal qualities of plant parts are just as variable, but a few generalizations can be made. This helps in understanding the healing action of the plant we wish to use—and may enhance our choice of herbs in a specific situation.

Bark

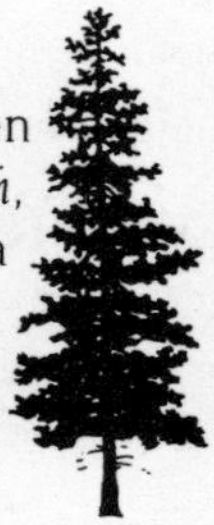

The barks of trees, shrubs, vines or other woody plants often contain the most active medicinal parts of the plant. P*rickly ash*, *willow* (*Salix*, i.e. aspirin), *cramp bark* (*Viburnum*), and *cascara* are a few of the famous healing herbs made from tree or stem bark. Barks are often high in tannins, making them astringent, but they can be spicy and warming, like *sandalwood* and *cinnamon*.

Root

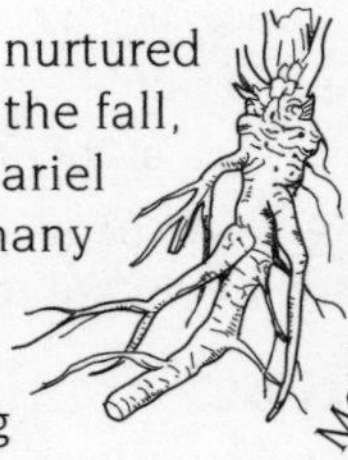

Roots frequently contain concentrated medicinal power, nurtured and held in the earth. Roots are generally collected in the fall, or after the first frost, when activity recedes from the ariel parts of the plant and dwells underground. Of the many examples of root herbs, we can mention *goldenseal* (*Hydrastis*), *ginseng*, *poke root*, *wild yam*, *marshmallow*, *ginseng* and *astragalus*. Traditionally, root plants carry a strong component of vitality and an earthy, detoxifying effect.

Marshmallow

Leaf

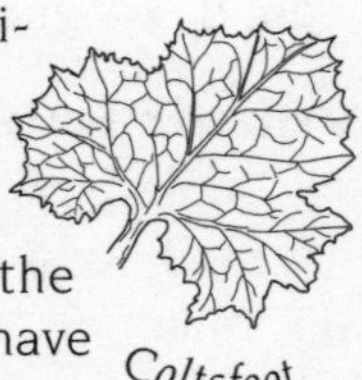

The leaf is at the center of plant metabolism and chemical transformation. As a result, this is the plant part most often imbued with healing properties and used as an herbal medicine. Leafy herbs include *coltsfoot*, *peppermint*, *plantain*, *vervain*, *uva ursi*, *buchu* and *green tea*. In spite of the diverse nature of these plants, leaves are considered to have a balancing, rhythmic effect on the nerves, lungs, heart, etc.

Coltsfoot

Fruit/Seed

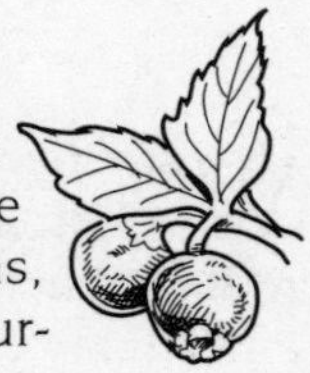

Seeds and the nourishing fruit around them contain the essence required to create a new plant, whether it be tree or tiny grass. Fruits often contain concentrated sugars, while seeds may contain oils or starches. Often high in vitamins, medicines made from fruits are traditionally considered nourishing and tonic. Seeds can be moist and lubricating, or may contain pungent or antiseptic essential oils. Herbal medicines composed of fruits include *anise, caraway, sesame* (these dry, hard herbs are actually fruits, not seeds), *hawthorn, schisandra* and *bilberry*.

Bilberry

Flower

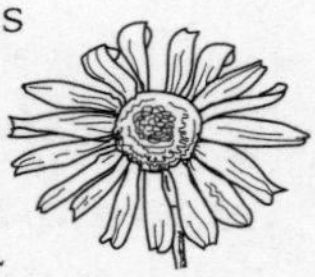

In spite of their beauty and fragrance, flowers are used less frequently than any other plant part in herbal medicine. Noticeable exceptions include *calendula, elderflower, clover* and *linden*. They are also the basis of the powerful system of healing Flower Essences and also figure largely into aromatherapy and perfumery, as a source of essential oils. Medicines made from flowers are often healing and detoxifying.

Calendula

Resins, Oils

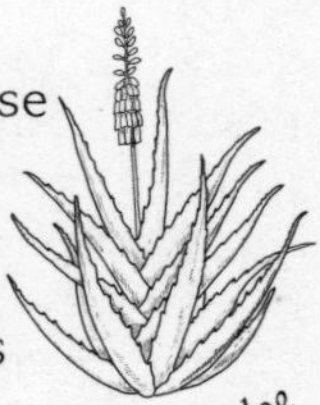

The most famous resinous herbs are biblical frankincense (*boswellia*) and *myrrh*, but also include *balm of gilead* and even *aloe*. *Tea tree oil, castor oil, eucalyptus, lavender* and many other plants yield concentrated essential oils that often have warming properties. The firey nature of many of these plants is astringent and expectorant and powerfully antiseptic.

Aloe

Whole Plant

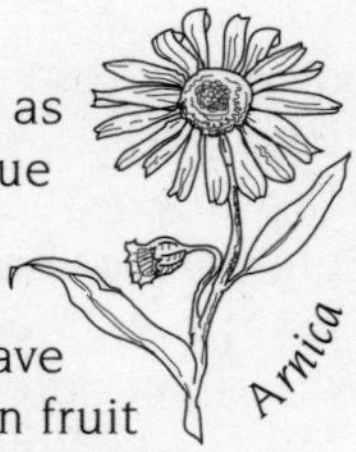

In an ideal world, each part of a plant would be available as a separate medicine and we would understand the unique differences in the healing properties of each one. As it is, it is sometimes useful to use all parts of the plant, to make sure the totality of its different healing properties have been captured. Plants in which root, leaf, flower and even fruit are often used together include *hawthorne* (flower and berry), *valerian* (root and leaf) and *arnica* (root, leaf and flower).

Arnica

HERBAL QUALITY

When purchasing something like an automobile, quality is relatively easy to discern, and what you pay for is what you get. Unfortunately, in herbal medicine, a pretty bottle or label is no guarantee of the value and vitality of the enclosed plant material. With herbs now a billion dollar industry and pharmaceutical companies entering the fray, the water has become further muddied. A few large-scale suppliers are behind many product lines, especially "house brands" in pharmacy chains and vitamin shop chains. These will work (just like junk food works), but will be on the lower rung of value and freshness. Buy products that are from a well-known, reputable company, with a track record of integrity and concern, with a commitment to the environment and to holistic and herbal medicine. For optimal results, look for products that are grown, harvested and processed according to the following general guidelines.

Organic Herbs

With literally dozens of dietary systems around, one size does not fit all. Yet there are a general principles that should be considered the single most important aspect of modern diet—eat organic. Similarly, a herb grown in healthy soil on organic farms or picked from the wild (i.e wild-crafted) can be expected to yield optimal healing benefits. However, for economic reasons, herbs that are in great demand may be grown using pesticides and herbicides, or be acquired from abroad where there is little environmental control. If imported from overseas, herbs may also be fumigated or even irradiated. While they will retain a certain chemical activity, their deeper healing capabilities are greatly diminished. They have a counterproductive effect, as toxic chemical residues can offset their benefits or interfere with their activity in the body.

Processing

The ultimate purpose of herbal preparations is to preserve all the freshness and vibrancy of the original plant, as well as concentrate their medicinal effects. To this end, plants that are to be processed for putting into capsules or tea bags should be dried and packaged as quickly as possible. Packaging that is airtight, and also light proof, will help preserve plant ingredients. Their subtle chemical ingredients can easily be oxidized, rendered rancid, or be destroyed by dampness, microorganisms (especially fungi) or enzymatic decay.

Fresh Plant Tinctures

Many tinctures are far more effective and vital when made directly from the freshly picked plant. The extra step of drying and storing may decrease the biochemical value of the plant, especially through the loss of its active enzymes systems. Moreover, a dried plant is in a sense a "dead" plant, devoid of a certain vitality and vibratory strength. It is for this reason that homeopathic remedies must be made from plants picked literally hours before. Such fresh or green plant tinctures are noticeably stronger and deeper in their effect. These *green tinctures*, made directly from fresh plants, will definitely preserve the vital life quality and vibrational fingerprint of the herb in a more precise way. However, barks and hard seeds may require drying so they can be powdered fine enough to make a tincture.

Organic Alcohol

Plants haven been extracted using alcohol since antiquity, creating medicinal wines and tinctures that could be preserved much better than raw plant material. Today, alcohol is created using commercial corn, wheat or other grains that receive more pesticide treatment than any other crop and contains residues of these poisons. Beginning with a company named Eclectic Research, organol or organic alcohol (made from organic grapes or apples) is being increasingly used to make herbal tinctures. This definitely improves the value and wholesomeness of organic herbs, and prevents chemical reactions that would destroy important healing ingredients, like bioflavonoids and alkaloids.

Manufacturing Process

Today, all FDA-approved herbal medicine manufacturers must follow good manufacturing practices (GMPs) for food products. While these are mandatory, some voluntarily follow the more strict GMPs required for drug manufacturing. Herbal Products Association guidelines are another standard followed by concerned manufacturers. Good companies provide full product disclosure on the label and offer considerable support literature, describing their manufacturing process and adherence to various guidelines for keeping herbs fresh and effective. There are dozens of systems in place at reputable herbal companies to ensure the quality of the final products. A few of the most important ones are listed below.

Identification

- Visual and microscopic inspection, along with an examination of the smell and taste of herbs, is the first step in any herb processing.
- A case of mistaken herbal identity at this stage would be increasingly difficult to catch once the herb is powdered, extracted or dissolved.

Purity Testing

- Before processing, herbs are quarantined and tested for contamination by insects, bacteria, fungi, chemicals, pesticides or heavy metals.

Chromatographic Testing

- Chromatography allows chemists to identify the unique chemical signature of each plant and to measure the strength of each batch.
- Variations, using gas (GC), thin layer (TLC) and high pressure chromatography (HPLC) provide ever more sophisticated information.

HERBAL FORMS

When we think of herbs, we may picture waving fields of fragrant flowers on a summer's day. Yet when we purchase a medicinal herb, it is in a bottle, box or carton. Thus, after the choice of herb, the next most important decision is the *form* of herb we wish to use. To clarify the choice between forms and their effects, the differences, advantages and disadvantages of the major types of products are outlined below. Following this is a description of external applications. The important topic of *standardization* deserves its own section.

Infusions

Infusions are the simplest and most ancient of herbal preparations, being none other than our familiar herbal teas. They can be made with fresh or dried plants, available as tea bags or in bulk. A general rule is to use one to two teaspoons of herb per cup of hot water, allowed to steep, covered, for 5 to 10 minutes. Excess heat or boiling can destroy their value.

ADVANTAGES

- Herb teas are a good substitute for black tea or coffee addiction.
- They may be absorbed better than dried herbs, tablets or capsules.
- They are a good choice for children, or when strong doses are not desired, i.e. for weakened or recuperating individuals.

DISADVANTAGES

- They have a short shelf life, lasting only a few days if refrigerated.
- Relatively large amounts must be taken for therapeutic effects.
- The strength and amount of each dose is quite variable.
- They are not particularly convenient to prepare, carry or store.
- Taste may be objectionable or unpalatable (i.e. *reishi mushrooms*).
- Only the water-soluble aspects of the plant are released, and with some plants it is only the fat-soluble part that is medicinal (i.e. *milk thistle*).
- Because of toxicity, some herbs are never taken in raw form (i.e. *ginkgo*).

Decoctions

Harder parts of plants—roots, seeds, dried berries or bark—may not yield their active ingredients to a simple infusion. With decoctions, these materials are simmered for 20 to 40 minutes, ideally in an earthenware or Pyrex pot, though stainless steel is acceptable. All the advantages and disadvantages of infusions apply, though decoctions are much stronger tasting and more concentrated. Traditional Chinese herbs are commonly prescribed and taken in this form.

Capsules

Capsules, containing dried herbs, represent the majority of herbal products sold today. They may also contain solid extracts or liquids (see below).

ADVANTAGES

- Their form is easy to take or to transport and needs no preparation.
- They maintain their freshness well and are very convenient to carry.
- They don't require the hard coatings and various compounding agents that are needed for tablets, and which make them less absorbable.

DISADVANTAGES

- Capsules may contain herbs that are old, outdated or simply not fresh.
- Unless using vegi-caps, one is consuming chemically treated gelatin.
- Capsules may contain filler or flow agents (often magnesium salts).
- They are not as well absorbed or digested as teas or tinctures.
- As with teas, fat-soluble components of the herb are not available. This can be overcome if fat-extracted substances are added back.

Tablets

Tablets are made by compressing the ground, powdered herb and adding binders and coatings to make them stable. Traditional Chinese patent medicines use waxes or hard casings.

ADVANTAGES

- They have similar advantages to capsules, but gelatin is not consumed.

DISADVANTAGES

- They require binders and stabilizing agents that may make them less absorbable by the body.

Freeze-Dried Herbs

A newer development is the use of freeze-dried herbs. As with similar foods, they are made by subjecting herbs to freezing, followed by evaporation at low pressure. This preserves the plant in a non-alcoholic form.

ADVANTAGES

- They are highly effective for certain conditions (i.e. *nettles* for allergy).
- They can store almost indefinitely if kept from moisture or high heat.
- They may provide better assimilation and absorption in certain herbs.

DISADVANTAGES

- Heat and especially moisture can cause rancidity and spoilage rapidly.
- Plants that are high in fatty acids are inappropriate for this form.
- As with capsules, they are not concentrated and potency is variable.

Tinctures

Tinctures are made by dissolving an herbal substance in alcohol, which effectively extracts both its water-soluble and fat-soluble components. Fresh or dried plants are ground and added to alcohol in a specific ratio. After sitting for up to two weeks, the resulting solution has a concentration of approximately 1 part plant to 9 parts of alcohol (1:10 ratio), but may be as concentrated as 1:5. Tinctures average about 50% alcohol content, but range from 25 to 80%, depending on the herb.

ADVANTAGES

- Both fat- and water-soluble compounds are extracted from the plants.
- Tinctures are often more potent than dried herbs in capsules or tablets.
- They are portable and easy to use and not required to be made fresh.
- They also have a shelf life of several years (especially if refrigerated).
- Combinations of herbs can be made up easily or altered as desired.

DISADVANTAGES

- Tinctures can be relatively weak or dilute, requiring larger doses.
- Taste aids the effectiveness of herbs, but may be too strong for some.
- Alcohol has to be consumed to get a therapeutic dose, though tinctures can be put in very hot (but not boiling) water to evaporate the alcohol.

Fluid Extracts and Solid Extracts

Fluid extracts (FE) are made by removing alcohol from a tincture, making it far more concentrated—usually 1:1. This can be done by low temperature methods. FEs are a common form used by practitioners. There are a number of sophisticated extraction and concentration methods in use today. Solid extracts go one step further, removing the alcoholic liquid and putting the remaining, highly concentrated solid in capsules.

ADVANTAGES

- FEs and solid extracts have all the above advantages of tinctures.
- Extracts are far more concentrated than tinctures, while still containing both fat- and water-soluble components, with far less alcohol.

DISADVANTAGES

- They still require a small ingestion of alcohol.
- The taste can be very strong, though they can be taken in juice.

Glycerates

Another innovation is the use of glycerine instead of alcohol. This is very useful for pets, children, the elderly or cancer patients. The taste is improved, and they may be flavored more easily this way. However, not all active ingredients are extracted and some preservatives are required.

Syrups

Syrups are made by adding honey or sugar to tinctures or extracts, typically for cough, sore throat or colds and flu medicines. They may contain significant amounts of alcohol, though putting them in freshly boiled water will evaporate much of this. They are palatable and easy to take. They do require ingesting a lot of sugar and contain some preservatives.

Essential Oils

Oils are heat distilled from plants or removed by cold extraction. They are mixed with vegetable oil or water and used as an inhalant, douche, or added to an eyewash, ear drops, mouthwash, massage oil or to treat cuts and abrasions. Essential oils absorb easily, but are extremely strong and can be irritating to the skin; many are lethal if ingested in excess.

External Usage

Topicals: External use of herbs can complement the use of internal ones or can be the sole method of treatment. Some herbs are effective in their raw form (*aloe*), or the extract can be applied directly or diluted with water (*witch hazel*). Herbs can be added to local or whole body baths. *Linden* or *valerian* baths are effective for sore muscles, stress, anxiety, etc.

Poultice: Fresh or dry herbs can be used directly on the skin. A hot, moist, soft mass of herbs, with the addition of oats, flour, mustard, etc. is spread on muslin or cloth. This is applied for one to eight hours to relieve pain, inflammation or infection. The cloth or muslin should be changed when cool. Poultices draw out infection and relieve congestion.

Compress: A compress is the simplest form of topical use. A cloth soaked in an infusion, warm tincture or extract can be applied directly to the skin for use on infections, bruises, and inflammations. A *succus*, or low-alcoholic plant extract, is sometimes available for this purpose.

Cream and Ointments: A powdered herb or tincture can be added to a fat or oil base to form a salve. These penetrate the skin easily and also provide a protective, healing barrier. *Calendula*, *comfrey*, *St. John's wort* and other typical external healers make excellent creams for treating wounds, strains and pains. These herbs can be put in a Vaseline base (petroleum is an ancient Native American skin healer) or a non-oily gel.

Liniment: When herbal creams, ointments or oils are made specifically to be rubbed deeply into the skin, they are called liniments. This is most useful for sore, tired muscles or strained ligaments, and not appropriate to irritated or infected tissue or inflamed skin rashes.

Douche: The application of an herbal infusion or decoction to the vagina is effective for local infections or to treat cervical dysplasia, with such herbs as *calendula*, *white cedar* or *goldenseal*.

Suppository: Like their medical counterparts, herbal suppositories can be designed to be inserted into body cavities for treating local problems. This includes rectal suppositories for hemorrhoids, while vaginal suppositories treat infections and inflammation in that area.

Inhalation: The breathing of steamed herbal mixtures through the oral or nasal cavity is a traditional and effective way to treat coughs, colds and asthma, with herbs like *eucalyptus*, *tea tree* or *peppermint*.

STANDARDIZATION

The Problem of Variability

An inherent problem in any medical treatment is dosage—providing a specific, quantified and consistent amount of healing substance. Herbs are part of the natural world, not artificial, manufactured products. Thus marked variations in the strength and potency of plants occur naturally. Variables such as different soil, temperature, sunlight and climate result in a striking difference in the content of essential plant chemicals, vitamins or minerals. The method of collecting, processing and storing can also vary widely, resulting in a different composition of active ingredients in each dose or bottle of a particular herb. It should be pointed out that, traditionally, this was much less of a problem, as herbs were harvested in the same areas for centuries. Local healers knew the potency of their herbs and were skilled at picking the most desirable plants.

Raising the Standards

A major innovation in the production of plant medicines is standardization. Standardization ensures that a given amount of herb has the same strength and potency in each capsule or bottle. To this end, a measurable marker substance and a desired concentration for it is chosen. This marker may be an active ingredient, or just one that is easily determined, but often, it is a compound that has been used in scientific research.

These products have generated both controversy and confusion among consumers and professionals. Unfortunately herbal manufacturers have done more than anyone to cloud the issue with new jargon and proprietary names. In fact standardization means different things to different people. The word "extract" is also confusing, since this term traditionally is associated with fluid extracts, which are highly concentrated tinctures made from the *whole plant*.

ADVANTAGES

- A consistent potency and dosage of active ingredients are available for the first time in the history of herbal medicine.
- Concentrated extracts may act more quickly and powerfully, and be effective where less invasive methods were not successful.
- Some plants, like *ginkgo*, require standardization, as other ingredients in the plant are poisonous and need to be discarded.
- Isolated ingredients can be patented and profited from in a way that nature's whole herbs never can be. This may be part of their allure for manufacturers.

DISADVANTAGES

- Thousands of natural compounds and co-factors in the herb are lost.
- This may reduce their effectiveness, broad scope and subtle effects, and eliminate compounds that could be essential and valuable.
- Standardized extracts may use solvents or acetone to extract the active ingredients (leaving residues) then destructive heat to evaporate them.
- Their nature is closer to pharmaceutical drugs than herbal medicine.
- They may be less gentle, with a greater tendency toward side effects.
- Confusion and errors occur regarding just what is the active ingredient or substance that is used as a marker for standardization. For example, *St. John's wort* is usually measured for *hypericin*, though it is now thought that *hyperforin* is the more active substance.
- Products may contain only one isolated ingredient, the remainder of the product being an inert filler and not the rest of the plant.
- Only a small number of plants are standardized. If different standardized and traditional whole herbs are used together, the one may overshadow the other or have unpredictable results.

Is a Chemical a Herb?

One well-known manufacturer tells us in its consumer literature that in standardized extracts "active compounds are natural compounds found in an herb that is proven to be responsible for its healthy benefits." Morphine is from opium, but it is not a herb! Citric acid is not an orange, and isoflavones are not a soy bean! An active compound is in fact an isolated chemical, and no longer belongs to the plant kingdom, but to the molecular world. Unfortunately, cheaper brands, like those routinely available now in pharmacies, corner stores and even airports, are usually standardized, yet do not contain the whole herb.

Whole Herb Extracts

There are several solutions to the problem of isolates and whole herbs.

- Blending: Some companies blend various herb batches to avoid variations and meet a standard, still using the whole herb.
- HPCL testing (chromatographic layering) provides a unique "fingerprint" of a herb's chemical constituents for creating consistent blends.
- The more concentrated a product is (i.e. the more water, alcohol and fiber is removed), the higher it will be in all important ingredients.
- Combining: A standardized single ingredient is added in with the whole herb. This provides the benefits of both whole herb and isolate.

Carefully examining labels will disclose whether the product contains the full spectrum of plant ingredients, aside from a single standardized isolate. There continues to be discussion and argument about the merits of the different approaches. Certainly, for those who want the full benefits of herbal medicine, the whole plant must be used. If a standardized isolate is added to this, this herbal "booster" may benefit certain illnesses.

THE HEALING PROCESS

The Healing Crisis

We are accustomed to a symptomatic form of health care and have become unfamiliar with the way the body and biology actually work when healing is initiated. Immune and metabolic resources spring into action, and this can entail what has been termed a "healing crisis."

Acute and chronic conditions sometimes entail a slight and short-lived intensifying of symptoms. Improvement should follow soon. In chronic conditions, however, acute symptoms can arise during the process of deep cure, and these can be both disturbing and confusing. This does not mean that worse is *always* better or that feeling bad is good. In fact, there are very specific signs to distinguish between just getting worse (a disease crisis) and a true healing crisis. In other words, healing follows very specific, recognizable patterns and pathways.

Healing as Process

The healing process does not proceed instantly nor in a simple progressive fashion. Like any living thing, our health unfolds in a highly unique way, according to a variety of factors, including age, duration of illness, genetic tendencies and the treatments used and the obstacles to cure. There are hills and valleys in the process that mirror the internal struggle and revolution of health that is taking place in the individual.

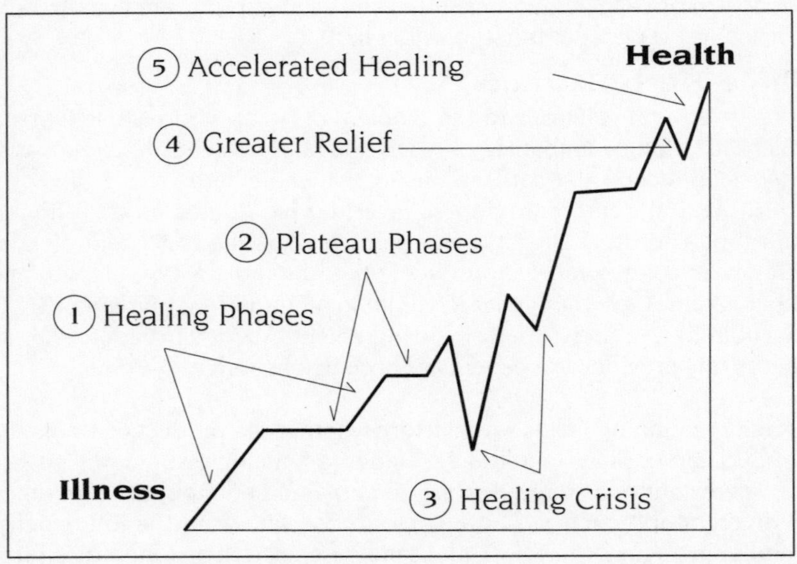

1. **HEALING PHASES.** These are periods of regular and marked improvement in the condition and in the person's overall level of well-being.
2. **PLATEAU PHASES.** These occur when, for a period of time, the body maintains an improved state, but goes no further. This is a time of consolidation, rest and gathering of biological strength and resources.
3. **HEALING CRISIS.** When the body has the strength and opportunity, it will throw off toxins from deeper tissues, while more superficial tissues like the skin or mucus membranes will discharge or erupt.
4. **GREATER RELIEF.** As toxicity lessens and vitality improves, healing crisis become shorter, and periods of complete relief become longer.
5. **HEALING ACCELERATES.** As obstacles lessen and immunity is strengthened, healing will proceed in an easier, streamlined way.

The Healing Hierarchy

- In its healing hierarchy, the body will always try to protect the organs that are most essential to life and cannot be regenerated.
- These take precedence over tissues that are easily replaced or can sustain considerable damage without endangering the whole.
- As in the diagram below, skin is the most superficial and easy to replace, while the heart and nervous system are the most crucial to survival.
- However, the skin can have a life-threatening disease like cancer, and a very vital organ (heart) can have a superficial condition (palpitations).
- It is the interplay of the depth of tissue and degree of pathology that makes a particular problem a top priority for the body.
- This is where the organism—body and mind—focuses its healing force in order to change and resolve the situation.

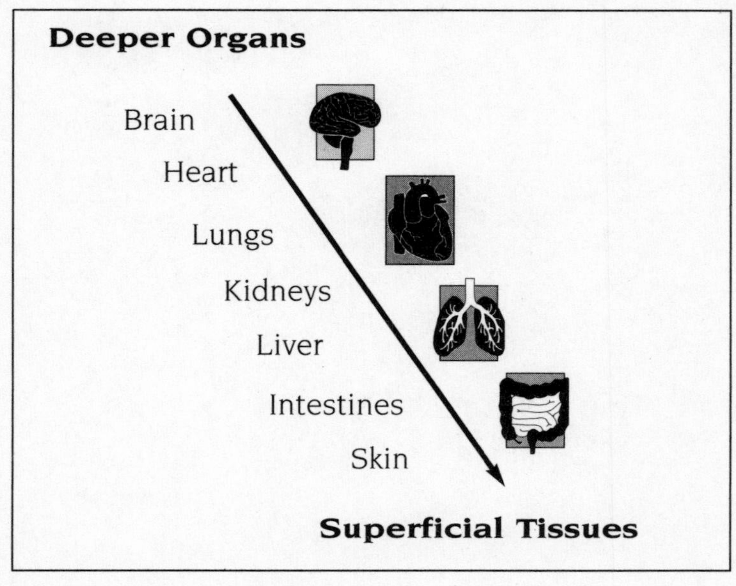

PART 2

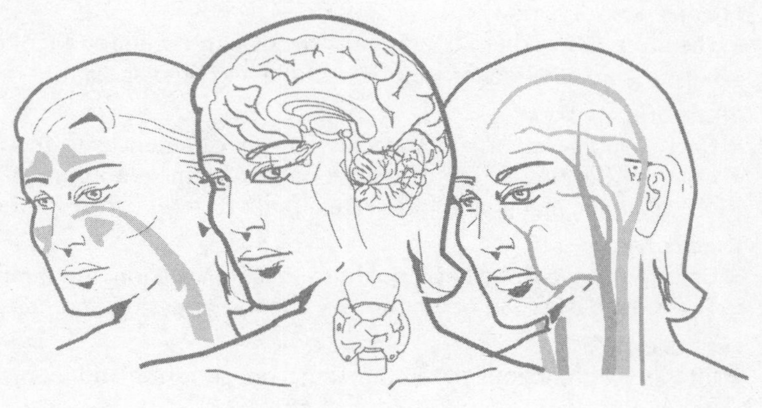

BODY SYSTEMS

PSYCHOLOGICAL CONDITIONS

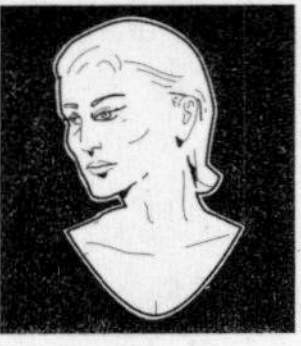

The System

Herbal medicine combined with psychotherapy is an excellent match. In spite of modern advances, our understanding of the "anatomy" of the mind is negligible. While there are specific body systems and brain areas relating to the mind, there is no easy physical map to our subtle experiences of thought and feeling.

HORMONAL SYSTEM

- The state of the thyroid, adrenals, ovaries and other endocrine glands have a marked effect on emotional tone and predispositions.

NERVOUS SYSTEM

- Nerves and sense organs transmit sensory experiences to the brain.
- Complex filtering and routing goes on in both the emotional parts (limbic, thalamic areas) and intellectual parts (frontal cortex) of the brain.

EMOTIONS

- Emotions have three basic qualities: desire, aversion and indifference.
- The most basic triad of emotions are fear, aggression and depression.

INTELLECT

- Intellectual functions entail thinking, concentration and memory.

WILL

- Though not a term popular in psychotherapy nowadays, the will is that part of us that gives direction, intent and force to our actions.
- The opposite of will is indifference, boredom and lack of motivation.

Herbal Solutions

ADD/ADHD

- Herbs should be a treatment of choice for attention deficit disorder.
- Toxic and symptomatic drugs like Ritalin should be a last resort.
- Nervines detoxify the brain and increase neurotransmitter production.

ANXIETY

- Numerous herbs have relaxant and anxiety-relieving properties.
- Nervines can reduce lactic acid and other fear-producing chemicals.

DEPRESSION

- Anti-depressant herbs are effective and much safer than their medical counterparts. Over time, herbs can offer deeper, more lasting change.

STRESS

- Adaptogen herbs have a unique ability to modify the stress response.
- Herbs provide a "pick up" that is not artificial, but based on promoting healthy neurological, metabolic and hormonal function.

Psychological Conditions

See the page references below for details on each condition and herb.

ADD/ADHD

- Bacopa
- California Poppy
- Catnip
- Ginkgo
- Grape Seed
- Hops
- Kava Kava
- Lemon Balm
- Oats
- Skullcap
- St. John's Wort
- Valerian

page 92

Anxiety

- California Poppy
- Chamomile
- Hops
- Kava Kava
- Lemon Balm
- Linden
- Motherwort
- Passionflower
- Skullcap
- St. John's Wort
- Valerian
- Vervain
- Wild Lettuce
- Wood Betony

page 102

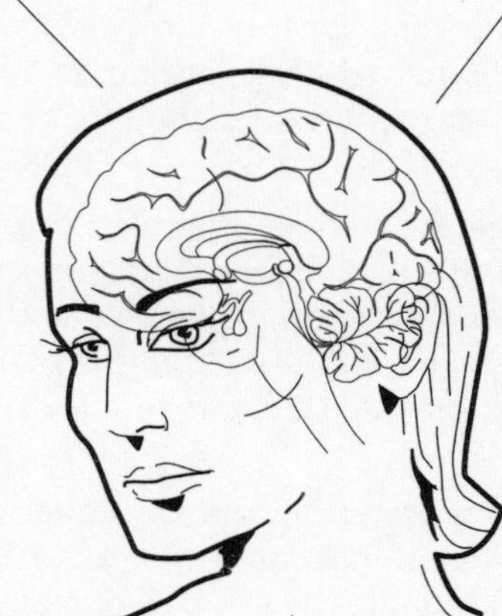

Depression

- Black Cohosh
- Ginkgo
- Ginseng
- Gotu Kola
- Kava Kava
- Lavender
- Lemon Balm
- Rosemary
- Schisandra
- Skullcap
- St. John's Wort
- Valerian
- Vervain

page 146

Stress

- Ashwaganda
- Cordyceps
- Ginseng
- Gotu Kola
- Holy Basil
- Licorice
- Maitake
- Oats
- Reishi
- Schisandra
- Siberian Ginseng
- Suma
- Wild Yam
- Yerba Mate

page 242

NERVOUS SYSTEM

The System

The intricate system of nerves that interweaves throughout the body provides constant surveillance and regulation of many thousands of body functions on a moment-to-moment and long-term basis.

BRAIN

- The brain handles incoming sensory and outgoing motor commands.
- A hierarchy of developmental layers regulates automatic acts, such as breathing, and complex pathways for thought and feeling.

SPINAL NERVES

- The spinal cord transmits signals from the periphery to the brain and vice versa, or travels directly in a reflex arc from sense organ to muscle.
- Sensory nerves transmit sensations like pain and heat to the brain.
- The motor nerves transmit impulses from the brain to muscles for conscious movement, but are also the medium for spasms or cramps.

AUTONOMIC SYSTEM

- The autonomic nervous system regulates all the "unconscious" systems of the body, such as breathing, circulation, digestion and elimination.
- It has two opposing systems: the sympathetic and parasympathetic.
- The sympathetic or "fight or flight" system shuts down digestion and prepares for action, increasing blood pressure and adrenal activity.
- The parasympathetic system promotes digestion, relaxes muscles and improves metabolism, reducing blood flow to the periphery.
- Imbalances between these two systems are part of many disease syndromes, including asthma, colitis, anxiety and stress disorders.

Herbal Approaches

HEADACHE

- Herbal treatment can provide non-toxic pain relief for tension or migraine headache and reduce the frequency and intensity of attacks
- They help address related toxic, circulatory or hormonal imbalances.

INSOMNIA

- Herbs are a gentle and non-addictive treatment for inducing sleep.
- With time, nervine plants can help underlying stress patterns.

MEMORY LOSS

- Herbs can improve brain circulation and metabolism in the aged.
- They also help with overall mental performance and concentration.

PAIN/NEURALGIA

- Herbal medicines have direct sedative and analgesic properties.
- They also help with related inflammation, muscle spasm and anxiety.

Nervous System

See the page references below for details on each condition and herb.

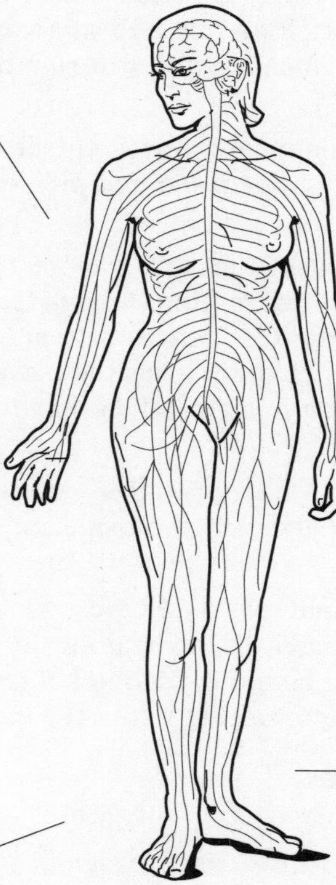

Headache

- Chamomile
- Feverfew
- Ginger
- Jam. Dogwood
- Kava Kava
- Lavender
- Linden
- Meadowsweet
- Petasites
- Skullcap
- Valerian
- Verbena
- Willow Bark
- Wood Betony

page 176

Memory Loss

- Bacopa
- Ginkgo
- Ginseng
- Gotu Kola
- Hawthorn
- Huperzine A
- Oats
- Periwinkle
- Rosemary
- Schisandra

page 210

Insomnia

- Catnip
- Chamomile
- Hops
- Kava Kava
- Lavender
- Lemon Balm
- Passionflower
- Skullcap
- St. John's Wort
- Valerian
- Wild Lettuce

page 204

Pain / Neuralgia

- Black Cohosh
- Cayenne
- Chamomile
- Ginger
- Jam. Dogwood
- Kava Kava
- Lavender
- Lobelia
- Meadowsweet
- Prickly Ash
- Skullcap
- St. John's Wort
- Valerian
- Willow

page 222

CIRCULATORY SYSTEM

The System

The cardiovascular system is designed to transport oxygen and nutrients to the tissues for a hundred years, but diet and free radical damage can destroy its function and structure by middle age.

HEART

- With three layers of overlapping muscles, the heart functions as a two-phase pump, with four chambers and its own electrical system.

ARTERIES

- From the heart, strong elastic tubes carry blood to all parts of the body.
- Arterial blood reaches its destination through the force of the heart. Ever smaller diameter arterioles convey oxygen to every tissue.
- A separate pulmonary circulation takes the blood back and forth from the lungs, picking up fresh oxygen and discharging carbon dioxide.

CAPILLARIES

- It is only at the level of tiny, thin-walled capillaries that oxygen and nutrients are discharged and carbon dioxide and wastes are picked up.

VEINS

- The blood leaves the capillaries as venules, connecting up to progressively larger veins, and finally to the heart again in this closed system.
- The veins depend on the pumping action of organs and muscles, along with a system of one-way valves, to return the blood to the heart.

Herbal Approaches

ARTERIOSCLEROSIS

- The lining of the arteries are subject to significant free radical damage and subsequent scarring and fatty deposits: hardening of the arteries.

CHOLESTEROL, HIGH

- Herbal treatment is dramatically effective in lowering cholesterol.
- It also corrects the ratio of "good" HDL to "bad" LDL cholesterol.

HEART CONDITIONS

- Herbs are critically important for heart health and rehabilitation.
- They both relieve symptoms and can actually strengthen heart tissue.

HIGH BLOOD PRESSURE (HBP)

- Herbal medicine plays a role in controlling HBP, whether due to arteriosclerosis or an imbalance in nervous regulation of the vessels.

VEINS/CIRCULATION

- Herbs can check inflammation and strengthen weakened veins.
- They also help when there is poor circulation due to arterial problems.

Circulatory System

See the page references below for details on each condition and herb.

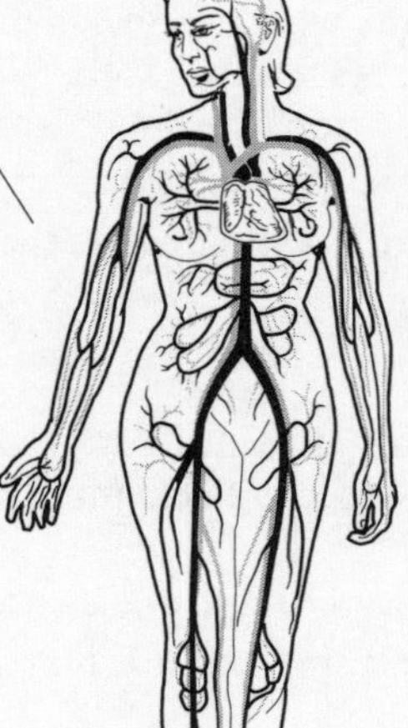

Arteriosclerosis

- Arjuna
- Bromelain
- Cayenne
- Curcumin
- Garlic
- Ginger
- Ginkgo
- Grape Seed
- Guggul
- Hawthorn
- Shiitake

page 104

Cholesterol, High

- Alfalfa
- Artichoke
- Curcumin
- Fenugreek
- Fo-Ti
- Garlic
- Ginger
- Green Tea
- Guggul
- Maitake
- Olive Leaf
- Red Rice Yeast
- Reishi

page 130

Heart Conditions

- Arjuna
- Bromelain
- Coleus
- Curcumin
- Dong Quai
- Ginkgo
- Green Tea
- Hawthorn
- Motherwort
- Olive Leaf
- Red Sage
- Reishi
- Shiitake

page 178

High Blood Pressure

- Cayenne
- Curcumin
- Garlic
- Ginger
- Ginkgo
- Hawthorn
- Linden
- Maitake
- Mistletoe
- Motherwort
- Olive Leaf
- Rosemary
- Siberian Ginseng
- Valerian

page 184

Veins / Circulation

- Bilberry
- Butcher's Broom
- Cayenne
- Coleus
- Daisy
- Garlic
- Ginger
- Ginkgo
- Gotu Kola
- Hawthorn
- Horse Chestnut
- Khella
- Stone Root
- Witch Hazel

page 250

EYE / EAR / MOUTH

The Systems

EYE

- The cornea, lens and retina are all precious and fragile organs.

EAR

- Sound vibrates the ear drum, which connects to a series of small bones and then to the cochlea, a resonant chamber with nerves to the brain.
- The inner ear contains the organ of balance, the semicircular canals.

MOUTH

- The mouth initiates digestion and provides the experience of taste.

Herbal Approaches

EAR INFECTIONS

- Herbs are effective for clearing up otitis caused by infection or allergy.
- Their gentleness and lack of side effects makes them ideal for children.

EYE CONDITIONS

- Herbs heal inflammation and help prevent blindness in conditions such as conjunctivitis, glaucoma and macular degeneration.

MOUTH AND GUMS

- Herbs treat canker sores caused by bacteria, while they rebalance a disturbed digestive system and increase immune resistance.
- Gingivitis is treated effectively with antiseptic and astringent herbs.

EAR INFECTION

- Astragalus
- Chamomile
- Echinacea
- Elder
- Eucalyptus
- Garlic
- Goldenseal
- Grapefruit Seed
- Larix
- Licorice
- Mullein
- Plantain
- St. John's Wort

page 158

EYE CONDITIONS

- Bilberry
- Bupleurum
- Calendula
- Cayenne
- Coleus
- Dusty Miller
- Eyebright
- Ginkgo
- Goldenseal
- Goldthread
- Grape Seed
- Lutein

page 160

MOUTH & GUMS

- Bloodroot
- Calendula
- Chamomile
- Echinacea
- Goldenseal
- Goldthread
- Grapefruit Seed
- Licorice
- Myrrh
- Neem
- Osha
- Peppermint
- Sage
- Tea Tree Oil

page 216

Respiratory system

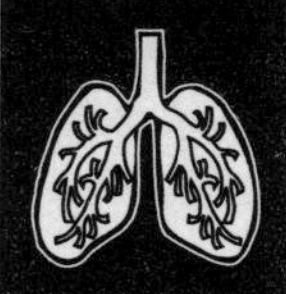

The System

Nose & Sinuses

- Air is warmed and filtered in the nasal passages, lined with mucous cells to trap foreign particles. The nose also houses the organs of smell.

Bronchi

- The main bronchi enter the right and left lung, and then branch into many secondary bronchi, leading into ever finer bronchioles.

Lungs

- The lungs contains tiny air sacs or alveoli, the core unit of breathing.
- Here the interface between the blood and inspired air takes place.
- The lungs expand 12 to 20 times a minute, with a surface area 40 times greater than that of the skin, allowing a tremendous exchange of gases.

Immune System

- The nose, sinuses, bronchi and alveoli are richly equipped with immune cells to absorb and eliminate inhaled toxins, such as air pollutants.

Herbal Approaches

Colds & Flu

- With both antiviral and immune-stimulating action, herbs can shorten the duration of respiratory infections and reduce the frequency of colds.

Hayfever/Allergy

- Typical allergy symptoms can be safely reduced with herbs, and in time, the immune weakness and oversensitivity behind them can be cured.

Sinusitis

- Herbs are an ideal treatment for acute or chronic sinusitis, often related, as it is, to allergy or long-standing yeast and viral infections.

Sore Throat

- Antibiotic and demulcent herbs are an effective treatment for sore throat, as well as tonsillitis, used internally and as a local gargle.

Cough

- Herbal medicine has dozens of remedies for helping the lungs and bronchi, relieving irritation, infection and healing the tissues.

Asthma

- Herbs help immensely with the symptomatic treatment of asthma.
- They also address underlying immune and hormonal causes.
- Even in advanced cases (i.e. emphysema) symptoms can be relieved.

Upper Respiratory System

See the page references below for details on each condition and herb.

Colds & Flu

- Andrographis
- Astragalus
- Boneset
- Cayenne
- Catnip
- Chamomile
- Echinacea
- Elder
- Eucalyptus
- Eyebright
- Garlic
- Ginger
- Goldenseal
- Ground Ivy
- Lomatium
- Meadowsweet
- Peppermint
- Siberian Ginseng
- St. John's Wort
- Wild Indigo
- Yarrow

page 132

Hayfever / Allergy

- Bromelain
- Chinese Skullcap
- Curcumin
- Dong Quai
- Echinacea
- Elder
- Ephedra
- Eyebright
- Garlic
- Ginkgo
- Goldenseal
- Horseradish
- Licorice
- Nettles
- Plantain

page 174

Sinusitis

- Cayenne
- Echinacea
- Elder
- Ephedra
- Eucalyptus
- Eyebright
- Garlic
- Ginger
- Goldenseal
- Horseradish
- Myrrh
- Osha
- Peppermint
- Tea Tree Oil
- Usnea

page 230

Sore Throat

- Echinacea
- Horseradish
- Isatis
- Kava Kava
- Licorice
- Lomatium
- Mullein
- Myrrh
- Oregano Oil
- Osha
- Poke Root
- Poplar
- Queen's Delight
- Sage
- Slippery Elm
- Wild Indigo

page 236

Lower Respiratory System

See the page references below for details on each condition and herb.

Asthma

- Elecampane
- Ephedra
- Ginkgo
- Grindelia
- Ivy Leaf
- Khella
- Licorice
- Lobelia
- Mullein
- Nettles
- P. Spurge
- Querbracho
- Spikenard
- Wild Thyme
- Yerba Santa

page 108

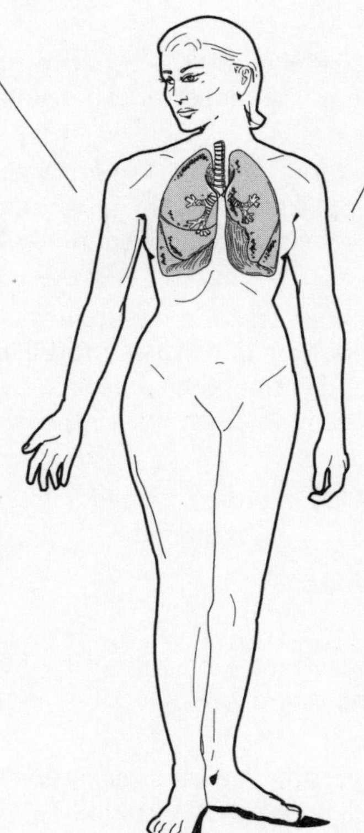

Cough

- Anise
- Coltsfoot
- Cowslip
- Elecampane
- Eucalyptus
- Grindelia
- Horehound
- Hyssop
- Irish Moss
- Licorice
- Lomatium
- Lungwort
- Maidenhair
- Mullein
- Osha
- Plantain
- Poplar
- Slippery Elm
- Thyme
- Usnea
- Wild Cherry Bark
- Yellow Dock
- Yerba Santa

page 142

UPPER DIGESTIVE
SYSTEM

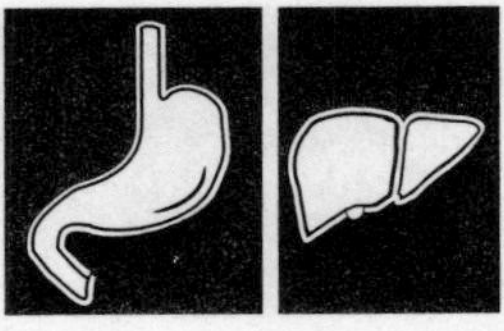

The System

The digestive system performs a long and complex series of reactions in order to extract essential nourishment from food. In this remarkable process, instead of spoiling (as it would outside the body), foodstuffs are broken down into their basic components. Both nutrients and energy are extracted and assimilated from food to maintain tissues and life.

ESOPHAGUS

- This simple tube or pathway, with a tough protective lining, leads through the diaphragm to the muscular expansion of the stomach.

STOMACH

- In the stomach, hydrochloric acid acts on foods and destroys bacteria, while the stomach lining is protected by tough mucus secretions.
- The stomach generates feelings of hunger, fullness, pain or pleasure.

LIVER

- The liver is the master chemical and metabolic factory of the body.
- It manufactures, metabolizes and stores proteins, starches, fats, vitamins and hormones, and is the body's largest detoxification organ.
- It also has important immune functions for the whole organism.

GALLBLADDER

- Bile produced in the liver, in order to digest fats, is stored here.

Herbal Approaches

NAUSEA

- Herbal medicine is excellent for eliminating nausea and vomiting, motion sickness and nausea of pregnancy.

STOMACH CONDITIONS

- Herbs can improve digestion and relieve gastritis and stomach ulcers.
- Antibiotic and anti-inflammatory, they help heal the stomach linings.

GALLBLADDER

- Herbal treatment can help control both inflammation and gallstones.
- Surgery is often unnecessary if herbal treatment is begun early enough.

LIVER CONDITIONS

- Herbs help in specific liver problems, like hepatitis or cirrhosis.
- They also tone the liver and help its metabolic and detoxifying work.
- This is crucial to improving many chronic, debilitating conditions.

Upper Digestive System

See the page references below for details on each condition and herb.

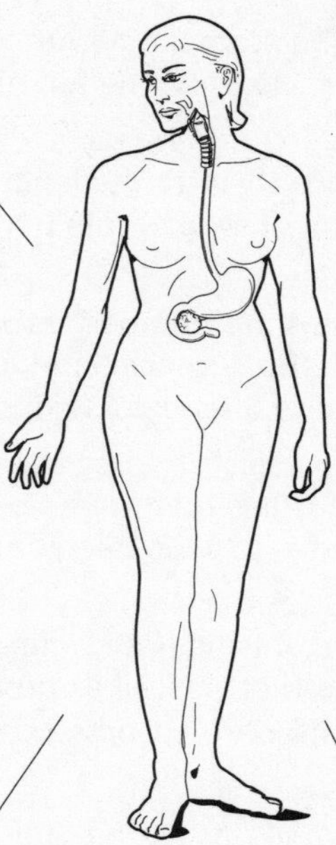

Gas / Bloating

- Anise
- Calamus
- Caraway
- Cardamom
- Chamomile
- Cinnamon
- Fennel
- Fenugreek
- Ginger
- Nutmeg
- Parsley
- Peppermint
- Sage

page 170

Stomach Conditions

- Anise
- Artichoke
- Calamus
- Cayenne
- Chamomile
- Gentian
- Geranium
- Ginger
- Goldenseal
- Licorice
- Marshmallow
- Meadowsweet
- Papaya
- Peppermint
- Slippery Elm

page 240

Nausea

- Cayenne
- Chamomile
- Cinnamon
- Cloves
- Curcumin
- Fennel
- Galangal
- Ginger
- Marshmallow
- Meadowsweet
- Patchouli
- Peppermint
- Raspberry Leaf

page 218

Gallbladder

- Artichoke
- Balmony
- Boldo
- Celandine
- Culver's Root
- Curcumin
- Dandelion
- Fringe Tree
- Garlic
- Milk Thistle
- Oregon Grape
- Peppermint
- Wild Yam

page 168

Liver Conditions

- Artichoke
- Astragalus
- Barberry
- Beet Leaf
- Black Radish
- Bupleurum
- Celandine
- Culver's Root
- Curcumin
- Dandelion
- Fringe Tree
- Milk Thistle
- Rehmannia
- Schisandra

page 208

LOWER DIGESTIVE SYSTEM

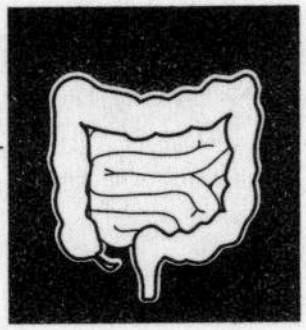

The System

DUODENUM

- Food enters here from the stomach and is mixed with powerful pancreatic enzymes and liver bile. Now the full digestive process begins.

ILEUM

- Enzymes break down foods through the length of the small intestine.
- Here the major absorption of food occurs in veins and lymph channels.

ILEOCECAL VALVE

- The liquefied food remains are dumped into the first part of the large intestine (colon) through the ileocecal sphincter.
- When weakened, this allows a reflux of toxins back into the intestines.

IMMUNE SYSTEM

- The lining of the intestines has many large patches of tonsil-like material, including the appendix, to keep bacteria down to a minimum.

LARGE INTESTINE

- With over 200 kinds of organisms (four pounds worth!), the colon flora helps break food down further, as well as produce certain vitamins.
- Here fluids and other matter are absorbed back into the blood stream.

Herbal Approaches

COLITIS/IBS

- Herbs work with these conditions through anti-inflammatory, antibiotic and astringent properties and address underlying immune weakness.

CONSTIPATION

- Herbal medicines work short-term to relieve spasms or soften stool.
- They can also correct underlying problems, such as enzyme deficiency.

CRAMPS/COLIC

- Anti-spasmodic herbs are effective for calming abdominal cramps.
- Their gentle nature makes them ideal for children and infantile colic.

DIARRHEA

- Herbal medicine is often effective for diarrhea when it is due to a recent upset/infection, but also when part of a chronic bowel disorder.
- Herbs help correct underlying dysbiosis, fermentation and toxicity.

HEMORRHOIDS

- Herbs can help this rectal problem, shrinking and soothing piles.
- Blood vessels may be strengthened and congested organs that are causing venous pressure (liver, uterus or colon) can be corrected.

Lower Digestive System

See the page references below for details on each condition and herb.

Colic / Cramps

- Anise
- Caraway
- Catnip
- Chamomile
- Cramp Bark
- Dill
- Fennel
- Kava Kava
- Lemon Balm
- Licorice
- Peppermint
- Valerian
- Wild Yam
- Yarrow

page 136

Colitis / IBS

- Aloe
- Bayberry
- Cat's Claw
- Chamomile
- Echinacea
- Goldenseal
- Myrrh
- Olive Leaf
- Peppermint
- Slippery Elm
- Triphala
- Valerian

page 138

Constipation

- Aloe
- Buckthorn
- Butternut
- Cascara
- Chinese Rhubarb
- Dandelion
- Flaxseed
- Peppermint
- Psyllium Seed
- Senna
- Yellow Dock

page 140

Diarrhea

- Bayberry
- Carob
- Chamomile
- Cinnamon
- Geranium
- Ginger
- Goldenseal
- Meadowsweet
- Oak
- Peppermint
- Potentilla
- Raspberry Leaf
- Sangre de Grado
- Yarrow

page 152

Hemorrhoids

- Aloe
- Butcher's Broom
- Comfrey
- Horse Chestnut
- Mullein
- Peony
- Plantain
- Psyllium Seed
- Slippery Elm
- Stone Root
- Witch Hazel

page 180

Urinary Tract

The System

Kidney

- The kidneys filter the blood continually, removing wastes and debris.
- Each kidney is made up of some one million filtering units (nephrons).
- At the center of each unit are tiny capillaries and a surrounding capsule where fluids, minerals, glucose, amino acids, etc., are filtered out.
- In miles of tiny tubules, water, minerals and chemical compounds are then absorbed back into the blood, according to the body's needs.

Ureters

- The ureters bring the filtered urine from the kidneys to the bladder.

Bladder

- The bladder is a muscular holding tank that has strong lining cells and tough secretions to protect it from the acidic and toxic urine.

Urethra

- The urethra exits from the bladder to the outside world. In men this is via the penis, while in women, the urethra has an opening separate from the vagina.
- Women are far more subject to bladder and kidney infections than men.

Herbal Approaches

Bladder Infection

- Herbal medicine is an effective, gentle and non-toxic treatment for cystitis, especially valuable in woman and children.
- It is also useful in childhood enuresis and adult incontinence.

Kidney Conditions

- Herbs are helpful for a wide range of kidney problems: infections, immune attack, nephritis, kidney stones and arteriosclerosis.
- Regular or annual detoxification programs should include herbs that help cleanse and rejuvenate the kidney tissue.

Urinary Tract

See the page references below for details on each condition and herb.

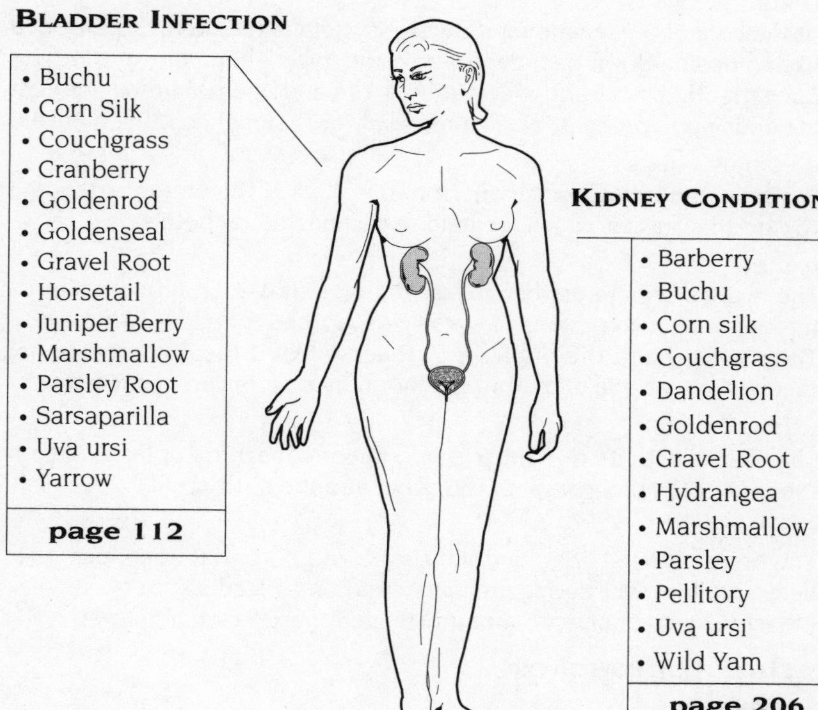

Bladder Infection

- Buchu
- Corn Silk
- Couchgrass
- Cranberry
- Goldenrod
- Goldenseal
- Gravel Root
- Horsetail
- Juniper Berry
- Marshmallow
- Parsley Root
- Sarsaparilla
- Uva ursi
- Yarrow

page 112

Kidney Conditions

- Barberry
- Buchu
- Corn silk
- Couchgrass
- Dandelion
- Goldenrod
- Gravel Root
- Hydrangea
- Marshmallow
- Parsley
- Pellitory
- Uva ursi
- Wild Yam

page 206

WOMEN'S HEALTH

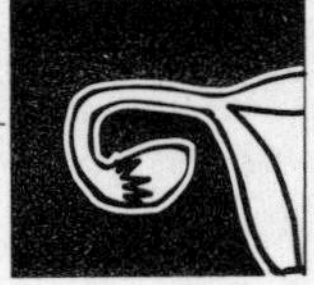

The System

Reproduction is at the center of all forms of life, from amoeba to plants, insects and animals. The complex requirements of growing a human child makes the female body far more intricate in form and function than that of the male. With this comes an increased risk and variety of illnesses.

UTERUS

- At the core of the female reproductive system is the uterus, positioned like an upside-down pear deep within the lower abdomen.
- Each month, from hormonal stimulus, the endometrial lining gradually builds up in preparation for pregnancy or is sloughed off at menses.

FALLOPIAN TUBES

- The fallopian tubes branch out from the sides of the uterus, extending toward the ovaries, which are held in suspension on both sides.

OVARIES

- The ovaries secrete estrogens (estriol, estradiol, estrone) and testosterone, while also producing eggs every month until menopause.
- The pituitary and the brain areas that control it (i.e. hypothalamus) regulate the waxing and waning of hormones produced by the ovaries.

VAGINA

- The vagina, with its own microenvironment of bacteria or flora, is both the route of impregnation of the ovum and the birth canal.

BREASTS

- The breast consists of glandular tissue and potential milk ducts that lie dormant except during pregnancy and breastfeeding.
- Breast tissue responds to monthly fluctuations in estrogen levels.

Herbal Approaches

AMENORRHEA

- Herbs are effective for missed periods caused by hormonal imbalance.

BREAST CONDITIONS

- Herbs can reduce or eliminate painful breast swelling during menses.
- Antibiotic herbs are effective mastitis, also detoxifying the tissues.
- Herbs are also useful for shrinking benign breast cysts or solid tumors.

BREASTFEEDING

- Herbal medicines have been used traditionally to improve the flow and quality of milk, while healing inflamed or irritated breasts or nipples.

DYSMENORRHEA

- Antispasmodic herbal medicines offer natural, rapid, reduction of menstrual cramps and pain, while correcting hormonal imbalances.

INFERTILITY

- Herbs should be a treatment of choice for infertility related to uterine weakness, hormonal dysfunction, infection and other common causes.

MENOPAUSE

- Herbal medicines are very effective for symptom relief in menopause.
- Long-term, they can rebalance pituitary, ovarian and thyroid hormones.

MISCARRIAGE

- Herbal medicines can prevent bleeding and cramping in miscarriage.
- They may be needed to correct a variety of toxic factors and underlying imbalances in thyroid, ovarian and pituitary function.

PMS

- Herbs offer short-term alleviation of symptoms like mood changes.
- They are also excellent for reducing excess estrogen build-up and underlying hormone imbalances in the pituitary, adrenals or thyroid.

VAGINITIS

- Vaginal infection can be successfully treated with herbs that act on candida, gardnerella, trichomonas and other typical organisms.
- Specific herbs help heal the vaginal linings, while changing the environment that invites infection, and boost immune resistance.

WOMEN'S HEALTH 1

See the page references below for details on each condition and herb.

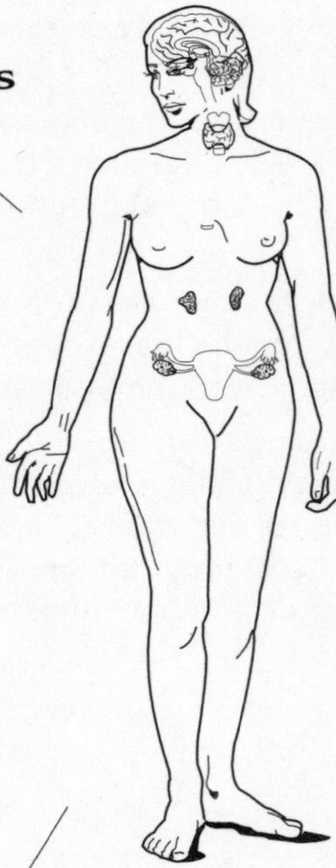

BREAST CONDITIONS

- Astragalus
- Black Cohosh
- Burdock
- Castor Oil
- Chamomile
- Chasteberry
- Cleavers
- Dong Quai
- Pipsissewa
- Poke Root
- Queen's Delight
- Red Root
- Saw Palmetto

page 118

BREAST-FEEDING

- Alfalfa
- Carrot Family
- Castor Oil
- Chamomile
- Chaste Tree
- Codonopsis
- Elder
- Fenugreek
- Goat's Rue
- Milk Thistle
- Nettles
- Poke Root
- Sage
- Vervain

page 116

DYSMENORRHEA

- Black Cohosh
- Black Haw
- Blue Cohosh
- Chamomile
- Cramp Bark
- Dong Quai
- Ginger
- Jam. Dogwood
- Kava Kava
- Meadowsweet
- Wild Yam
- Valerian

page 156

PMS

- Black Cohosh
- Bupleurum
- Chamomile
- Chaste Tree
- Dandelion
- Dong Quai
- Licorice
- Maca
- Skullcap
- Vervain
- Wild Yam

page 226

VAGINITIS

- Calendula
- Echinacea
- Garlic
- Goldenseal
- Myrrh
- Oregano Oil
- Oregon Grape
- Pau D'Arco
- Slippery Elm
- Tea Tree Oil
- Usnea
- Yarrow

page 248

WOMEN'S HEALTH 2

See the page references below for details on each condition and herb.

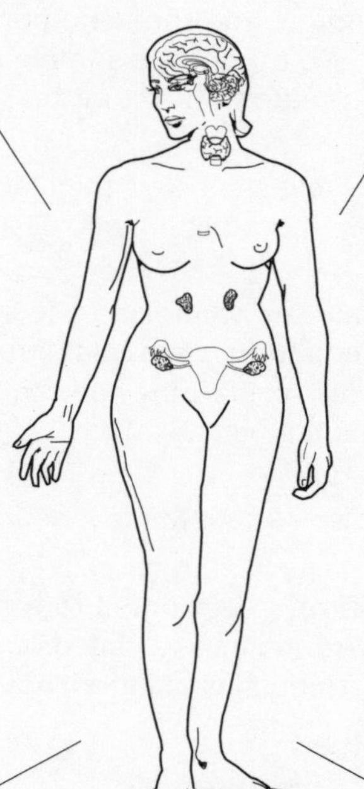

AMENORRHEA

- Black Cohosh
- Blue Cohosh
- Chaste Tree
- Dong Quai
- False Unicorn
- Kelp
- Lady's Mantle
- Licorice
- Maca
- Rehmannia
- Shativari
- True Unicorn

page 96

MISCARRIAGE

- Black Cohosh
- Black Haw
- Blue Cohosh
- Chamomile
- Cramp Bark
- False Unicorn
- Partridge Berry
- Savine Juniper
- Trillium
- True Unicorn
- Wild Yam

page 214

INFERTILITY

- Black Cohosh
- Chasteberry
- Dong Quai
- False Unicorn
- Fo-Ti
- Licorice
- Maca
- Motherwort
- Partridgeberry
- Red Clover
- Shativari
- Siberian Ginseng
- Wild Yam

page 196

CHILDBIRTH

- Black Cohosh
- Black Haw
- Blue Cohosh
- Chamomile
- Feverfew
- Motherwort
- Partridgeberry
- Raspberry Leaf
- Shepherd's Purse
- Trillium
- Vervain

page 128

MENOPAUSE

- Black Cohosh
- Chaste Tree
- Dandelion
- Dong Quai
- False Unicorn
- Fo-Ti
- Licorice
- Maca
- Motherwort
- Oatstraw
- Red Clover
- Wild Yam

page 212

MEN'S HEALTH

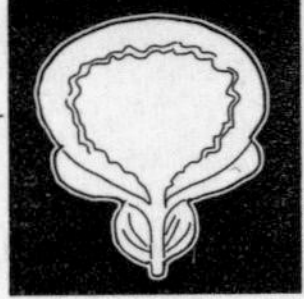

The System

While less complex than the female, the male genital system has its own unique set of problems. Both male infertility and erectile dysfunction are common, and the male hormonal system also has cyclic fluctuations. Men also experience a "male menopause" in mid-life, as levels of testosterone produced by the testes and adrenals diminish.

PROSTATE

- The chestnut-sized prostate sits below the bladder, secreting both prostatic fluid necessary for reproduction and as-yet-unknown hormones.

TESTES

- The testes produce male sex hormone, testosterone, which gives men their characteristic hair patterns, muscular structure—and aggression.
- They also produce sperm, containing half the DNA sequence required for producing a new human organism.

SEMINAL VESICLES

- The seminal vesicles also secrete fluids that are mixed with the sperm.

PENIS

- The penis functions as an exit channel for urine accumulated in the bladder, as well as sperm and its associated seminal and prostatic fluid.
- Erection occurs solely through circulation, not via muscular action.

Herbal Approaches

IMPOTENCE

- A number of non-toxic herbs can help to improve blood flow through the penis, like many drugs (e.g. Viagra), but without their risks.
- These herbs also have the advantage of elevating male hormone levels.
- Penile function is also dependent on a healthy prostate gland.

MALE INFERTILITY

- Male fertility can be increased by herbs that promote elevated hormone levels and cleanse the tissues of pesticides and other toxins.

PROSTATE CONDITIONS

- Herbs are effective in 90% of cases of benign prostate enlargement.
- Other herbal medicines are excellent for acute or chronic prostate inflammation, relieving infection, swelling and hardening.

Men's Health

See the page references below for details on each condition and herb.

Impotence & Male Infertility

- Ashwaganda
- Astragalus
- Chaste Tree
- Cordyceps
- Damiana
- Ginkgo
- Ginseng
- Maca
- Muira Puama
- Oats
- Sarsaparilla
- Schisandra
- Siberian Ginseng
- Tribulus
- Yohimbe

page 192

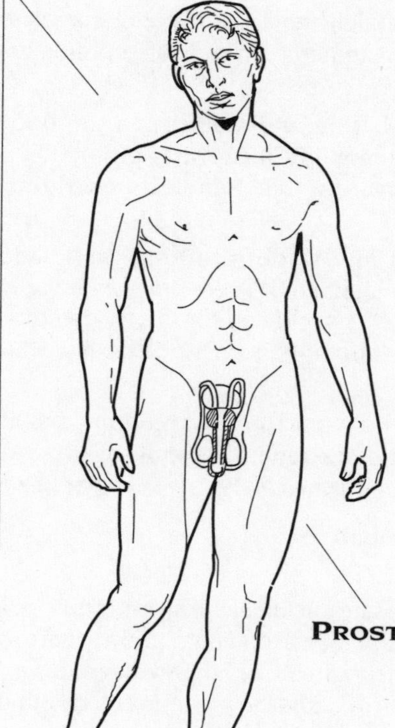

Prostate Conditions

- Goldenseal
- Lycopene
- Nettles
- Pipsissewa
- Pollen
- Pumpkin Seed
- Pygeum
- Red Clover
- Saw Palmetto
- Tribulus

page 228

MUSCULOSKELETAL SYSTEM

The System

Stress, tension, poor posture and prolonged immobility make musculoskeletal problems familiar to everyone. Repetitive activities, including the type performed in many sports, occupations, computer use, etc., put undue stress on specific joints. Combined with nutritional deficiencies and genetic weakness, the whole spectrum of joint problems emerge, from acute sprains to chronic arthritis.

BONE

- Bone provides structure and stability to the body, yet allows for its incredible range of mobility. It provides protection of soft inner tissues.
- It also houses the marrow that manufacturers white and red blood cells.

JOINTS

- Joints are covered with smooth cartilage and banded together with a variety of powerful ligaments. There are a wide variety of types of joints.
- In the legs, mobility is sacrificed for increased stability and strength.
- In the upper limbs, mobility is enhanced, yet with less stable joints.

MUSCLES

- Muscles attach to bony fulcrums via tendons, providing powerful leverage to perform feats of strength, as well as extraordinary subtlety.
- The level of muscular tone can result in either flexibility or tension.

Herbal Approaches

ARTHRITIS

- The most common chronic disease, arthritis can be benefited immensely by herbal medicine, for both acute and chronic symptom relief.
- Damage to joint structures can be prevented or healed to some extent.
- In rheumatoid arthritis, underlying immune dysfunction can be helped.

FIBROMYALGIA

- This difficult immune and neurological problem can be treated successfully by natural medicine, with herbal medicine as a key factor.
- A variety of anti-inflammatory, antiviral and immune-boosting herbs are needed to successfully reverse this condition and regain health.

BACK PAIN

- Herbal medicines provide anti-inflammatory and joint healing effects.
- They work hand in hand with chiropractic care, massage and body work.

SPORTS FITNESS

- Herbal medicines are perfect aids to enhancing physical performance.
- They can reduce fatigue, increase stamina and accelerate growth of muscle mass, while improving circulation and enhancing hormones.

Musculoskeletal System

See the page references below for details on each condition and herb.

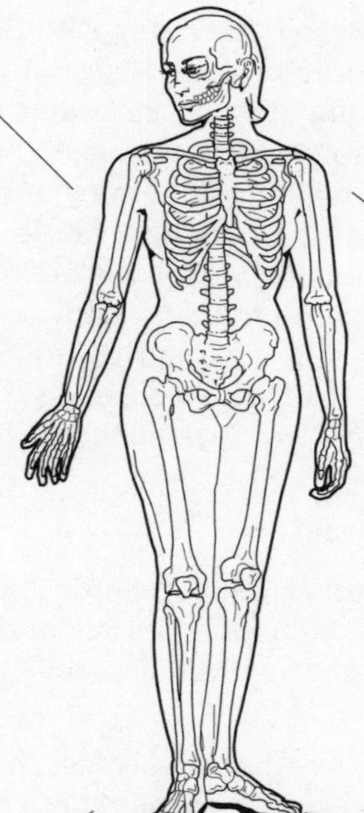

Arthritis

- Angelica
- Black Cohosh
- Bogbean
- Boswellia
- Bromelain
- Cayenne
- Curcumin
- Devil's Claw
- Feverfew
- Ginger
- Guaiacum
- Licorice
- Meadowsweet
- Willow Bark
- Yucca

page 106

Fibromyalgia

- Astragalus
- Black Cohosh
- Bromelain
- Burdock
- Cat's Claw
- Curcumin
- Devil's Claw
- Feverfew
- Flax/Psyllium
- Ginger
- Kelp
- Licorice
- Milk Thistle
- Olive Leaf
- Pau D'Arco
- Poke Root
- Prickly Ash
- Shiitake
- Siberian Ginseng

page 164

Back Pain

- Barberry
- Black Cohosh
- Black Haw
- Bromelain
- Boswellia
- Corydalis
- Devil's Claw
- Dong Quai
- Horse Chestnut
- Jam. Dogwood
- Kava Kava
- Meadowsweet
- Valerian
- Wild Yam

page 110

Sports Fitness

- Amalaki
- Ashwaganda
- Codonopsis
- Cordyceps
- Ginseng
- Jianogulan
- Maca
- Rhodiola
- Sarsaparilla
- Schisandra
- Siberian Ginseng
- Suma
- Tribulus
- Yerba Mate

page 238

SKIN

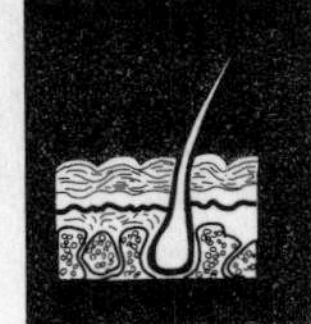

The System

SKIN

- The skin is the largest organ in the body, with the greatest surface area.
- The epidermis and dermis provide a mechanical, protective barrier against injury, temperature fluctuations, water, infection and drying.
- It has special nerve receptors for touch, pain, heat, cold and pressure.
- It is also essential for regulating our temperature and fluid balance.
- The skin is a mirror of one's health as a whole, reflecting the metabolic, hormonal and nutritional status of the entire individual.
- Skin is a major detoxification route for body wastes and debris.
- It works overtime when other detoxifying organs, like the liver, kidney and intestines are overloaded or weakened. Thus all dermatological problems should be considered systemic, not just local or superficial.

Herbal Approaches

ACNE/ABSCESS

- Herbs have powerful antibacterial properties for treating infections.
- Detoxifying herbs drain the tissues of cellular debris and poisons.
- Herbs also work on underlying liver, intestinal and hormonal toxicity.

HERPES

- Herpes virus infections, whether cold sores, shingles or genital herpes, can be helped or even cured by powerful antiviral herbal medicines.

HIVES

- Antihistamine and anti-inflammatory herbs work without side effects.
- Used long term, plant medicines reduce the tendency to allergic reactions and environmental sensitivities by strengthening immunity.

SKIN CONDITIONS

- In eczema herbs can soothe irritation and change underlying allergies.
- A number of herbs have been shown, through both research and clinical practice, to markedly reduce or eliminate psoriasis.

WARTS

- Herbal medicines are a safe and effective method to remove warts.
- They can also destroy the tissue viruses that cause these growths in the hands, feet, genitals or elsewhere.

Skin

See the page references below for details on each condition and herb.

Skin Conditions

- Aloe
- Bitter Melon
- Burdock
- Calendula
- Cardiospermum
- Cayenne
- Chamomile
- Chickweed
- Coleus
- Elder
- Evening Primrose
- Gotu Kola
- Licorice
- Lycium
- Neem
- Olive Leaf
- Oregon Grape
- Red Clover
- Sarsaparilla
- Tea Tree Oil
- Wild Pansy
- Witch Hazel
- Yellow Dock

page 232

Acne / Abscess

NOTE: see *Infection* on page 81

Hair Loss

- Amala
- Arnica
- Bay Oil
- Fo-Ti
- Gotu Kola
- Horsetail
- Lavender Oil
- Neem
- Nettles
- Pygeum
- Rosemary
- Sage
- Saw Palmetto
- Tea Tree Oil
- Yarrow

page 172

Hives

- Aloe
- Bromelain
- Burdock
- Chinese Skullcap
- Curcumin
- Echinacea
- Ginger
- Goldenseal
- Green Tea
- Licorice
- Nettles
- Quercetin
- Schisandra
- Yarrow

page 188

Herpes

- Cayenne
- Chaparral
- Echinacea
- Goldenseal
- Grapefruit Seed
- Lavender Oil
- Lemon Balm
- Licorice
- Lomatium
- Olive Leaf
- Passionflower
- Pau D'Arco
- St. John's Wort
- Tea Tree Oil

page 182

Warts

- Aloe
- Birch Bark
- Bittersweet
- Bloodroot
- Castor Oil
- Celandine
- Ginger/Garlic
- Houseleek
- Juniper
- Lemon Peel
- Milkweed
- Olive Leaf
- Protelolytics
- White Cedar

page 252

METABOLIC CONDITIONS

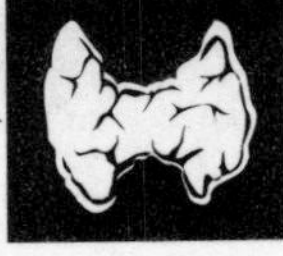

Herbal Approaches

While they encompass a wide range of problems, metabolic conditions share the fact that they affect the body globally. Their causes may be straightforward (anemia, diabetes) or highly complex (cancer, aging), but each involves multiple systems and requires unique herbal approaches.

ANEMIA

- Specific herbs deliver bioavailable iron while enhancing its absorption and utilization in the body. Others directly increase hemoglobin levels.

ANTI-AGING

- Longevity herbs have traditional and proven effects for prolonging life.
- They are also able to halt or even reverse many of the effects of aging.

CANCER

- While there is no easy answer to cancer, herbs can play a primary role, with their powerful and unequalled immune-enhancing capabilities.

(continued on page 80)

ANEMIA

- Alfalfa
- Ashwaganda
- Codonopsis
- Dong Quai
- Gentian
- Hawthorn
- Kelp
- Nettles
- Raspberry Leaf
- Red Root
- Siberian Ginseng
- Yellow Dock

page 98

CANCER

- Astragalus
- Black Cumin
- Cat's Claw
- Celandine
- Chapparal
- Curcumin
- Garlic
- Ginseng
- Goldenseal
- Green Tea
- Maitake
- Mistletoe
- Noni
- Pau D'Arco
- Poke Root
- Red Clover
- Reishi
- Rosemary
- Shiitake

page 122

INFLAMMATION

- Boswellia
- Bromelain
- Chamomile
- Curcumin
- Flaxseed
- Ginger
- Hawthorn
- Licorice
- Meadowsweet
- Quercetin
- Willow Bark
- Yarrow

page 198

METABOLIC CONDITIONS

See the page references below for details on each condition and herb.

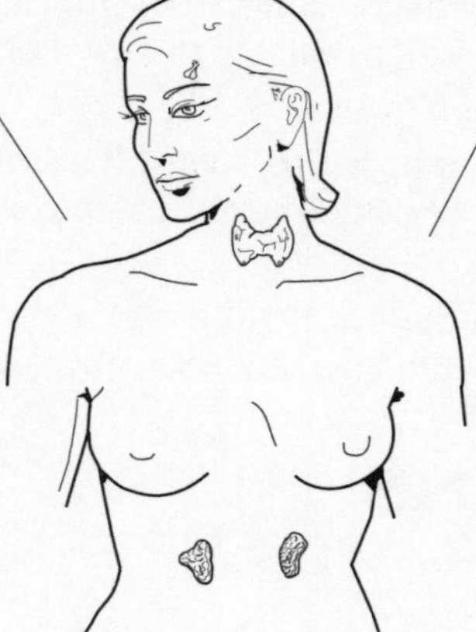

ANTI-AGING

- Ashwaganda
- Fo-Ti
- Garlic
- Ginseng
- Gotu Kola
- Green Tea
- Hawthorn
- Licorice
- Maca
- Reishi
- Rhodiola
- Siberian Ginseng
- Suma

page 100

DIABETES

- Bilberry
- Bitter Melon
- Dandelion
- Devil's Club
- Fenugreek
- Ginkgo
- Ginseng
- Gymnema
- Holy Basil
- Jumbul
- Licorice
- Siberian Ginseng
- Stevia

page 150

FATIGUE

- Alfalfa
- Astragalus
- Cordyceps
- Ginseng
- Gotu Kola
- Licorice
- Maitake
- Oats
- Schisandra
- Siberian Ginseng
- St. John's Wort
- Yerba Mate

page 162

THYROID CONDITIONS

- Bitter Herbs
- Bugleweed
- Coleus
- Gotu Kola
- Guggul
- Hai Zao
- Irish Moss
- Kelp
- Meadowsweet
- Motherwort
- Myrrh
- Siberian Ginseng

page 244

OVERWEIGHT

- Bitter Orange
- Cayenne
- Chickweed
- Coleus
- Dandelion
- Ephedra
- Garcinia
- Gotu Kola
- Guar Gum
- Guggul
- Kelp
- Maitake
- Stevia
- Yerba Mate
- Yohimbe

page 220

DIABETES
- Herbs have an essential place in treating this widespread disease.
- Many can lower blood sugar or even help regenerate the pancreas.

INFLAMMATION
- There are scores of effective anti-inflammatory herbal medicines.
- They work more broadly than similar drugs, without their side effects.

FATIGUE/EXHAUSTION
- Herbal medicine is perfectly suited to "burn-out" and boosting adrenal and nerve energy, as well as raising the level of vitality as a whole.

OVERWEIGHT
- Herbs help normalize appetite, liver function and hormonal disturbance that results in obesity. They can also control emotional factors.

THYROID CONDITIONS
- Herbs are very useful for low thyroid function, which is both very common and frequently undiagnosed. Hyperthyroidism is also benefited.

INFECTIONS

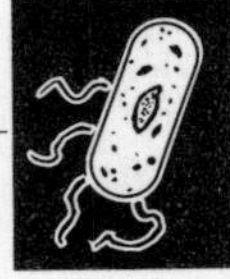

Herbal Approaches

Infectious organisms are mankind's oldest and most constant foe. Fortunately, evolution has also equipped humans with a whole host of inherent defense mechanisms, and these can be ably assisted by healing herbs.

ACNE/ABSCESS
- Antiseptic herbs help skin infections, using internal and local treatment.
- Detoxifying and immune-enhancing herbs address background causes.

CANDIDA/YEAST
- Antifungal plants, taken on a rotating basis, can destroy candida.
- Herbal treatment should be continued for some time, even when medical drugs have been used to eliminate the more superficial infection.

HIV/AIDS
- Herbs have shown good results in relieving and slowing HIV/AIDS.
- Viral replication may be halted and the progression to AIDS stopped.

IMMUNE WEAKNESS
- Herbs are the primary way to enhance immunity, which plays a role in every conceivable form of illness, whether acute or chronic.
- Disease prevention is synonymous with immune health.

PARASITES
- Anti-parasitic herbs have been used effectively since remote antiquity.
- Prolonged and repeated treatment is necessary to eradicate worms.

Infections

See the page references below for details on each condition and herb.

Acne / Abscess

- Burdock
- Calendula
- Cleavers
- Dandelion
- Echinacea
- Figwort
- Myrrh
- Oregon Grape
- Red Clover
- Red Root
- Tea Tree Oil
- Wild Indigo
- Yellow Dock

page 90

Candida / Yeast

- Black Walnut
- Cat's Claw
- Celandine
- Garlic
- Goldenseal
- Grapefruit Seed
- Holy Basil
- Larix
- Maitake
- Olive Leaf
- Oregano Oil
- Pau D'Arco
- Spilanthes
- Tea Tree Oil
- Usnea

page 126

Infection

- Bayberry
- Echinacea
- Garlic
- Goldenseal
- Grapefruit Seed
- Lemon Grass
- Lomatium
- Myrrh
- Neem
- Olive Leaf
- Oregano Oil
- Osha
- Pau D'Arco
- Tea Tree Oil
- Usnea

page 194

HIV/AIDS

- Astragalus
- Cat's Claw
- Curcumin
- Garlic
- Ginseng
- Isatis
- Licorice
- Maitake
- Milk Thistle
- Olive Leaf
- Pau D'Arco
- Reishi
- Shiitake
- Siberian Ginseng
- St. John's Wort

page 186

Immune Weakness

- Astragalus
- Cat's Claw
- Cordyceps
- Echinacea
- Ginseng
- Larix
- Licorice
- Maitake
- Pau D'Arco
- Reishi
- Schisandra
- Shiitake
- Siberian Ginseng

page 190

Parasites

- Black Walnut
- Elecampane
- Garlic
- Goldenseal
- Grapefruit Seed
- Male Fern
- Olive Leaf
- Papaya Seed
- Pomegranate
- Pumpkin Seed
- Quassia
- Tansy
- Wood Sage
- Wormwood

page 224

TRAUMA

The System

Injury is a constant fact of life, with our bodies vulnerable to every manner of bump, fall, bruise and sprain. Injury is actually a global event that galvanizes a response from the nervous, hormonal and immune systems. Pain, inflammation and swelling after injury are part of a defensive reaction that seeks to return the body to a normal state. But this action may be ineffective and at times even slight injuries can create far-reaching effects and long-term pain and dysfunction.

- Trauma can result in physical misalignments, tensions or tissue damage on a microscopic level, as well as adhesions and scars.
- Trauma leaves an imprint on the nervous system and cellular memory.
- This can create maladaptive patterns that predispose to further injuries.
- Traumatic medicine as practiced in hospitals is, by far, the most advanced and effective part of modern medicine.
- Every use should be made of emergency medical care, combined with appropriate herbs and other natural therapies for accelerating healing.

Herbal Approaches

BLEEDING

- Styptic herbs are a well-proven treatment for excess bleeding.
- Specific herbs are excellent for external bleeding, while others treat blood loss from internal organs, such as the uterus, stomach or colon.

BURNS

- Apart from well-known first-aid treatments for burns, internal herbal remedies can quickly alleviate pain and accelerate tissue healing.

INJURY/WOUNDS

- Vulnerary herbs promote healing of cuts, scrapes and deeper wounds.
- Herbal medicine also works extremely well for bruises; discoloration and swelling can be negligible or prevented altogether.
- Sprains to ligaments and joints are perfect candidates for herbal anti-inflammatories that also stimulate connective tissue repair.

Trauma

See the page references below for details on each condition and herb.

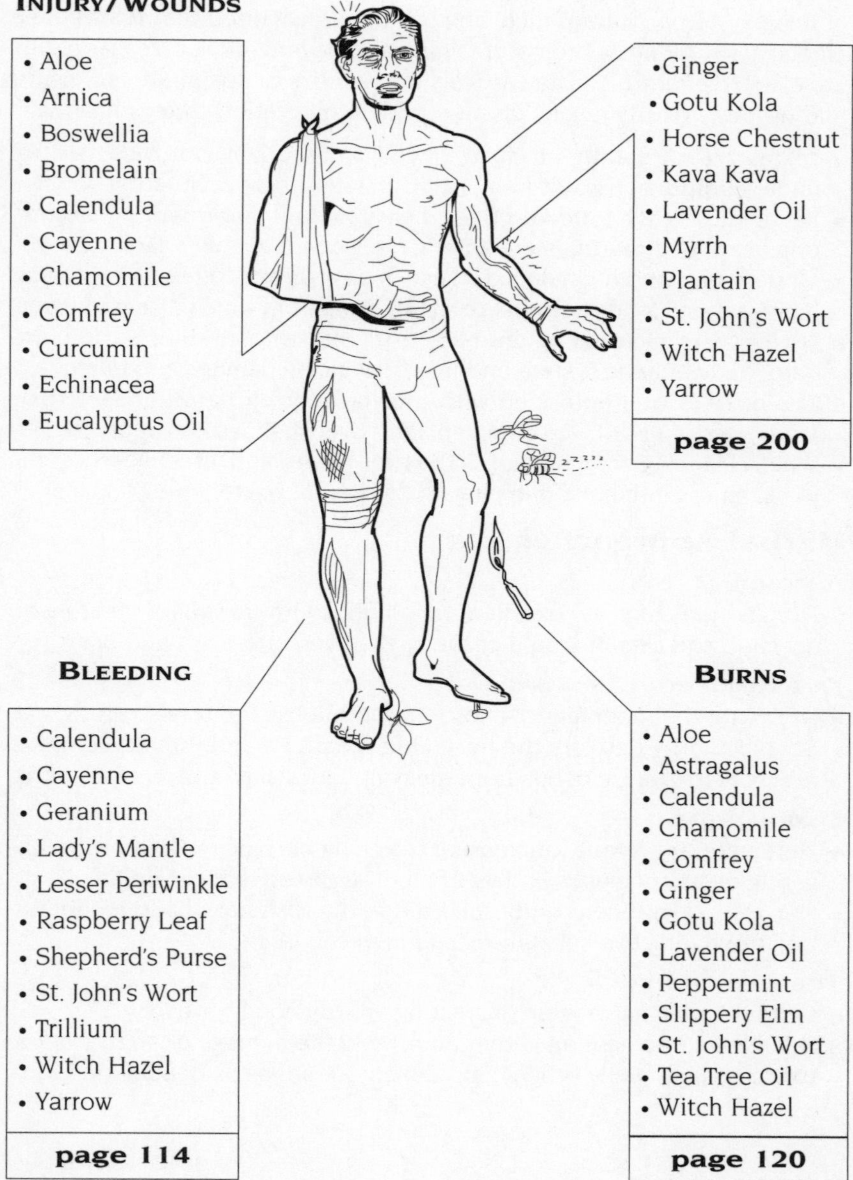

DETOXIFICATION

The System

Toxins are chemical and biological substances that are harmful to normal tissue and interfere with the function of cells and enzyme systems. Natural medicine has long recognized that toxins are a chief cause of illness, premature aging and degenerative disease. Toxins are also "free radicals," the particles that oxidize or coagulate molecules and tissues. Toxicity means disease, and detoxification creates healing.

- Toxins are normal by-products of cell metabolism, but today we are under additional assault from artificial, man-made pollutants.
- Pesticides, PCBs, food additives, heavy metals, fluoridation, vaccinations and medical drugs are among the worst toxic offenders.
- Modern diet and lifestyle habits, such as alcohol, coffee, tobacco and highly refined foods help create a toxic soup from which disease begins.
- Highly toxic bacterial by-products from intestinal dysbiosis can inundate the lymphatic system and liver, producing damage and allergy.
- The body is well-equipped with mechanisms to handle heavy toxic loads, but can easily become deficient, overwhelmed or suppressed.
- When cleansing organs, such as the liver, kidney and intestines, become weak, an essential link in the chain of internal waste removal is lost.

Herbal Approaches

ALCOHOL DETOX

- Herbal medicines are excellent for alcohol withdrawal, for creating an aversion and cleaning up damage to the liver, intestines and brain.

DETOXIFICATION

- Herbs are the treatment of choice for both local and total body detox.
- Specific herbs detoxify the liver, kidney, spleen and intestines, while others help cleanse debris from the lymphatics and intercellular matrix.

DRUG DETOX

- Herbs are important for clearing the body of toxic resides or the lingering effects of a wide variety of medical or recreational drugs.
- Nervines, adaptogens and tonics aid in the withdrawal and rehabilitation from addictive substances and medical drugs.

TOBACCO DETOX

- Certain herbs are capable of creating an aversion to tobacco.
- Demulcent and healing herbs can reverse the damage done to respiratory passages, while others help the emotional basis of addiction.

Detoxification

See the page references below for details on each condition and herb.

Detoxification

- Burdock
- Chickweed
- Cleavers
- Dandelion
- Nettles
- Poke Root
- Red Clover
- Red Root
- Queen's Delight
- Triphala
- Wild Indigo
- Yellow Dock

page 148

Alcohol Detox

- Acorn
- Angelica
- Calamus
- Cayenne
- Celandine
- Hops
- Khella
- Kudzu
- Milk Thistle
- Oatstraw
- Passionflower
- Quassia
- Schisandra
- Wild Lettuce

page 94

Drug Detox

- California Poppy
- Chaparral
- Chamomile
- Ginger
- Ginseng
- Goldenseal
- Gotu Kola
- Holy Basil
- Milk Thistle
- Oats
- Passionflower
- Schisandra
- Skullcap

page 154

Tobacco Detox

- Cayenne
- Coltsfoot
- Ephedra
- Ginger
- Licorice
- Lobelia
- Mullein
- Oats
- Plantain
- Skullcap
- Spikenard
- Valerian
- Yerba Santa

page 246

Part 3

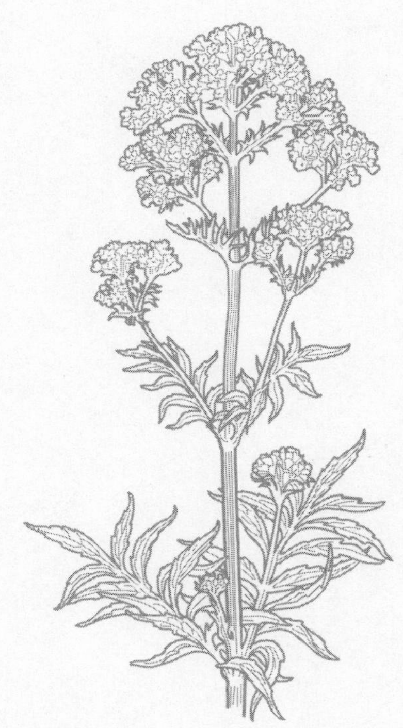

A-Z Herbal Prescriber

A-Z Condition Index

A Note on Grading

In the descriptions of the conditions and herbs that follow, a personalized system of grading has been used. Each herb has a "usefulness" rating of good (*), very good (**) and superior (***). Obviously, every herb that is worthy of being listed is a valuable medicine. Yet from a practical standpoint, one has to judge some herbs as more clinically effective for a particular condition than others. Additional factors influencing the herbal rating are its availability, its palatability and, of course, its safety.

ACNE/ABSCESS

Select the herbs that are most suitable for your condition.

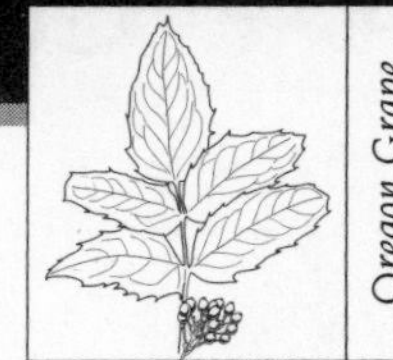
Oregon Grape

The Herbal Approach

Infections within the pores and sebaceous glands of the skin can manifest as abscesses, boils and pimples. In acne, hormone imbalance overstimulates the skin's oil glands, making it particularly common during infancy, adolescence, menses and menopause. Underlying factors include nutritional deficiencies, hypoglycemia, stressed adrenals, food allergies and environmental toxins. Though these skin infections are caused by bacteria, they indicate a toxic overload in this, the body's largest detoxification organ. Eliminating as much waste per day as the kidneys, the skin must take over when other detox organs, such as the colon and liver, are not functioning up to par. Poor liver function also increases the build-up of acne-producing steroids in the body. Suppression with antibiotics or topical treatments have significant side effects and are hardly a cure.

Herbs with natural antibacterial effects can be used alongside those that strengthen the immune system and improve various detoxification pathways—especially the liver and intestines. Elimination of dairy, coffee and individual dietary allergens is crucial. Appropriate plants are also needed to restore hormonal balance. Locally, *calendula, witch hazel, tea tree oil* or *Hauschka* or *Weleda* products are beneficial and non-suppressive. See also ■ Detoxification ■ Liver Conditions ■ Skin Conditions.

Burdock***—Arctium lappa
- A traditional detoxifier and blood cleanser; treats acne, boils, eczema.
- Cleanses the lymphatics, blood, liver and kidneys of toxic build-up.
- Antiseptic, with antibacterial, antifungal and antiviral capabilities.
- Diuretic; tones the kidney and stomach, promotes perspiration.
- Stimulates immunity and white cell production. Cancer-protective.

Calendula**—Calendula officinalis
- Use externally as an antiseptic wash; effective even in long-standing, deep infections. Anti-inflammatory, promotes rapid wound healing.
- Helps heal skin ulcers, erysipelas, prevents excess scar formation.

Cleavers**—Galium aparine
- One of the most versatile lymphatic restoratives and tonifiers.
- Facilitates elimination of cellular and tissue wastes, toxins, fluids.
- Reduces tissue inflammation, congestion and enlarged glands.

Dandelion***—Taraxacum officinalis
- One of the best detoxifying herbs, gentle and balancing in nature.
- Works on the liver, gall bladder, colon and kidneys to help clear waste

products more efficiently. Helps balance body's hormone ratios.

Echinacea***—Echinacea angustifolia
- Powerful short-term immune stimulant, increasing toxin removal.
- Internal use as an antibacterial and to accelerate wound healing.
- External use as a poultice or local compress, applied several times daily.

Figwort**—Scrophularia nodosa
- An herb with a broad range of applications in treating skin disorders.
- Promotes lymphatic cleansing, restores body's elimination pathways.
- Combines well with dandelion and burdock roots.

Myrrh**—Commiphora myrrha
- Antiseptic, antimicrobial, anti-inflammatory and astringent herb.
- Use externally to treat boils, abscesses, pressure sores and wounds.

Oregon Grape***—Berberis aquifolia
- An excellent herb for chronic acne and rosacea, as well as psoriasis, eczema and other skin disorders. Helps prevent pitting scars.
- Antimicrobial, like goldenseal, against candida, strep and staph, etc.
- Stimulates the liver, gall bladder, and heals the digestive membranes.

Red Clover***—Trifolium pratense
- Specific for skin disorders and safe to use in children and the elderly.
- Immune-enhancing, blood-purifying herb with hormone-balancing effects.
- Treats ulceration and sores. Used in traditional cancer formulas.
- Particularly for acne on forehead, scalp, nose. Treats rosacea, oily skin.

Red Root***—Ceanothus americanus
- A traditional detoxifying herb and important blood and spleen tonic.
- Rids the body of excess heat and assists in tissue waste removal.
- Used internally to treat fevers and congested tissues of the body.

Tea Tree Oil***—Melaleuca alternifolia
- Used externally, will destroy a broad range of invading microorganisms.
- As effective as benzol peroxide solutions, but without their side effects.
- Improves skin dryness, redness, itching, stinging. Gentle on the face.

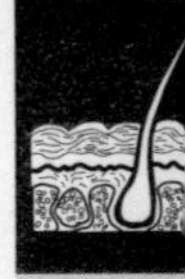

Wild Indigo**—Baptisia tinctoria
- Immune-stimulating and antimicrobial, reduces enlarged lymph nodes.
- Internal use for deep tissue cleansing and for generalized toxicity.
- Use externally to bathe infected wounds, or as a gargle or compress.

Yellow Dock***—Rumex crispus
- External compress used to discharge pus and infection from the skin.
- Eliminates wastes and toxins from the skin and deeper tissues.
- Combine with burdock and dandelion for blood and liver detoxification.
- Mild laxative effect that corrects sluggish and congested intestines.

ADD / ADHD

Select the herbs that are most suitable for your condition.

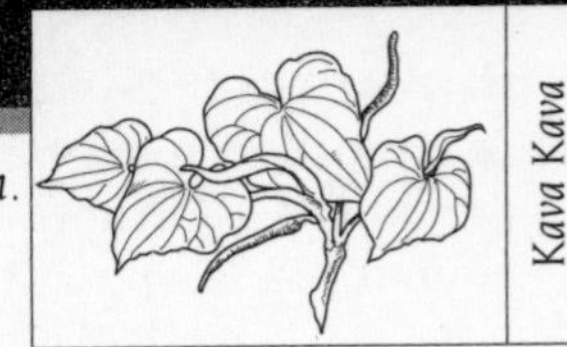
Kava Kava

The Herbal Approach

Attention deficit disorder and hyperactivity are the epidemic of our age, but current treatment is woefully inadequate. While our society wages an ongoing "war on drugs," millions of children are hooked on "speed" in the form of Ritalin and amphetamines. Apart from serious and permanent side effects, these do not remotely address underlying causes and can in no way be regarded as a cure. Diagnoses such as learning disability, hyperactivity and poor impulse control are usually attributed to a brain chemistry imbalance. A better term might be "toxic brain syndrome," since the overriding factor is a constant bombardment of the child's nervous system with pesticides, mercury, lead, food additives, artificial sweeteners, vaccines, antibiotics and allergenic foods. Each one of these factors has been shown to significantly and profoundly impact developing brain cells and combine together with devastating effects.

A full-scale assault on these problems requires a homeopathic, herbal and nutritional program to undo the developmental and biological damage caused by chronic exposure to toxins. Herbs have the short-term gain of relaxing and calming, while improving brain function and neurotransmitter production. In the long run, nervine and adaptogenic plants can protect, detoxify and heal the nervous system—all without the significant toxicity or side effects of drugs. See also ■ Anxiety ■ Fatigue ■ Insomnia ■ Depression ■ Memory ■ Stress.

Bacopa**—Brahmi/Bacopa monnieri
- Calming and sedative. Improves anxiety; important for hyperactivity.
- Improves intellectual capacity, acuity, clarity of thought, concentration.
- Improves memory, especially in the elderly; shortens learning time.

California Poppy***—Eschscholtzia californica
- A gentle sedative that relieves psychological and emotional disturbances in kids. Soothes and balances an overactive nervous system.
- Reduces anxiety and tension in overactive states, decreases spasms.
- Effective for difficulty in falling asleep or frequent, regular waking.

Catnip*—Nepeta cataria
- Relieves anxiety, restlessness, tension, stress and hyperactivity.
- A mild relaxant that promotes restful sleep. Helps diarrhea, headache, colic or stomach ache due to stress. Balances mood swings or hysteria.

Ginkgo**—Ginkgo biloba
- Improves focus, memory, cognition, knowledge retention, perception.
- Increases neurotransmitters, boosts the brain's ability to use oxygen.
- Increases circulation to brain; high in nutritive antioxidants that protect the brain and nervous system from damage by various toxins.

Grape Seed Extract***—Vitis vinifera
- Contains bioflavonoids with the most potent antioxidant effects known.
- Able to cross the blood brain barrier and directly protect the brain against a wide variety of toxins and damaging free radicals.
- Improves brain blood flow, strengthens brain capillaries.

Hops**—Humulus lupulus
- Indicated for nervous tension, excitability, restlessness and irritability.
- Excellent for insomnia, taken orally or as a hops and lavender pillow.
- Calms and improves the mood, but should be avoided in depression.
- Strengthens and stimulates digestion, relieves intestinal discomfort.

Kava Kava**—Piper methysticum
- Valuable in attention deficit disorder; relieves anxiety without any cognitive or mental impairment. Reduces insomnia, tension and stress.
- Produces a sense of tranquility and softens angry or violent feelings.
- Significantly improves mood, tension level and sleep patterns.

Lemon Balm**—Melissa officinalis
- A gentle, safe and calming children's herb for depression and anxiety.
- Relaxes the nervous system; eases agitation while soothing digestion.

Oats***—Avena sativa
- Nervous system nutritive and tonic for mental stress, nervousness, overwork, exhaustion, weakness. Improves mental concentration, focus.
- Eases stress, tension, depression, insomnia—but improves clarity.
- Excellent for transitioning and weaning off neurological medications.

Skullcap**—Scutellaria laterifolia
- Helps anxiety, restlessness, crying spells, irritability and nervousness.
- A useful daytime sedative, with no mental impairment or drowsiness.
- Nervine action relieves frequent headaches, relaxes muscular spasms.

St. John's Wort***—Hypericum perforatum
- An herb of choice for attention deficit or hyperactive children.
- Calms an agitated nervous system, yet safe for long-term usage.
- Regulates mood and attention, relieves feelings of sadness, apathy, low self-esteem, isolation, anger, guilt, shame. Good for nervous exhaustion.

Valerian***—Valeriana officinalis
- Relaxing and sedating, reduces restlessness, nervousness, improves sleep; should be taken for 2–4 weeks to improve mood and sleep.
- Shows improvements in learning skills, with less aggressive behavior.

Alcohol Detox

Select the herbs that are most suitable for your condition.

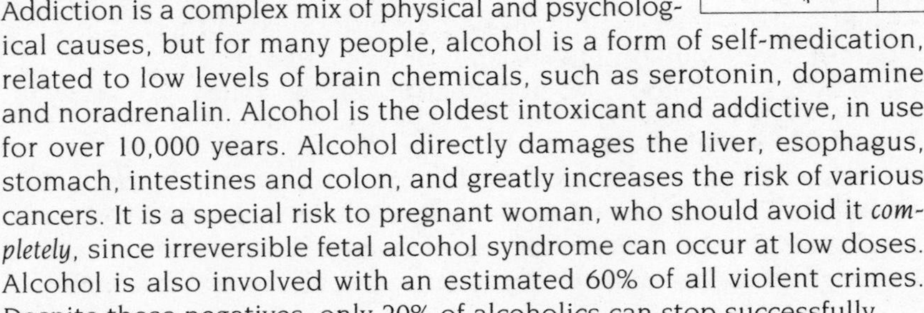

The Herbal Approach

Addiction is a complex mix of physical and psychological causes, but for many people, alcohol is a form of self-medication, related to low levels of brain chemicals, such as serotonin, dopamine and noradrenalin. Alcohol is the oldest intoxicant and addictive, in use for over 10,000 years. Alcohol directly damages the liver, esophagus, stomach, intestines and colon, and greatly increases the risk of various cancers. It is a special risk to pregnant woman, who should avoid it *completely*, since irreversible fetal alcohol syndrome can occur at low doses. Alcohol is also involved with an estimated 60% of all violent crimes. Despite these negatives, only 20% of alcoholics can stop successfully.

Herbal medicines offer a valuable resource for the effects of, and addiction to, alcohol. Initially, there are herbs to detoxify and lessen cravings, while reducing the symptoms of withdrawal. *Acorn* tincture (*Quercus glandis*) or *angelica* can be used in all cases to create a powerful aversion to alcohol. Other plant medicines help repair the damage done, including liver herbs like *milk thistle*. Adaptogenic and tonic herbs can correct biochemical and neurological imbalances that contribute to drinking, by doing such things such as increasing the manufacture of neurotransmitters like serotonin. Others herbs can help underlying anxiety or depression. See also ■ Anxiety ■ Depression ■ Drug Detox ■ Fatigue ■ Headache ■ Immune Weakness ■ Liver Conditions ■ Stress.

Acorn***—Quercus robur glandium

- Diminishes alcoholic craving, antidotes its effects, such as enlarged spleen and liver. *Diarrhea may appear during treatment as a curative effect.*
- Available as a homeopathic liquid under the name Quercus glandis.

Angelica**—Angelica atropurpurea

- Reduces craving or creates dislike for alcohol; use 5 drops, 3 times daily.
- A warming circulatory tonic that relieves gas, bloating, colic, headache.
- Helps with enlarged spleen; anti-inflammatory and antispasmodic.

Calamus*—Acorus calamus

- Reduces the craving for alcohol; restorative for brain, nervous system.
- Relieves gas, cramps, distention. Improves appetite, helps exhaustion.

Cayenne***—Capsicum frutescens

- Helps stop morning vomiting and gnawing stomach, reduces intense cravings for alcohol and promotes appetite; use in single drop doses.

- Reduces irritability, anxiety and tremor and induces calm sleep.
- Delirium tremens, chills, exhaustion can often be speedily relieved.

Celandine***—Chelidonium majus
- Specific for liver problems from alcohol; extreme sensitivity to, and bad effects from, drinking. Liver healer and detoxifier, even for cirrhosis.
- Calms emotions (i.e. anger, depression) during withdrawal or cravings.
- For general sluggishness, difficulty concentrating and mental dullness.

Hops**—Humulus lupulus
- Sedative that relieves anxiety-related withdrawal symptoms; aids DTs.
- Helps irritability and restlessness, promotes healthy digestion.
- Relieves insomnia, frequent wakings; not suitable during depression.

Khella**—Ammi visnaga
- Ayurvedic herb that alleviates the acute and chronic effects of alcohol.
- Powerful antispasmodic and pain remedy. Used for asthma, angina.

Kudzu***—Pueraria lobata
- Traditional use in China to sober a drunk person and for various side effects of alcohol (hangover, thirst, gastric bleeding, loss of appetite).
- Recent research shows it can dramatically reduce craving for alcohol.

Milk Thistle**—Silybum marianum
- Protects against damage to the liver by alcohol, drugs and toxins.
- Powerfully regenerates damaged liver tissue; essential for cirrhosis.

Oats***—Avena sativa
- Excellent for weaning off alcohol, drugs, opiates, narcotics. Invigorating without intoxication or overstimulation. Improves clarity, focus.
- Restores proper nerve functioning; eases a racing heart or palpitations.

Passionflower*—Passiflora incarnata
- Treats insomnia, delirium tremens or spasms related to withdrawal.
- Useful to induce restful sleep without producing hangover effects.
- Combines well with kava, skullcap, valerian, hops or Jamaican dogwood.

Quassia*—Picrasma/Quassia excelsa
- Antidotes effects of alcohol, rejuvenates the spleen. A bitter that stimulates appetite and digestive function; tonifies a weak digestive system.

Schisandra**—Schisandra chinensis
- Controls anger and aggression without sedation; combats depression.
- A liver tonic for hepatitis and an adaptogen that assists the body in balancing stress; effective for nervous exhaustion, weakness, insomnia.

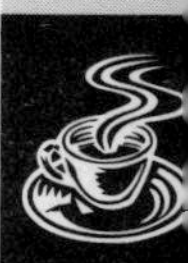

Wild Lettuce*—Lactuca virosa
- Produces a general sense of well-being, calms excitability, relieves pain.
- Mild sedative and cure for insomnia; safe for both young and old.

AMENORRHEA

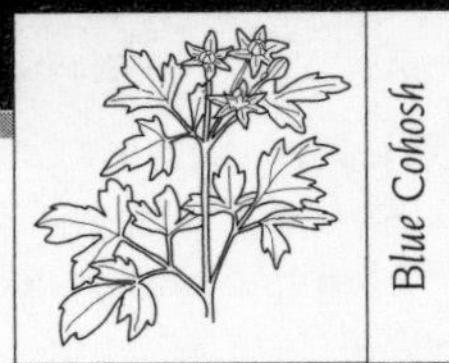

Select the herbs that are most suitable for your condition.

The Herbal Approach

Primary amenorrhea refers to delayed onset of menses at puberty. *Secondary amenorrhea* is defined as a loss of menses for three months or more. This commonly occurs due to an imbalance in the coordinated functioning of the pituitary gland and ovaries, which secrete estrogen and progesterone. This kind of imbalance can be caused by intense athletic activity, nutritional deficiency, sudden weight loss, hormone or drug therapies, or psychological shock or stress. It can also be related to disorders of other endocrine glands, notably the adrenals or thyroid. On the other hand, amenorrhea is a normal occurrence during periods of breast-feeding.

Separate herbal traditions from China, India, Europe and North America all have plants that show excellent results in rebalancing the estrogen/progesterone ratio and reestablishing a normal menstrual cycle. Many of the herbs listed below are also used for infertility and for hormonal disruption during menopause. These can be used singly or in combination. One famous American formula, which has been used for centuries as an herbal "Mother's Cordial," is prepared from the tinctures of *blue cohosh, true unicorn root, false unicorn root, cramp bark* and *partridge berry*. The use of this mixture helps with menstrual regularity and fertility, as well as in preventing miscarriage in the first trimester. In most cases, several months of use may be required to produce a stabilized hormonal balance. See also ▪ Anemia ▪ Infertility ▪ Menopause ▪ Miscarriage.

Black Cohosh***—Cimicifuga racemosa
- Helps delayed, irregular or absent menses; normalizes cycles.
- For amenorrhea after emotional upset, colds, chilling or infections.
- Antispasmodic effective for dysmenorrhea; helps dark, clotted menses.
- Stimulates endocrine activity, which mimics estrogen in the body.

Blue Cohosh**—Caulophyllum thalictroides
- Uterine tonic and stimulant; promotes menses when late or suppressed.
- Regulates cycle, reduces pain and excess bleeding during menses.
- Strong antispasmodic, relieves cramps, ovarian and uterine pains.

Chaste Tree***—Vitex agnus castus
- Works via the pituitary to increase progesterone, decrease prolactin.
- Regulates menstrual cycle, where the cause is hormonal imbalance.
- For suppressed menses from the pill, emotional upset, exercise, illness.
- Valuable for PMS or excess bleeding. Requires several months of use.

Dong Quai**—Angelica sinensis
- Has overall balancing, regulating effect on female hormones and cycles.
- Helps the body regain its normal menstrual cycle after use of the pill.
- Helpful in anemia, regulates blood sugar and lowers blood pressure.

False Unicorn***—Chamaelirium luteum/Helonias dioica
- For recurrent miscarriage or amenorrhea from prolapse or a weak uterus.
- Balances hormones and menstrual cycle, stimulates onset of menses.
- Antispasmodic, tonifies and tightens weak tissue, helps low back pain.

Kelp**—Bladderwrack/Fucus vesiculosis
- For amenorrhea due to subclinical thyroid or adrenal dysfunction.
- Contains trace minerals and iodine for thyroid function, weight control.
- Increases vitality, helps edema, weight loss and symptoms of fatigue.

Lady's Mantle*—Alchemilla vulgaris
- Promotes menstrual flow, regulates cycle; helps during menopause.
- Relives menstrual cramping and excess bleeding at or between menses.
- Used for fibroids, endometriosis. Astringent effects, useful in vaginitis.

Licorice**—Glycyrrhiza glabra
- Aids adrenal and corticosteroid production. Synergistic herb, increasing action of others; found in 1/3 of all Chinese female formulations.
- Estrogen and steroid-like compounds help balance endocrine glands.

Maca***—Lepidium meyenii
- Increases fertility, the number of pregnancies and the birth weight of offspring. Decreases fatigue, increases libido, combats anemia.
- Regulates the relationship between the pituitary, ovaries and adrenals.
- Reestablishes normal rhythms, regulates cortisol and melatonin levels.

Rehmannia**—Rehmannia glutinosa
- A woman's Chinese tonic for "blood deficiency," anemia, exhaustion.
- For irregular menses, amenorrhea or abnormal menstrual bleeding.
- Restorative after childbirth, helps in menopause. Liver-protective herb.

Shativari**—Asparagus racemosa
- Main Ayurvedic herb for women; promotes estrogen production.
- Helps irregular menses, infertility, loss of libido, threatened miscarriage.
- Promotes lactation. A digestive tonic for hyperacidity, ulcers.

True Unicorn Root**—Star Grass/Aletris farinosa
- Uterine tonic that promotes menses; tones a weak or displaced uterus.
- Effective for habitual miscarriage, prolapse, sterility, excess bleeding.
- Balances menstrual cycle; acts as a synergist for other uterine herbs.

ANEMIA

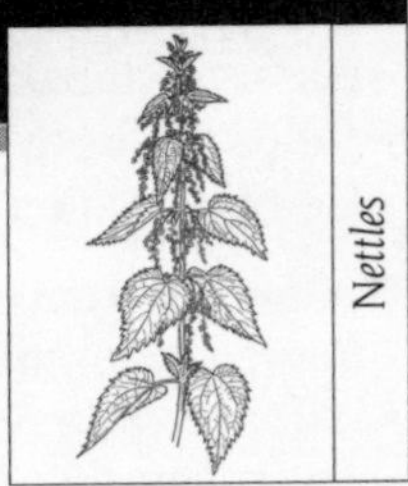

Select the herbs that are most suitable for your condition.

The Herbal Approach

Anemia is a blood disorder, in which the red blood cells are no longer able to carry oxygen to the tissues. This is a common nutritional problem, when inadequate iron (the carrier of oxygen in the blood) is taken in the diet, or excess blood is lost, typically via menses or uterine bleeding. Vitamin B12 or folic acid deficiency results in pernicious anemia—a developmental defect where the deformed red cells are not able to retain iron. Many other more serious conditions can cause anemia, including various kinds of leukemias, thalassemia, toxins or poisons that destroy blood cells, and medical drugs or radiation that affects the home of blood cells—the bone marrow.

Once a cause is diagnosed, various herbs provide a highly absorbable and bioavailable form of iron. This is often more effective than iron supplements or can be used to supplement or increase their effectiveness. Iron sulphate, for example, is a commonly prescribed form of iron that is very poorly absorbed, causing constipation. Other herbs act more centrally, promoting blood cell production, and aiding different aspects of iron and blood metabolism in the liver, spleen and marrow. Traditionally, these herbs also boost overall body chi, prana or life force. See also ▪ Bleeding ▪ Detoxification ▪ Liver Conditions.

Alfalfa***—Medicago sativa

- Nutritive herb, promotes digestion/assimilation of vitamins, minerals.
- Excellent source of nutrients that improve iron absorption and blood clotting, including B6, E, K, iron, calcium, potassium, zinc, magnesium.
- High in hemoglobin-building chlorophyll, protein and amino acids.

Ashwaganda**—Withania somnifera

- Tonic strengthening herb, high in iron content; increases hemoglobin.
- Berries are a blood tonifier that improves circulation and absorption of nutrients by cells. Used as a liver and kidney tonic in Chinese medicine.

Codonopsis**—Codonopsis pilosula

- A nourishing Chinese herb to "build strong blood" in nursing mothers.
- Increases red blood cells and hemoglobin levels in research studies.
- Similar, but gentler than ginseng; increases stamina and vitality in exhaustion or fatigue. Tonifying to the blood and digestive system.

Dong Quai***—Angelica sinensis

- Rich in B12 and folic acid, treats pernicious or iron deficiency anemia.
- Increases red blood cell production, combats weakness and fatigue.

- Protects the liver, improves the body's oxygen metabolism.
- Balances, replenishes female hormones (i.e. estrogen, progesterone).
- Traditionally combined with astragalus for greater effect.

Gentian*—Gentiana lutea
- A bitter digestive stimulant, improving gastric secretions; increases the proper absorption of many nutrients, especially protein, iron and B12.
- Treats debility and anemia caused by iron deficiency or blood loss.
- Regulates and strengthens overall digestion, increasing vitality.

Hawthorn**—Crataegus oxycantha
- Most useful in anemia associated with heart disease or at puberty.
- Tonifying to the blood, heart and circulatory system; strengthens heart.
- Helps with anemic weakness, rapid heart beat, effects of exhaustion.

Kelp**—Bladderwrack/Fucus vesiculosus
- Contains bioavailable iodine for thyroid function, as well as iron.
- Protects against ionizing radiation and radioactive iodine 129 and 131, potent causes of bone marrow disruption and subsequent anemia.

Nettles***—Urtica dioica
- Traditional blood tonic for debility, exhaustion. Diuretic and detoxifier.
- Contains high amounts and highly absorbable forms of iron.
- A natural source of essential vitamins and minerals, such as magnesium, silicon, chlorophyll, niacin, pantothenic acid and vitamin C.
- Increases hemoglobin, tissue oxygenation and blood coagulation.

Raspberry Leaf***—Rubus idaeus
- Rich in iron and calcium; particularly effective for anemia before or after childbirth or blood loss from excess menstruation. Useful uterine tonic.
- Helps with excess bleeding and hormone imbalances.

Red Root**—Ceanothus americanus
- Tonifies and regenerates the spleen, which is crucial for immune and blood cell health. Used for anemia with an enlarged or diseased spleen.
- Has been used in pernicious anemia, Hodjkin's disease, malaria.

Siberian Ginseng**—Eleuthrococcus senticosus
- Increases stamina, stress adaptation and cold tolerance in anemia.
- Tonic for weakness, recovery and convalescence, increasing immunity.

Yellow Dock***—Rumex crispus
- A blood tonic that assists in the assimilation of dietary iron, while itself absorbing available iron from the soil and providing rich iron salts.
- Releases the liver's iron stores into the circulation for use by cells.
- Traditional liver tonic, aiding metabolism of iron and blood proteins.

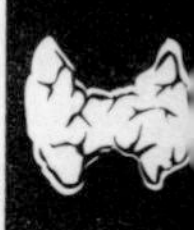

ANTI-AGING

Reishi

Select the herbs that are most suitable for your condition.

The Herbal Approach

Life span is ultimately determined by the fact that cells can only replicate a certain number of times—a genetically predetermined cut-off point that prevents physical immortality. Understanding this, most researchers still believe that humans should live 120 years or more. Why then is the average life span hovering around age 70? We deteriorate mainly due to damage from free radicals, produced as a by-product of normal metabolism, or created by various toxins, pollutants, allergens, heavy metals, etc. Additionally, 75% of Americans are not getting enough free radical fighting antioxidants, such as vitamin E, selenium or even vitamin C. These are quickly used up under stress, while hormonal, immune and neurological imbalances further accelerate aging.

A number of herbs are highly prized and renowned for their anti-aging and longevity-promoting effects. Science has extensively verified that these complex plant medicines have the definite ability to prolong the duration and quality of life. Many of these anti-aging herbs are adaptogens and tonics, normalizing metabolic, hormonal and neurological systems and stimulating cellular regeneration. Others have more focused effects on the brain, heart or immunity. They are safe for long-term use and disease prevention. See also ■ Arteriosclerosis ■ Fatigue ■ Heart Conditions ■ Immune Weakness ■ Memory ■ Stress.

Ashwaganda***—Withania somnifera
- Tonic that slows aging, rejuvenates tissues throughout the body.
- Clears the mind, strengthens the nerves, promotes restful sleep.
- Improves memory, cholesterol, sexual ability; lessens hair graying.

Fo-Ti***—Polygonum multiflorum
- Chinese tonic herb that promotes longevity, strengthens the blood, improves vitality, sexual vigor and fertility and can reduce hair graying.
- Lowers cholesterol, improves arteriosclerosis, regulates blood sugar.

Garlic**—Allium sativa
- Protects nervous system, improves brain function, memory, learning.
- Prevents/treats arteriosclerosis, reduces clotting, lowers cholesterol.
- Increases life span in animal tests; inhibits viruses, bacteria, parasites.

Ginseng***—Panax ginseng
- Rejuvenating, stimulating adaptogen, yet helps calm nerves, increases vitality; reduces exhaustion; increases stamina, speeds wound healing.
- Enhances immune system; balances metabolism and stress response.

Gotu Kola***—Centella asiatica
- Rejuvenating, longevity herb in the Ayurvedic and Chinese traditions.
- Increases intelligence, memory, creativity, learning ability, reduces mental fatigue. Strengthens nervous system, adrenals and immune system.
- Improves wound healing, reduces scar tissue, increases circulation.

Green Tea**—Camellia sinensis
- High in vitamins, minerals, antioxidants and flavonoids and especially polyphenols; decreases cellular and tissue damage incurred with aging.
- Protective against cancer, heart diseases and is an immune stimulant.

Hawthorn**—Crataegus oxycantha
- Heart and circulation tonic; normalizes blood pressure, heart rhythm.
- Slows aging process, protects connective tissue and blood vessel walls.
- Reduces atherosclerosis, helps adaptation to physical and mental stress, protects against radiation, improves digestion and assimilation.

Licorice**—Glycyrrhiza glabra
- Traditional Chinese longevity herb; stimulates adrenal glands, balances and conserves cortisol and energy during stress. Anti-inflammatory.
- Has potent antioxidants that protect the digestive tract, liver and other tissues from the damaging effects of aging. Inhibits atrophy of thymus.

Maca**—Lepidium meyenii
- Ancient Peruvian herb that increases vitality, strength and stamina.
- Invigorates libido and is a sexual restorative in both men and women.
- Alleviates signs of decreasing hormones in middle age and menopause.

Reishi***—Ganoderma lucida
- A traditional "elixir of immortality" in Traditional Chinese Medicine.
- Treats a wide range of conditions, including heart disease and cancer.
- Normalizes blood pressure, cholesterol, platelet stickiness. Enhances immune and liver health, helps indigestion, eases tension, improves sleep.

Rhodiola**—Golden Root/Rhodiola rosea
- Increases immunity, prolongs life span, increases exercise capacity.
- Clears toxins, strengthens nervous and digestive system. Reduces fatigue.

Siberian Ginseng**—Eleuthrococcus senticosus
- Called the "king of adaptogens," has a wide range of vitalizing effects.
- Increases hearing, improves eyesight, supports immunity and stress adaptation. Increases mental and physical work capacity.

Suma**—Pfaffia paniculata
- An adaptogen that is antiviral, antibacterial and immune stimulating.
- Increases muscle mass, protein production, overall physical endurance.
- Balances hormones, reduces blood sugar, cholesterol, triglycerides.
- Reduces fatigue, promotes liver and kidney regeneration, skin healing.

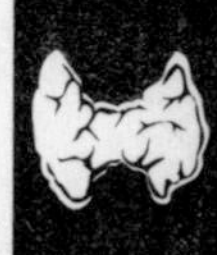

ANXIETY

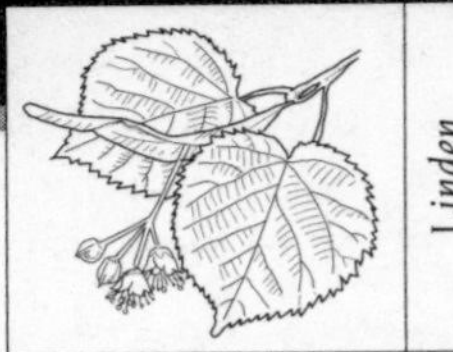

Select the herbs that are most suitable for your condition.

The Herbal Approach

Anxiety is the second most common psychological problem, yet remains undiagnosed 75% of the time. In our anxious age, doubts and fears can manifest as simple worries, free-floating anxiety, phobias (agoraphobia, social phobias, etc.), panic disorders and obsessive-compulsive tendencies. The latter may affect as many as 7 million Americans. Physical aspects of anxiety include stomach upsets, colitis, migraines, palpitations, hypertension and sweating. Anxiety after trauma, *post traumatic stress syndrome* (PTSD), is also increasingly common. Underlying, contributing factors are low blood sugar, food allergy, nutrient deficiency (fatty acids, B complex, etc.) and imbalances of the thyroid, ovaries or adrenals.

Many of the herbs that help anxiety work on the same brain receptor sites as drugs like Valium, Xanax and Halcion. Herbs however, tend to be gentler, safer and non-addictive. They have relaxant properties but also nourish and strengthen the nervous system. See also ■ ADD/ADHD ■ Fatigue ■ Immune Weakness ■ Liver Conditions ■ PMS ■ Stress.

California Poppy**—Eschscholtzia californica
- A tension-relieving, sedative, anti-anxiety and antispasmodic herb.
- Helps sleeplessness, quells headache and muscular spasm from stress.
- Gentle, non-addictive action that is safe for children and the elderly.

Chamomile***—Matricaria recutita
- Tranquilizing effects, with action similar to drugs, i.e. Halcion, Valium.
- Reduces effects of stress-induced chemicals in the brain, while promoting healthy adrenal hormones (e.g. cortisol). Relieves pain and spasms.
- Aids digestion, cramping and back pain. Promotes restful sleep.

Hops**—Humulus lupulus
- Calms nerves, eases anxiety, restlessness and tension. For headaches from stress, insomnia / sleep loss, indigestion or effects of alcohol.
- Its sedative properties are not appropriate for use during depression.

Kava Kava***—Piper methysticum
- Reduces anxiety, fear, tension; alleviates stress from many emotional, interpersonal and career factors. Improves performance; no grogginess.
- Relaxes muscles, relieves pain, insomnia and promotes restful sleep.
- Compares favorably to tranquilizers and benzodiazepines for anxiety.

Lemon Balm*—Melissa officinalis
- Relaxing and tonic herb, reduces anxiety, restlessness and nervousness.

- Helps with panic disorder, palpitations, racing heart, overactive thyroid.
- For digestive upset from stress or anxiety; nausea, indigestion, colic.
- Anti-depressant. Good in synergistic combination with other herbs.

Linden**—Tilia europaea
- Reduces tension, promotes relaxation; mild mood-elevating qualities.
- Protects against illness due to stress, anxiety and overactive adrenal glands, including high blood pressure, palpitations, gastric ulcers.

Motherwort**—Leonarus cardiaca
- A relaxing, tonic herb and mild sedative that gently relieves tension, anxiety when feeling under pressure. A heart, uterine and thyroid tonic.
- Relieves symptoms like a racing heart, shallow breathing.

Passionflower**—Passiflora incarnata
- Sedative herb that relieves anxiety, tension, spasms, pains, neuralgia.
- Promotes restful, refreshed sleep; induces relaxation, mild euphoria.
- Gentle action, suitable for nervousness in children and the elderly.

Skullcap***—Scutellaria laterifolia
- Relaxes, yet tones and renews the nervous system. Calms oversensitivity.
- Helps hysteria, depression and exhaustion, eases stress during PMS.
- Pain reliever and antispasmodic, decreases restlessness, nervousness.

St. John's Wort***—Hypericum perfoliatum
- Effective long-term action for anxiety and tension, as well as irritability and depression. Also for mood changes during menopause and for pain syndromes, including fibromyalgia, arthritis and neuralgia.

Valerian***—Valeriana officinalis
- Sedative and muscle relaxant; for anxiety, stress, muscle tension and pain, nervous cramps, restlessness, insomnia, overwork or overstudy.
- For easing off drug dependency (both medical and recreational drugs).
- For after effects of chronic flu. Improves poor concentration.

Vervain**—Verbena officinalis
- Relaxing nervine; reduces tension, strengthens the nervous system.
- Reduces anxiety due to stress, PMS or menopause, calms hysteria.
- Useful for lingering depression after a cold or flu. Tones the liver.

Wild Lettuce*—Lactuca virosa
- Gentle tranquilizer, calming an overactive, excitable nervous system.
- Very suitable for anxious children or adolescents. Helps with insomnia.
- General pain reliever and antispasmodic, especially for irritable coughs.

Wood Betony**—Stachys officinalis
- Sedative action, relieves tension, anxiety and nervous exhaustion.
- Calms an overactive, edgy state. Relieves headaches and neuralgic pain.
- Strengthens neurological function and improves memory, clarity.

Arteriosclerosis

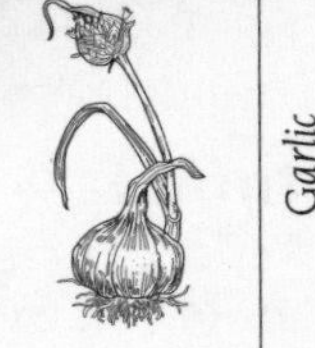

Select the herbs that are most suitable for your condition.

The Herbal Approach

Hardening of the arteries is the leading cause of disease and death in America, causing heart disease, stroke, kidney disease and problems with circulation in the limbs. Arteriosclerosis occurs due to oxidative damage to the lining of the arteries, infiltration with fat-filled cells and formation of plaques and clots. Risk factors include smoking, blood sugar disorders, obesity, an excess of "bad" cholesterol or LDL and high homocysteine levels, as well as a diet high in refined carbohydrates and trans fatty acids (i.e. processed oils). Damage to the arterial wall may also be due to chronic viral or bacterial infection. Supplementation with folic acid, B12 and B6, CoQ10, selenium, omega 3 oils and antioxidants would cut the risk of heart disease to a fraction of its current rate.

Herbal treatment for hardening of the arteries relies upon the strong antioxidant power of many plants, preventing the arterial damage that acts as a site for the development of plaque. They also prevent oxidation of LDL cholesterol, which leads to arterial deposits. Some herbs can remove existing arteriosclerosis, returning elasticity to arteries. Such plants have multiple benefits, such as toning the heart, reducing cholesterol and preventing blood cell clumping and clot formation. The central herb for the heart is *hawthorn*, while a combination or rotating schedule of several other healing plants will maximize their long-term benefit. See ■ Bleeding ■ Cholesterol, High ■ Heart Conditions ■ Veins/Circulation.

Arjuna**—Terminalia arjuna
- Main Ayurvedic heart tonic, normalizes the heart's rhythm, improves blood flow in coronary arteries. Reduces cholesterol; antibacterial.
- Improves symptoms of congestive heart failure and reduces angina pain.

Bromelain**—Pineapple/Ananas comosus
- A proteolytic enzyme derived from the stem of the pineapple plant.
- Reduces blood platelet "stickiness" and subsequent clot formation.
- Decreases the inflammatory response to artery injury or irritation.

Cayenne**—Capsicum frutescens
- Stimulates blood flow, lowers cholesterol; may affect arteriosclerosis.
- Reduces risk of blood clotting, increases heart output.
- Increases capillary resistance, strengthens blood vessels in the limbs.
- Improves peripheral circulation and warms the hands and feet.

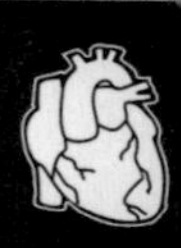

Curcumin***—Turmeric/Curcuma longa
- Antioxidant power eight times more potent than Vitamin E; prevents damage to blood vessel walls to prevent onset of arteriosclerosis.
- Improves blood flow in arteries, while strengthening blood vessels.
- Significantly reduces cholesterol, serum lipids, blood clot formation.

Garlic***—Allium sativa
- In one two-year study, reduced the size of arterial plaque by 20%.
- Blocks the formation of new plaque.
- Lowers cholesterol and triglycerides (by 10–20%), lowers LDL and raises HDL cholesterol; prevents oxidation and thus damage to arteries.
- A natural anti-coagulant; helps dissolve potential clots (fibrinolysis).

Ginger**—Zingiber officinale
- Thins the blood, decreases platelet aggregation and lowers cholesterol.
- Decreases blood pressure and reduces hardening of the arteries.
- Antioxidant, contains potent proteolytic enzymes; prevents clots.

Ginkgo***—Ginkgo biloba
- Increases microcirculation to all parts of the body, heart, limbs, brain.
- Blood-thinning activity, inhibits clot formation and inflammation.
- Antioxidant; strengthens, tones arteries, improving their elasticity.

Grape Seed Extract***—Vitis vinifera
- Antioxidant power 20 times that of vitamin C, 50 times vitamin E.
- Prevents arteriosclerosis and improves circulation in arteries, veins.
- Lowers cholesterol and actually shrinks existing deposits in arteries.
- Reduces blood cell agglutination, preventing clots, heart attack, stroke.
- Proanthocyanidins (OPCs) strengthen vessel walls, capillaries.

Guggul***—Commiphora gulgul
- Prevents arteriosclerosis, while reducing existing plaque in arteries.
- Lowers cholesterol and triglycerides as well as medical drugs. Lowers total cholesterol up to 30% in 3 months, raising HDL and lowering LDL.

Hawthorn***—Crataegus oxycantha
- Traditionally used over a long term to remove arteriosclerotic deposits.
- Essential cardiotonic that strengthens the heart muscle (myocardium).
- Prevents cardiovascular disease by dilating the coronary vessels.
- Improves blood and oxygen to the heart, coronary arteries and tissues.
- Strengthens contraction of the heart muscles, regulates blood pressure.

Shiitake**—Lentinus edodes
- Protective antioxidant, inhibits the formation of arteriosclerotic plaque.
- Helps prevent cardiovascular disease, stroke and diabetes.
- Lowers cholesterol up to 15%, prevents clots, regulates blood sugar.

ARTHRITIS

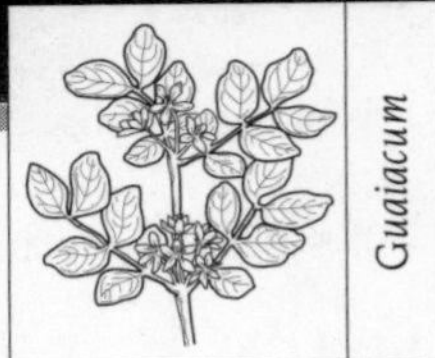

Select the herbs that are most suitable for your condition.

The Herbal Approach

Affecting some 40 million people, including 200,000 children, arthritis is the most common chronic disease in America. Osteoarthritis, the "wear and tear" arthritis, is by far the most frequent type. On the other hand, rheumatoid arthritis is part of an autoimmune syndrome and can be far more destructive and progressive. Its more serious nature also needs careful professional attention. There are a further 100 kinds of arthritic joint diseases, most related to immune dysfunction. Underlying causes for these conditions include long-term deficiencies and free radical damage, which undermines the body's structural tissues. Note too that chronic infections anywhere in the body can be a contributing cause.

Many herbs have been shown to surpass even cortisone in their ability to relieve pain and inflammation. Over time they also have the potential for stopping and reversing these crippling conditions. Glucosamine sulphate, MSM, omega 3 oils and various antioxidants are essential for promoting cartilage maintenance and repair. Ironically, a major side effect of aspirin and other anti-inflammatory drugs is cartilage damage. By promoting the health of the hormonal and immune systems, arthritis can be prevented, as well as treated on a deep level. See also ■ Fibromyalgia ■ Inflammation ■ Injury / Wounds ■ Low Back Pain.

Angelica*—Angelica archangelica
- Traditional anti-inflammatory for relieving arthritis and rheumatism.
- Warming herb, stimulates digestion, liver function, balances hormones.

Black Cohosh**—Cimicifuga racemosa
- Anti-inflammatory herb for both osteoarthritis and rheumatic pain.
- Salicylic acid inhibits enzymes responsible for pain; reduces swelling and the muscular spasms that accompany many arthritic symptoms.

Bogbean***—Menyanthes trifoliata
- Anti-inflammatory specific for rheumatoid arthritis and osteoarthritis.
- Promotes digestion and action of liver and gall bladder. Laxative effect (not for use in colitis or diarrhea). Helps fatigue, weakness, weight loss.

Boswellia***—Boswellia serrata
- In osteo- and rheumatoid arthritis, has anti-inflammatory action similar to NSAIDs, without stomach irritation. Improves circulation to joints.
- Improves pain, stiffness, inflammation; tonic and immune effects.

Bromelain**—Pineapple/Ananas comosus
- Contains protein-digesting enzymes; blocks inflammatory chemicals.
- Inhibits swelling, pain and tissue damage in affected joints.

Cayenne*—Capsicum frutescens
- Increases circulation, depletes nerves of pain-transmitting chemicals.
- Used as an external ointment for pain, inflammation and muscle spasm.
- Effective for symptomatic relief; does not affect underlying disease.

Curcumin***—Turmeric/Curcuma longa
- Powerful antioxidant, anti-inflammatory herb for rheumatoid and osteo.
- Stimulates body's cortisone production; equal to, or more effective than cortisone and anti-inflammatory drugs. Both internal and external use.

Devil's Claw**—Harpagophytum procumbens
- Effective anti-inflammatory in chronic arthritis (osteo or rheumatoid).
- Reduces pain, increases range of motion in 90% of research subjects.
- Useful blood purifier and tonic. Causes very little digestive irritation.

Feverfew*—Tanacetum parthenium
- Inhibits inflammation, lessening pain, swelling, tenderness of joints.
- Anti-inflammatory action has similar properties as COX-2 inhibitor drugs, Vioxx or Celebrex. Decreases migraine pain, thins blood.

Ginger***—Zingiber officinale
- Superior to NSAIDs as a potent anti-inflammatory in relieving muscle pain, swelling, stiffness; may be taken internally and applied externally.
- Reduces arthritic inflammation and associated bursitis, tendonitis.

Guaiacum**—Lignum Vitae/Guaiacum officinale
- Anti-inflammatory effects, reducing joint pain and swelling, gout.
- Helps contraction, shortening of tendons, joint stiffness and deformity.
- Specific affinity to the wrist, knee, limbs, spine. Diuretic / laxative effects.

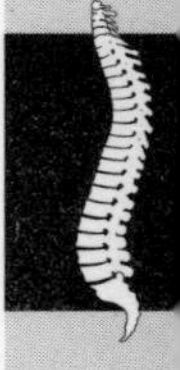

Licorice**—Glycyrrhiza glabra
- Anti-inflammatory and adrenal supportive, with cortisone-like effects.
- Is beneficial in gastric ulcers and possesses antiviral properties.

Meadowsweet**—Filipendula ulmaria
- Anti-inflammatory pain reliever, containing natural salicylates.
- Reduces stomach acidity, helps ulcers, the opposite of regular aspirin.

Willow*—Salix alba/fragilis/purpurea
- Similar to meadowsweet. Slower acting, but longer lasting than aspirin.

Yucca**—Yucca filamentosa
- Anti-inflammatory for arthritis and joint pain; non-toxic to intestines.
- Helps break up and remove inflammatory and mineral deposits from tissues. Effective for 60% of people for reducing pain, stiffness, swelling.

ASTHMA

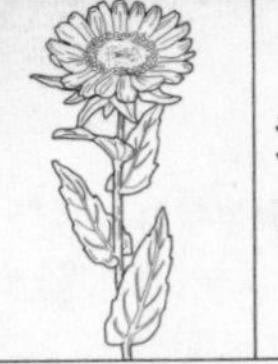

Select the herbs that are most suitable for your condition.

The Herbal Approach

Affecting over 14 million Americans (one-third of them children), asthma statistics have doubled in the last 20 years. The mechanism of asthmatic attacks is the release of inflammatory chemicals, such as leukotrienes and prostaglandins. Yet the underlying causes are nutritional and toxic, including pollutants and chronic food allergies. Other complicating factors are repeated or chronic viral infections, vaccine side effects and emotional stress. Suppression of skin problems or respiratory infections is also a basis for later development of asthma. Like so many chronic illnesses, this condition reflects the health of the entire immune and nervous systems. Though drugs and inhalers may be needed acutely, long-term cure lies in eliminating causes and rebuilding the immune system.

Herbs used to treat asthma are for both acute care and long-term benefit. Some act similarly to medical drugs by relaxing bronchial tubes and interrupting inflammatory pathways. However, herbs often do so more effectively and without side effects. Others are expectorants, liquefying and clearing the mucus from clogged respiratory pathways. Immune boosters, antioxidants and antimicrobial herbs complete the picture. See also ■ Anxiety ■ Coughs ■ Immune Weakness ■ Liver Conditions ■ Stress.

Elecampane**—Inula helena

- A tonifying lung herb used in respiratory ailments and disorders.
- Used in bronchitis, asthma, tuberculosis, emphysema and pneumonia.
- A stimulating and anti-inflammatory expectorant; dries up secretions.

Ephedra**—Ma Huang/Ephedra sinica

- Contains adrenaline-like substances that dilate the bronchioles.
- Antihistamine effect, reducing hayfever symptoms, nasal congestion.
- See Dosage; do not use with steroids, inhalers or anti-depressants.

Ginkgo**—Ginkgo biloba

- Though widely used for increasing mental acuity and brain blood flow, also inhibits factors that cause spasm of the bronchial tubes.
- Decreases hypersensitivity symptoms of allergy and inflammation.

Grindelia***—Grindelia squarrosa/Gum Plant

- For chronic asthma, bronchitis, hayfever or emphysema, with difficult breathing, shortness of breath, a rattling chest, panting or wheezing.
- Antispasmodic, relaxing the bronchi and expectorant, clearing phlegm.
- Slows the heart rate and decreases irritability of the bronchial passages.

Ivy Leaf*—Hedera helix
- Used for symptoms of bronchitis, emphysema; reduces airway obstruction of asthma in children ages 6–15, with no side effects or interactions.

Khella**—Ammi visnaga
- Relieves bronchial spasm; the basis of the common asthma drug Intal.
- Bronchial tube relaxation lasts up to six hours with no side effects.

Licorice**—Glycyrrhiza glabra
- Supports adrenal glands to produce natural cortisone and adrenaline.
- Demulcent that soothes and coats the irritated respiratory channels.
- Excess can weaken the heart and adrenals; use DGL form (see Dosage).

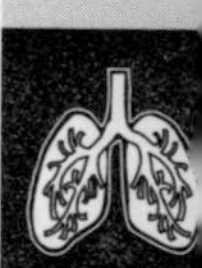

Lobelia**—Lobelia Inflata
- Traditional use and effectiveness to clear mucus, reduce spasms.
- Stimulates adrenal function; also lessens craving for tobacco.
- Dilates bronchi in asthma through adrenal action (see Dosage).

Mullein**—Verbascum thapsus
- A soothing demulcent, reduces mucus, encouraging expectoration.
- Benefits inflamed mucus membranes, reduces asthmatic wheezing.
- Eases tonsillitis, sore throats, bronchitis, tracheitis and emphysema.

Nettles*—Urtica dioica
- Nettles have powerful antihistamine effects in their freeze-dried form.
- Effective for symptoms of hayfever and relief of mild asthma.

Pill-Bearing Spurge** —Euphorbia harta
- Specific for bronchial asthma. Relaxes bronchial tubes, eases breathing.
- Mild sedative, expectorant. Treats bronchitis and other infections.

Querbracho*—Aspidosperma
- Antispasmodic "digitalis of the lungs" that dilates constricted bronchial tubes in asthma and emphysema; relieves tightness in the chest.

Spikenard*—Aralia racemosa
- Useful for asthma with irritating coughs or hay fever and sneezing.
- An adaptogenic herb known for its balancing effects during stress.

Wild Thyme*—Thymus vulgaris
- Prescribed for allergic asthma in children and adults; antimicrobial.
- A stimulating antispasmodic. Provides relief for allergy and hayfever.

Yerba Santa**—Eriodictyon californicum
- A bronchodilating herb indicated for asthma with chest tightness.
- Antibacterial and tonifying to a weakened respiratory system.
- A sweet-tasting tonic also used for chronic bronchitis, flus and colds.

BACK PAIN

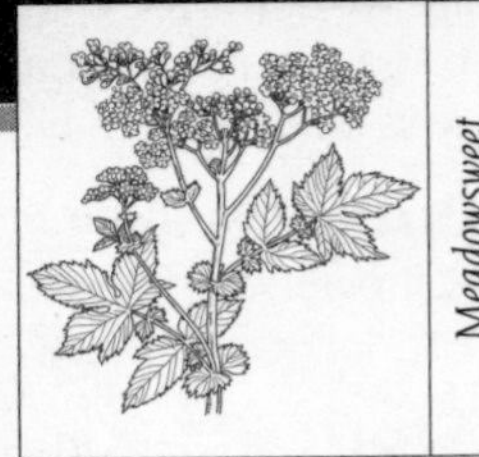

Select the herbs that are most suitable for your condition.

The Herbal Approach

Back pain affects at least 80% of people at some time, and most often concentrates in the low back. This results in an estimated 40 million days of lost work, at a cost of $70 billion. Poor postural habits are a major contributing cause, while other factors include repeated strains or microtrauma, muscle tension, nutritional deficiencies and reflex irritation from related internal organs. When repeated episodes of injury are added to this mix, the discs become subject to thinning, deterioration or rupture. These events can also gradually lead to arthritic changes. With nerves close by, swelling or compression in the spine often results in neuritis, lumbar neuralgia or sciatica.

Herbal medicines are used similarly to medical drugs in this type of condition, though with far more safety. Both the anti-inflammatory and pain-relieving qualities of plants can be used effectively and taken for prolonged periods of time. Other benefits are relief of muscle spasm and repair of connective tissue and cartilage tissue. Bioflavonoids and other healing factors contained in herbs, along with well-known nutritional substances like glucosamine sulphate, can complete deeper repair and strengthening of tissues. The herbs listed under Arthritis can provide further help for chronic joint dysfunction. If nerves become inflamed or compressed, additional sedative and nerve-repairing herbs may be needed. See also ■ Arthritis ■ Injury/Wounds ■ Pain/Neuralgia.

Barberry**—Berberis vulgaris

- For low back pain, often related to kidney weakness or congestion.
- For sciatica and neuralgia with radiating pain and weakened muscles.
- Use in rheumatic disorders, sciatica, bursitis, neuralgia and gout.

Black Cohosh**—Cimicifuga racemosa

- Anti-inflammatory effects, relaxing muscle spasms in low back and neck.
- Suitable for wry neck (torticollis), sciatica, neuralgia and intercostal (rib) neuralgia. Treats muscle pain associated with fibromyalgia, arthritis.

Black Haw***—Viburnum prunifolia

- With aspirin-like ingredients, relieves spasms and neuralgia of back and neck, sciatica, leg cramps, tension headache, wry neck, digestive spasm.
- A nervous system tonic and sedative, helps back pain during menses.

Boswellia***—Boswellia serrata

- Strong anti-inflammatory effects, reduces stiffness and pain.
- Works for acute problems, but needs 2–4 weeks for maximal effects.
- Improves circulation around inflamed joints, ligaments, tendons.

Bromelain**—Pineapple/Ananas comosus
- Enzyme found in pineapple stem, helps resolve late stages of inflammation, speeding healing and reducing the potential for scar tissue.

Corydalis*—Corydalis soldida
- Chinese herb that relieves pain of all kinds, especially from injury.
- Sedative, analgesic, relives spasm and abdominal pain, dysmenorrhea.
- Often used in combination with other complementary herbs.

Devil's Claw**—Harpagophytum procumbens
- Anti-inflammatory and pain-relieving herb, with rapid results.
- Useful for low back pain, arthritis and chronic rheumatic disorders, neuralgia and headaches. The whole herb preparation works best.

Dong Quai**—Angelica sinensis
- Reported to possess 1.5 times the analgesic activity of aspirin.
- Relieves back pain, cramping, muscular spasms and inflammation.
- Also for menstrual cycle regulation, anemia; a liver and heart tonic.

Horse Chestnut*—Aesculus hippocastanum
- Low back, *sacrum*, and sacroiliac pain. Stiff, weak back that "gives out."
- Helps with arthritic and rheumatic back pain with heaviness, swelling.

Jamaican Dogwood***—Piscidia erythrina
- Strong sedative, pain-relieving and antispasmodic effects.
- Especially valuable for muscular back spasms and pain, but also used in asthma, menstrual pain, insomnia, toothache or nervous conditions.

Kava Kava**—Piper methysticum
- Relaxes muscles, reduces internal and external spasms and cramps.
- Pain reliever, plus enhances pain-reducing effects of aspirin and drugs.
- No hangover, tolerance, build-up or addiction, typical of medical drugs.

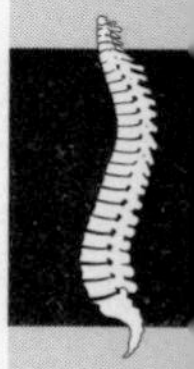

Meadowsweet*—Filipendula ulmaria
- Herbal forerunner of aspirin provides anti-inflammatory pain relief.
- No gastric irritation like medical NSAIDs; neutralizes stomach acids and general internal acidity.

Valerian**—Valeriana officinalis
- Relaxing and sedative effects, reduces transmission of pain signals.
- Muscle relaxant, relieves muscle spasms and contractures due to stress and tension; eases menstrual pain, colic, asthma, irritable bowel spasm.

Wild Yam**—Dioscorea villosa
- Indicated for back pain characterized by sharp, knife-like sensations.
- A relaxant used for pain originating in the digestive system, gall bladder, nervous system, uterus. Supplies precursors for adrenal cortisol.

BLADDER INFECTION

Select the herbs that are most suitable for your condition.

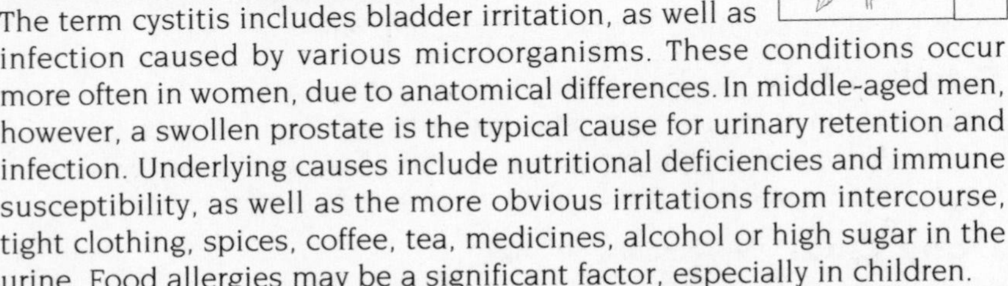

The Herbal Approach

The term cystitis includes bladder irritation, as well as infection caused by various microorganisms. These conditions occur more often in women, due to anatomical differences. In middle-aged men, however, a swollen prostate is the typical cause for urinary retention and infection. Underlying causes include nutritional deficiencies and immune susceptibility, as well as the more obvious irritations from intercourse, tight clothing, spices, coffee, tea, medicines, alcohol or high sugar in the urine. Food allergies may be a significant factor, especially in children.

Herbs for the urinary tract generally have diuretic effects, to flush out infection and inflammation by-products. Many are also antimicrobial, either destroying microorganisms or stimulating the body to do so. Along with quelling inflammation, other plants help heal irritated mucus membrane linings of the bladder, urethra and ureter, and the kidney tubules. In most cases, simple bladder infection can be easily and effectively dealt with using the herbs below. In cases where antibiotic resistant bacteria are involved, or where no bacteria are detected, as in interstitial cystitis, herbs become even more important and uniquely effective. See also ■ Detoxification ■ Infection ■ Kidney Conditions.

Buchu**—Agathosma or Barosma betulina
- A diuretic and urinary antiseptic for cystitis, urethritis, prostatitis.
- Tones the urinary tract and helps prevent stones; treats bedwetting.
- Helpful for prostate enlargement and resulting bladder infections.

Corn Silk**—Zea mays
- A soothing diuretic for irritation of the bladder, urethra and prostate.
- Relieves urinary tract inflammation and bedwetting in children.
- Effective for difficult and scant urination, cystitis and kidney stones.

Couchgrass*—Agropyron repens
- A soothing urinary demulcent, useful for infection or inflammation of the prostate, urethra or bladder. Useful in kidney stone and gravel.

Cranberry***—Vaccinium macrocarpon
- Reduces bacteria and prevents them from adhering to the bladder walls.
- Can be taken as a preventive in people with recurring infections.
- Safe and effective during pregnancy, for children and the elderly.
- Mildly acidifies the urine, eliminating alkaline bacteria, (i.e. E. coli).
- Reduces effectiveness of uva ursi; should not be used together.

Goldenrod**—Solidago virgaurea
- Diuretic, anti-inflammatory and antiseptic effects for cystitis, urethritis.
- Pain-relieving and antifungal, tones the bladder, soothes irritation.
- Safe and mild action; does not deplete body's electrolytes/potassium.

Goldenseal***—Hydrastis canadensis
- Anti-inflammatory and antimicrobial; destroys many types of bacteria.
- Especially effective for chronic cystitis or stubborn urinary mucus.
- Healing effect on bladder linings, stops bleeding, heals ulcerations.

Gravel Root*—Joe Pye Weed/Eupatorium purpureum
- For bedwetting in kids with bad dreams, hold their urine in too long.
- For irritable bladder with frequent desire, always feels full, uneasy.
- For incontinence in women, old age, children, enlarged prostate.

Horsetail**—Equisetum arvense
- Acute urinary tract infection; safe during pregnancy or weakened states.
- For bed-wetting or enuresis in children or weak bladder in the elderly.
- Diuretic effects, but does not deplete the body of salts or electrolytes.

Juniper Berry*—Juniperus communis
- A powerful diuretic, antispasmodic and strong antibiotic for cystitis.
- Must not be used for prolonged periods or in kidney infections.

Marshmallow***—Althea officinalis
- A soothing demulcent to the lining of the urinary tract.
- Use for acute inflammation, typical of bladder infections.
- Decreases inflammation in the respiratory, digestive or urinary tract.

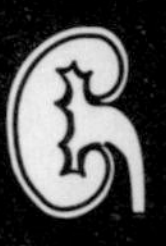

Parsley Root*—Petroselinum crispum
- Diuretic effects for cystitis, kidney stones. Soothes burning, itching, crawling in the urethra. Avoid in kidney disease or pregnancy.
- Helps symptoms of pain, frequent desire, urging, mucus discharges.

Sarsaparilla***—Smilax officinalis
- For cystitis, kidney infections, bladder stones, kidney colic, bedwetting.
- A blood purifier that is antiseptic, anti-inflammatory; controls itching.
- Diuretic. Rheumatic or skin problems (psoriasis) with urinary irritation.

Uva ursi***—Arctostaphylos uva ursi
- Urinary disinfectant and antiseptic, effective for many types of bacteria.
- Diuretic and astringent for chronic and acute urinary problems.
- Avoid acidic foods—and cranberry—which decrease its effectiveness.

Yarrow**—Achillea millefolium
- Increases urination, has antimicrobial effects, stops bleeding.
- Anti-inflammatory properties, while soothing bladder spasms.
- Tones the urinary tract and acts as a mild pain reliever in infections.

BLEEDING

Shepherd's Purse

Select the herbs that are most suitable for your condition.

The Herbal Approach

While any excessive or unusual bleeding is certainly a medical emergency, herbs can also be very effective for bleeding from a wide variety of causes. Traditionally these anti-hemorrhagic herbs are called *styptics*. Indeed, their unique ability to both prevent and arrest bleeding should make them part of every emergency kit. Botanical medicines can work speedily for bleeding from injuries or wounds. They are also very effective for ruptures of capillaries or small veins in the nose, gums or around hemorrhoids. Several herbs are particularly effective as a compress, wash or lotion for these types of external bleedings, especially *calendula*, St. *John's wort* and *witch hazel*. These *vulnerary* herbs also have the advantage of accelerating wound healing, while being antiseptic. Additionally, herbs rich in collagen-building nutrients, bioflavonoids and vitamin C can strengthen blood vessels to prevent excess bruising or bleeding. Other plants are effective for internal bleeding as well, affecting organs that include the stomach, intestines and bronchial tubes. *Geranium, lesser periwinkle* and *lady's mantle* are good examples. Excess menstrual bleeding (menorrhagia) or bleeding between periods (metrorrhagia) require attention and specific herbs such as *trillium* and *shepherd's purse*. Naturally, any underlying causes of bleeding, such as hormonal imbalance, need to be discovered and dealt with. See also ■ Anemia ■ Injury/Wounds ■ Menopause ■ Miscarriage.

Calendula**—Marigold/Calendula officinalis
- Stops bleeding from wounds, or from the scalp, mouth or gums.
- For external use on wounds, scrapes, cuts. Antiseptic and disinfectant, while accelerating tissue healing and prevents secondary infection.

Cayenne***—Capsicum frutescens
- Extract or powder applied externally stops bleeding in small wounds.
- Speeds healing by improving circulation and has antiseptic effects.
- Capsules or tea reduce internal bleeding. Useful for nosebleeds.

Geranium**—Cranesbill/Geranium maculatum
- An astringent and styptic; decreases clotting time in external wounds.
- Especially for bleeding in the digestive tract, including stomach ulcers, bleeding and diarrhea in irritable bowel syndrome or Crohn's disease.
- May also be used in excess menstrual or vaginal bleeding.

Lady's Mantle*—Alchemilla vulgaris
- Promotes blood coagulation and is a strong astringent for internal bleeding, heavy menstrual flow or bloody diarrhea.
- Useful as a rinse after dental surgery or as a douche for vaginitis.

Lesser Periwinkle**—Vinca minor
- Astringent/styptic for internal bleeding, bloody diarrhea or heavy menses.
- Reduces bleeding from nose, gums, mouth or after tooth extractions.
- Useful for arteriosclerosis and insufficient blood flow to the brain.

Raspberry Leaf*—Rubus idaeus
- Traditional use to prevent or treat bleeding during pregnancy or labor.
- Used to stop bleeding from skin ulcers, wounds, gums or sore throat.
- An effective astringent used to treat conjunctivitis, diarrhea, vaginitis.

Shepherd's Purse***—Thlaspi bursa pastoris
- A strong styptic; stops bleeding from external wounds, nosebleeds.
- Internally for bloody diarrhea and dysentery or urinary tract bleeding.
- Used for heavy uterine bleeding during or between menses or due to fibroids, miscarriage, menopause or post-partum bleeding.

St. John's Wort***—Hypericum perfoliatum
- Stops bleeding from injuries and open wounds, puncture wounds, abrasions, irritated gums or hemorrhoids (take internally and externally).
- Internally: effective for various kinds of bleeding or bleeding tendency.
- Externally: antiseptic and antiviral, speeds healing of wounds, burns.

Trillium***—Birthroot/Trillium erectum or pratense
- Excellent for excess bleeding associated with fibroids, too frequent or prolonged periods, bleeding between periods or uterine prolapse.
- Specific benefit for excess blood loss during menopause.
- Uterine tonic; relieves pain in the back, hip and pelvis.

Witch Hazel***—Hamamelis virginiana
- Apply to wounds, cuts, nosebleeds, or for injury to veins, eyes.
- Good for chronic effects of trauma, for bruising; relieves pain, soreness.
- Stops bleeding, prevents infection, promotes healing in ragged wounds.

Yarrow***—Achillea millefolium
- An astringent healing herb, effective for hemorrhage from wounds, internal injuries, hemorrhoids, after surgery or childbirth, nosebleed.
- Internal use to staunch bleeding from lungs, bladder, bowels, uterus.
- Specifically benefits endometriosis, bleeding from varicose veins.

Note: Other astringents that arrest bleeding include *oak*, *bistort* and *plantain*. For hormone-related bleeding, consider *vitex*, *maca* and especially *dong quai* to regulate menses.

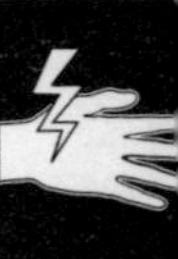

BREAST-FEEDING

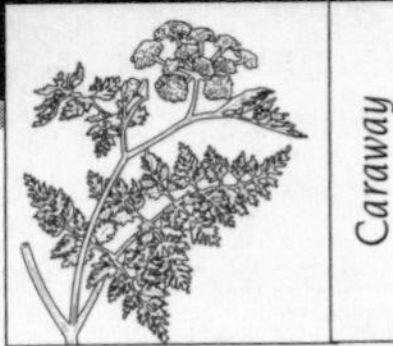

Select the herbs that are most suitable for your condition.

The Herbal Approach

A simple deficiency of milk production is a surprisingly common problem in nursing mothers. Important helpers for midwives, healers and physicians of all times and places, herbs have had a central role in promoting the healthy flow of milk since antiquity. The mechanism of action of many of these herbs is now known, as they balance the endocrine glands and the output of estrogen, progesterone and prolactin. Many herbal liver tonics, notably *milk thistle*, have a positive effect on lactation. The quality of the milk may also be a problem. Several herbs, like *alfalfa* and *elderflower*, can rectify this situation. For the mother, there may be difficulty or pain with breast-feeding, or the risk of breast inflammation or infection (mastitis). Antibiotics contaminate the milk, while many of the herbs below provide a safe anti-inflammatory treatment for mastitis. Additional problems may occur with cessation of breast-feeding (i.e. weaning), especially if done too quickly. Here, the tried and true herbal medicines, like *sage*, can help stop milk flow and return the breasts to their former health. A*ll* nursing mothers should have a 100% pesticide-free diet, since these poisons become highly concentrated in breast milk. See also ■ Acne/Abscess ■ Breast Conditions ■ Infection ■ Inflammation.

Alfalfa**—Medicago sativa
- Stimulates lactation and improves quality and quantity of milk.
- A nutritive herb, high in vitamins and minerals, used as both a food and medicine. Nourishing to the female reproductive system and breasts.

Carrot Family Herbs**—Umbelliferae species
- A number of members of the carrot or celery family of plants have estrogen-like effects and are traditionally used to increases the flow of milk, including fennel (*Foeniculum vulgare*), caraway (*Carum carvi*), anise (*Pimpinella anisum*) and dill (*Anthem graveolens*).

Castor Oil*—Ricinus communis
- Helps with deficiency of milk or poor quality. Brings milk into breasts.
- Use as an external poultice only, to reduce swelling, inflammation.
- Internally, causes vomiting, rumbling, colic and green, slimy, diarrhea.

Chamomile***—Matricaria recutita
- For inflamed breasts, sore nipples, suppressed or cheesy milk.
- Reduces negative effects of coffee in breast milk for infant and mother.
- Counters the effects of anger, including suppressed milk, cramps, colic.

Chaste Tree***—Vitex agnus castus
- Increases flow of breast milk by affecting pituitary's prolactin secretion.
- Balances the ratio of estrogen/progesterone. Can be taken long term.
- Helps to re-regulate menstrual cycle after pregnancy and childbirth.

Codonopsis**—Codonopsis pilosula
- Widely utilized in China to increase lactation and strengthen the blood.
- Revitalizes the body in a similar manner to ginseng, but gentler action.
- Increases energy; relieves symptoms of fatigue and digestive weakness.

Elder**—Sambucus nigra
- Increases the flow of milk; corrects "bad" or spoiled milk. Reduces breast swelling. Chest tonic, effective for allergies, candida. Reduces anxiety.

Fenugreek**—Trigonella foenumgraecum
- Increases milk production, stimulates hormones, return of menses.
- Safe for infant use and assists digestive disorders in suckling infants.
- Increases breast development or rejuvenation after breast-feeding.

Goat's Rue***—Galega officinalis
- A traditional "galactogogue" used for centuries by midwives.
- Shown to increases breast milk production by as much as 50%.
- Is known to regulate blood sugar levels and is a gentle diuretic.

Milk Thistle**—Silybum marum
- Promotes production of breast milk; safe for nursing mothers.
- Helps with pelvic congestion, stasis and prolapse after childbirth.
- Decreases pesticide residues in breast and found excreted in the milk.

Nettles**—Urtica dioica
- Traditional herb for promoting the flow of milk in nursing mothers.
- A blood-builder, rich in chlorophyll, iron, proteins, vitamins, minerals.
- Used to stop postpartum bleeding and decrease size of hemorrhoids.

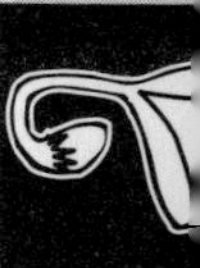

Poke Root**—Phytolacca decandra
- Corrects milk that has becomes cheesy, bad, lumpy. Helps pains during nursing. Reduces swollen breasts, heals cracks in the nipples.
- For mastitis right after childbirth or chronic discharges after weaning.
- Potential toxicity; supervised doses advisable in breast-feeding.

Sage*—Salvia officinalis
- Use to decrease the amount and flow of breast milk during weaning.
- An herb for galactorrhea or reducing excessive breast milk production.
- Beneficial for revitalizing weakened circulation and for excess sweating.

Vervain***—Verbena officinalis
- Encourages milk secretion and flow; excellent restorative for exhaustion following childbirth. Mood enhancing for postpartum depression.
- Increases absorption of nutrients from food and stimulates digestion.

BREAST CONDITIONS

Select the herbs that are most suitable for your condition.

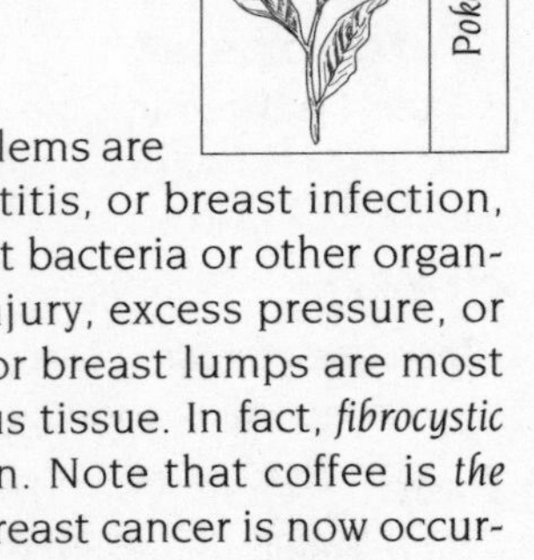

The Herbal Approach

The most common and most benign breast problems are premenstrual or menopausal breast pain. Mastitis, or breast infection, can happen during breastfeeding or anytime that bacteria or other organisms spread upward through the milk ducts. Injury, excess pressure, or lymphatic congestion can contribute. Tumors or breast lumps are most often benign, made of fluid-filled cysts or fibrous tissue. In fact, *fibrocystic breast disease* occurs in almost half of all woman. Note that coffee is *the* major cause of benign breast lumps. However, breast cancer is now occurring in one woman in six, and incidence rising steeply. For prevention, CoQ10, selenium and lycopene are essential, and no commercial pesticide-laden foods should be used. Rather than x-ray mammograms, which themselves are cancer-inducing, infrared mammography should be used.

A variety of herbs help breast problems. Hormone-balancing plants can help normalize breast tissue and monthly pain. Anti-inflammatory and infection-fighting herbs are very effective in mastitis. For cysts and tumors, blood cleansers and detoxifying herbs are essential. *Poke root* is one of the most useful herbs for the breast, though its toxicity limits its overuse. For underdeveloped breasts, *saw palmetto* and *pygeum* may be effective for increasing breast size, especially at puberty. See also ■ Acne/Abscess ■ Breast-feeding ■ Cancer ■ Detoxification ■ Infection ■ Inflammation ■ Menopause ■ PMS.

Astragalus*—Milk Vetch/Astragalus membranaceous
- Increases circulation to the surface of the skin, enabling greater blood flow to clear out toxins and heat. An adaptogen and lymphatic tonic.
- Restores immune function in immunosuppressed conditions.

Black Cohosh**—Cimicifuga racemosa
- Hormonal balancer; regulates menstrual cycle to reduce breast cysts.
- Anti-inflammatory; effective for breast pain, especially with menopause.

Burdock**—Arctium lappa
- Classic liver herb that stimulates the detoxifying channels of the body.
- Drains lymphatic fluid and promotes the excretion of toxins and waste.
- Improves the metabolism of liver hormones, acts as a mild laxative.

Castor Oil*—Ricinus communis
- A traditional therapy for shrinking cystic tumors and softening tissues.
- Use a warm oil compress over the affected breast tissue.
- Safe for daily applications; may take months before changes are seen.

Chamomile**—Matricaria recutita
- For inflamed, tender breasts, sore nipples, cramps when child nurses.
- Used for suppressed or thickened milk. Treats tender breasts in children.
- Helps when there is suppressed milk, inflamed breast after anger or rage.
- Antidotes the effects of coffee on the body, or in the breast milk.

Chasteberry***—Vitex angus castus
- Rebalances progesterone-to-estrogen ratio (or excess of estrogen).
- Particularly for cyclic breast tenderness or hormonally responsive cysts.
- Must be used over several months for maximum effectiveness.

Cleavers**—Galium aparine
- Used mostly to treat enlarged lymph glands of a soft and pliable nature.
- Specific for swellings and growths resulting from blocked lymph channels and toxin build-up. One of the safest and gentlest lymph cleansers.

Dong Quai**—Angelica sinensis
- Decreases breast tenderness, clears stagnation and congested tissue.
- Improves and balances liver functioning and hormonal metabolism.
- Regulates the hormonal cycle; especially good for PMS symptom relief.

Pipsissewa**—Chimaphila umbellata
- For retracted nipple, breast ulcers or atrophy; breast problems in sexually inactive women. Effective for tumors, cysts in large-breasted women.
- A mild lymphatic stimulant, gentle diuretic and tissue detoxifier.

Poke Root***—Phytolacca decandra
- Taken internally and applied to breasts and nipples in mastitis.
- Help swollen breast tissue, hard glands in neck, underarm or groin.
- For sore, cracked or inverted nipples, premenstrual or nursing pain.
- Lymphatic cleanser, to clear abscess, infection, toxin accumulation.

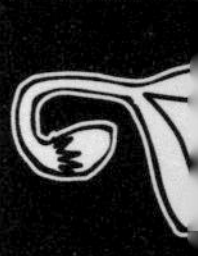

Queen's Delight**—Stillingia sylvatica
- Fresh poultice or internal/external tincture is alterative and detoxifier.
- Clears congestion of lymphatic vessels, swollen lymph glands, stimulates white blood cells to respond to infection. Mild anti-inflammatory.

Red Root**—Ceanothus americanus
- Specific action for breast pain and for decreasing size of cysts.
- Drains lymph fluid from congested areas and in chronic illnesses.
- Astringent that helps dry and clear fluids from cysts, tumors, growths.

Saw Palmetto**—Seronoa repens
- Anti-inflammatory effects for swollen, tender breast tissue.
- Hormone regulator, reduces build-up of male hormones in the tissues.
- Can help increase breast size if underdeveloped, especially at puberty.

BURNS

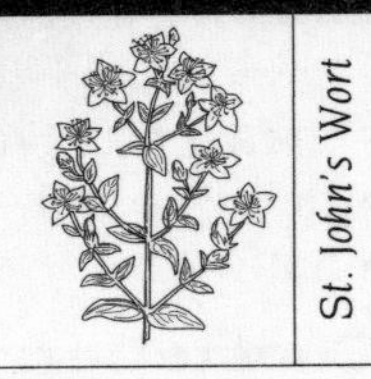

Select the herbs that are most suitable for your condition.

The Herbal Approach

Whether through fire, hot air, hot surfaces, steam, scalding water, electricity or chemicals, the effects of burns or thermal injuries are the same. Skin protein becomes coagulated or even carbonized, releasing many toxic by-products into the tissues and setting up an inflammatory response. *First degree burns* have redness, intense heat, pain and swelling, while *second degree burns* produce blisters and may ooze fluids from the skin. *Third degree burns* happen when the skin is charred into its deeper layers. Second and third degree burns, chemical burns or whole body first degree burns require emergency medical care.

Herbs for burns are usually prescribed externally and have the ability to provide soothing pain relief, prevent infection and stimulate tissue healing. Apart from obvious anti-inflammatory effects, many of these herbs can reduce skin damage and minimize the tendency toward scarring. *Do not* use butter, oils, creams or gels, since they keep the heat in the tissues. *Calendula* and *hypericum* tincture, used singly or mixed in equal parts, can be diluted with water in a ratio of approximately 1:5 and applied hourly or more often. Follow-up treatment may require herbs to clear toxins from the tissues and major detoxification organs and rebuild immunity. See also ■ Detoxification ■ Injury/Wounds ■ Immune Weakness.

Aloe***—Aloe vera/barbadensis
- Important for thermal injuries like sunburn; used on 2nd or 3rd degree burns; speeds tissue healing. Effective against staph, strep, candida.
- Anti-inflammatory, antiseptic, pain-relieving and anti-aging skin effects.
- Important for external use during radiation therapy.

Astragalus***—Milk Vetch/Astragalus membranaceous
- Used in China to speed the healing of burns. Bolsters immune function, especially if suppressed; prevents infection by viruses and bacteria.
- Increases skin circulation, facilitating removal of burn toxins and heat.

Calendula***—Marigold/Calendula officinalis
- Applied as a wash externally, gives immediate relief, prevents blisters.
- Prevents scarring. For chemical burns to eye, scalds to mouth, ulcers.
- Antiseptic action, preventing infection; speeds healing of tissues.

Chamomile**—Matricaria recutita
- A compress of strong tea applied to the skin speeds healing in burns.
- Prevents wound infections; antibacterial against staph organisms.
- Anti-inflammatory, decreases swelling as it soothes burned tissues.

Comfrey**—Symphytum officinale
- Used externally, accelerates tissue repair and cell growth. Can be applied as a poultice, cream, lotion, or as a diluted tincture or extract.
- Do not use where there is redness, puffiness or oozing.
- Important remedy for preventing scar formation in skin injuries.

Ginger**—Zingiber officinale
- The juice from the fresh rhizome helps first and second degree burns.
- Anti-inflammatory, inhibits bacterial growth and provides pain relief.
- Encourages skin circulation, relieving swollen tissues and carrying away waste products that accumulate at the site of thermal injury.

Gotu Kola***—Centella asiatica
- Used internally and as an external compress, helps burns heal faster.
- Lessens and optimizes scar tissue formation, prevents ulceration.
- Antiseptic that prevents infection, strengthens local blood vessels.

Lavender Oil**—Lavandula officinalis
- Stops pain of burns, promotes rapid healing of tissues, reduces pain.
- Antiseptic and antibacterial, helps prevent infection, stops spasms.
- Stimulates the superficial circulation to bring nutrients to the affected areas, while relieving the tissue of waste fluids. Not for internal use.

Peppermint**—Mentha piperta
- Provides relief from pain and burning through its analgesic effect.
- Volatile oils, like *menthol*, are antibacterial, antiseptic, and antifungal.
- Reduces subsequent hypersensitivity that may ensue as the burn heals.

Slippery Elm*—Ulmus fulva
- Forms a soothing paste or gel that protects and heals skin after burns.
- Traditionally used as a salve, poultice, or ointment for skin irritation.
- Soothing emollient that softens the skin and prevents chaffing.

St. John's Wort***—Hypericum perforatum
- Good externally for first and second degree burns, especially sunburn.
- Relieves nerve pain. Useful for radiation burns or tissue x-ray damage.
- Prevents blistering, stops infection, quickly soothing, speeds healing.

Tea Tree Oil**—Melaleuca alternifolia
- In burns/sunburn; use after applying ice packs, then several times daily.
- Excellent antiseptic oil for infected burns; well tolerated topically.
- Stimulates the immune system, as it heals burns and infected tissues.

Witch Hazel***—Hamamelis virginiana
- External anti-inflammatory, provides pain relief after burns, wounds.
- Excellent for first degree burns, scalds, burns of tongue, mouth or lips.
- Reduces scarring tendency. For burn injuries to the cornea or eye itself.
- Also very effective for associated bruising or stopping wound bleeding.

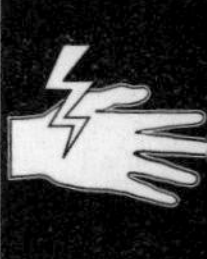

CANCER

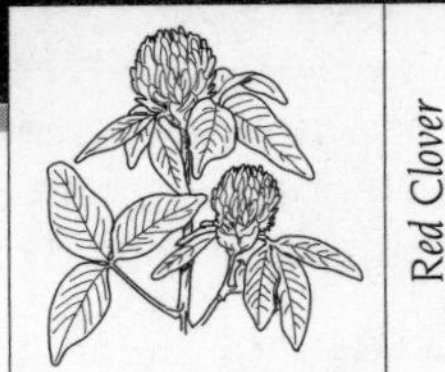

Select the herbs that are most suitable for your condition.

The Herbal Approach

Many traditional cancer remedies are adaptogenic herbs, plants that improve the body's healing capacities in a global way. Often they also function as immune stimulants and biological response modifiers (BRMs). Such herbs assist the intricate relationship between our response systems—the nervous and immune system—and various health stressors that damage or weaken the organism. The result is improvement in the body's ability to fight disease and maintain strength and vitality. These herbs also reduce uncomfortable and damaging side effects of cancer drugs, while increasing their effectiveness. Many of the herbs below also strengthen detoxification organs, like the liver and kidneys. These plants also provide very real protection against the development of various cancers, taken as an occasional course of treatment for a month or more, annually or semi-annually.

Actual or suspected cancer is obviously not suitable for "home treatment." Though the use of herbs as an adjunct to mainstream therapies, such as radiation, surgery or chemotherapy, is becoming more common, there is the potential for negative interactions with these treatments. Ideally, an herbal expert should be part of one's health team. Alternatively, one can provide their current doctor with information supporting the scientific use of these herbs and their possible interactions. Single or multiple herbs can then be combined as part of an individualized treatment program. See the Herbal Reading List for suggested information sources. See also ■ Detoxification ■ Drug Detox ■ Immune Weakness ■ Injury/Wounds (both before and after surgery) ■ Liver Conditions.

Astragalus***—Milk Vetch/Astragalus membranaceous

- Energy tonic, equivalent to ginseng, useful for exhaustion, wasting.
- Normalizes immune function, tones the liver, has diuretic action.
- Increases numerous cancer-fighting immune cells and chemicals.
- Patients recover faster and live longer after radiation or chemotherapy, showing better bone marrow and immune system recovery.

Black Cumin**—Nigella sativa

- Studies show the seed extract, a traditional cancer remedy, to be toxic to cancer and tumor cells, including those resistant to anti-cancer drugs.
- Stimulates immunity and reduces toxic effects of cancer drugs on liver.

Cat's Claw*—Uncaria tormentosa

- Strengthens weakened cancer patients after chemotherapy or radiation.

- May decrease spread of cancer; most claims not yet verified.

Celandine***—Chelidonium majus
- Traditional cancer cure, a powerful liver detoxifier and antibiotic.
- Used in an anti-cancer drug called Ukrain, which shows good immune stimulation as well as destruction and shrinkage of cancer tissue.

Chaparral**—Larrea tridentata
- A powerful antioxidant that has, clinically, cured cancers and shrank tumors. Scientifically, it remains controversial for cancer treatment.
- Antibiotic and anti-inflammatory: kills bacteria, viruses, parasites.
- Also used for colds, flu, cystitis, diarrhea, as well as eczema, acne.
- Excess or prolonged use purported to cause liver damage or hepatitis.

Curcumin***—Turmeric/Curcuma longa
- Prevents and reduces cancer growth in mouth, stomach, duodenum, colon.
- Inhibits growth and promotes death of cancer cells in breast cancer.
- Inhibits growth of various lymphomas, including virus-induced types.
- Antioxidant and free radical activity prevents cancer if used daily.

Garlic***—Allium sativa
- Cancer-preventive effects shown with just one ounce of garlic a week.
- Neutralizes carcinogens and prevents DNA damage, inhibiting stomach, colon, breast, prostate, esophagus, liver, lung and brain cancers.
- Reduces side effects of cancer treatment and the potential of liver damage; protects from radiation. Reduces tumor growth in animal studies.

Ginseng**—Panax ginseng
- Adaptogenic and immune-modulating herb, increases overall vitality.
- Boosts many immune cells, including tumor-destroyed killer T cells,
- Increases various cancer-fighting chemicals, like interleukin-2.
- Caution: increases platelets, may cause bleeding during chemotherapy.

Goldenseal***—Hydrastis canadensis
- Powerful antibacterial and antifungal herb that strengthens and powerfully detoxifies the liver. Heals ulcerated tissue, stops bleeding.
- Traditional use in cancer of various mucus membranes; lips, throat, stomach, liver cancer, lung cancer. Traditionally for breast cancer.
- Counters the wasting (cachexia) of cancer; helps maintain vitality.

Green Tea***—Camellia sinensis
- While known to be a cancer preventive, also inhibits spread of cancer.
- Enhances effects of chemo in shrinking tumors; yet decreases toxicity.
- Specific protection against colon and rectal cancers (use decaf forms).

Maitake***—Grifola frondosa
- Immune stimulant; aids destruction of cancer cells in blood, lymph; inhibits spread and growth of tumor cells (up to 70%), protects healthy cells.

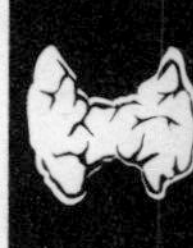

- Works on cancers of lung, liver, breast, ovary, uterus, some leukemia.
- Combines well with and augments chemo, radiation; reduces side effects of vomiting, appetite loss, white blood cell deficiency.
- Highest anti-tumor effect of any mushroom and most easily absorbed.

Mistletoe***—Viscum album
- Stabilizes DNA, is toxic to cancer cells and stops growth of new blood vessels to tumors. May increase survival of cancer patients.
- Increases white blood cell production; offsets cancer drug side-effects.
- Injectable form needed; only available through health care providers.

Noni*—Morinda citrifolia
- May reduce toxicity of chemotherapy and increase its effectiveness.
- Shown to stimulate immune system, but many unsubstantiated claims.

Pau D'Arco**—LaPacho/Tabebuia avellanedae
- Antioxidant and immune-stimulating, fights bacteria, fungi, parasites.
- Some anti-cancer activity, but curative effects yet to be substantiated.

Poke Root**—Phytolacca decandra
- Lymphatic cleanser, rids the body of infection and toxin accumulation.
- Traditionally for swollen nodes, benign and cancerous breast tumors.

Red Clover***—Trifolium pratense
- Laboratory effects against leukemia, breast, colon and prostate cancers.
- Only plant with all 4 isoflavones (plant estrogens); 10 times that of soy.
- Estrogen-balancing and cancer-preventing effects, even in melanoma.

Reishi***—Ganoderma lucidum
- An ancient longevity tonic; now an official cancer-treating herb in Japan.
- Increases immunity in a variety of ways; improves T cells, interleukin 2 production, protects against radiation and free radical damage.
- Antiviral, anti-inflammatory; improves the liver, increases endurance.
- Success has been shown in stomach, breast, lung and stomach cancers.

Rosemary*—Rosmarinus officinalis
- Potent antioxidant, effective against a wide range of carcinogens.
- Shown to protect against development of various cancers and tumors.
- Detoxifies the liver, increases enzymes that protect against cancer.

Shiitake**—Lentinus edodes
- Increases immune function, helps shrink existing tumors. Used in Japan as an adjunct to chemotherapy, improving its effectiveness. antiviral.
- Increases cancer survival times and outcomes. Increases interferon.

For an excellent overview of Essiac, Hoxsey, *and other historical and current herbal cancer formulas, consult* Ralph Moss's Herbs Against Cancer, *listed in the* Herbal Reading List *at the end of this book.*

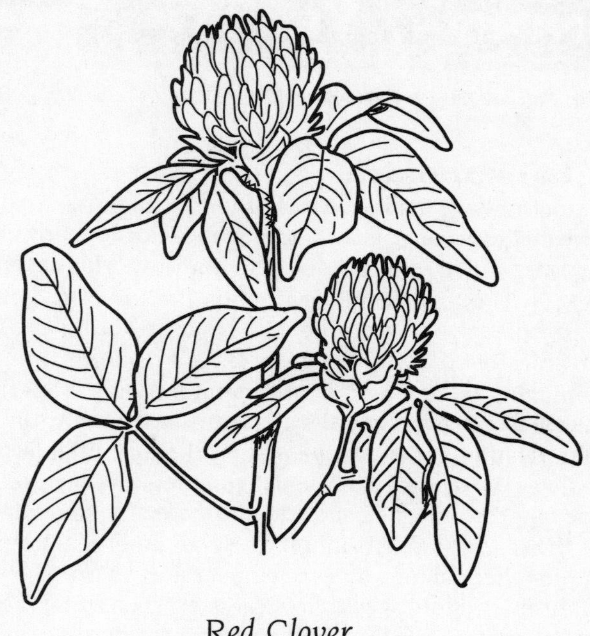

Red Clover

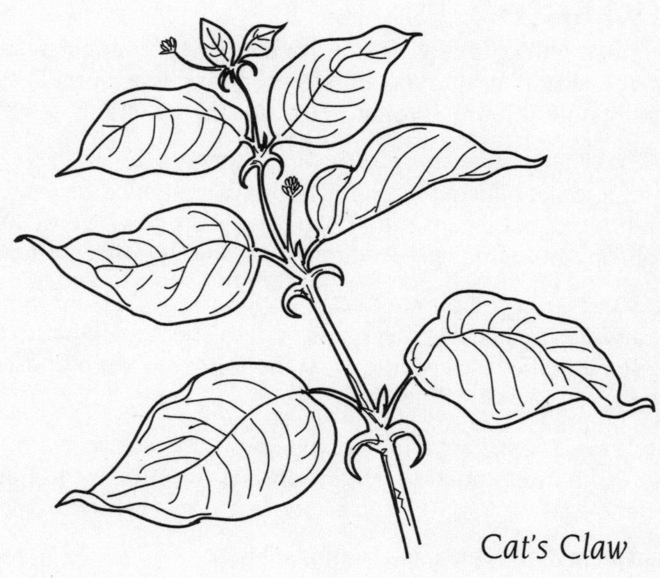

Cat's Claw

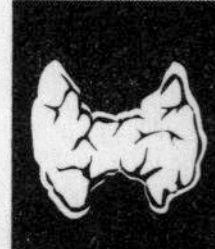

CANDIDA / YEAST

Tea Tree

Select the herbs that are most suitable for your condition.

The Herbal Approach

Systemic infection with candida and other strains of yeast is epidemic today and is an underlying factor in many chronic conditions (e.g. migraines, colitis, obesity, fibromyalgia, chronic fatigue, sinusitis, PMS). This is a result of immune failure and contributes to immunity's progressive weakening. Other contributing causes include antibiotics, which destroy protective intestinal bacteria, and a variety of immune-damaging factors and environmental toxins. Sugar and carbohydrate excess, or estrogen imbalance (hormone therapy, the pill, PMS), sweetens the tissues, creating a yeast breeding ground. Food allergies and a toxic digestive system (dysbiosis) complete the picture.

Antifungal herbs must be used and alternated for some time. An integral part of treatment is yeast die-off or Herxheimer reaction, which can produce fatigue, headaches, digestive upset and so on. The side effects can be minimized by starting with low dosages, increasing gradually, and helping detoxification. A low-carb, high-protein diet, digestive enzymes, liver detoxification and immune-strengthening herbs are essential. See also ■ Detoxification ■ Fatigue ■ Immune Weakness ■ Infection.

Black Walnut**—Juglans nigra
- Unripe, green hulls contain juglone, an effective antifungal agent.
- Assists with systemic candida, athlete's foot and ring worm infections.
- Also inhibits other fungi, cryptococcus, salmonella, staph, E. coli.

Cat's Claw***—Una de gato/Uncaria tormentosa
- Has antimicrobial effects for fungi, viruses, bacteria, parasites.
- Important intestinal cleanser for dysbiosis, leaky gut, diverticulitis, colitis, Crohn's. Anti-aging, anti-inflammatory, immune strengthening.

Celandine*—Chelidonium majus
- Treats candida effectively; powerful liver detoxifier and hepatic strengthener; helps in removal of candida metabolites from the bloodstream.

Garlic***—Allium sativa
- Contains several antifungal ingredients; rapidly destroys yeast.
- Stimulates immune function. Highly antiseptic, effective in infections, and is beneficial for long-term use against chronic candida syndromes.

Goldenseal***—Hydrastis canadensis
- Strong antifungal effects, while healing intestinal mucus linings.
- Strengthens and detoxifies the liver; immune and white cell stimulant.

Grapefruit Seed Extract***—Citrus paradisi
- A powerful, non-toxic antifungal and yeast killer, used internally for systemic infection and externally for mouth, skin and vaginal yeast.
- Use in capsules or as a liquid gargle, as a douche, or as a suppository.

Holy Basil**—Ocimum sanctum
- Traditional Ayurvedic herb for chronic yeast infection.
- Anti-inflammatory, anti-ulcer and anti-cancer herb.
- An adaptogen that improves immunity and revitalizes the body.

Larix**—Larch/Larix decidua
- Contains chemicals also found in echinacea, astragalus, shiitake.
- Immune stimulation to combat the candida infection systemically.
- Treats respiratory and urinary tract infections, psoriasis, eczema.

Maitake*—Grifola frondosa
- Increases immune and white cell function, interleukin, T cells, killer cells.
- Helps protect immune system from effects of toxic substances.
- Adaptogen, improving response to stress. Anti-tumor and antiviral.

Olive Leaf***—Olea europaea
- Broad-spectrum antimicrobial against viruses, bacteria, yeasts, fungi.
- Inactivates and eradicates candida and yeast, locally and system wide.
- Immune-boosting effects, promotes removal of toxic cellular wastes.

Oregano Oil**—Origanum vulgare
- Strong antiseptic, effective as an anti-candida herb, taken in capsules.
- Shown to inhibit *Candida albicans* to a greater extent than caprylic acid.

Pau D'Arco**—LaPacho/Tabebuia avellanedae
- A popular anti-yeast herb with broad spectrum antimicrobial effects.
- Rebuilds immune system, while undergoing candida treatment.

Spilanthes*—Spilanthes oleracea
- Used to heighten the response capability of the immune system.
- Antifungal, antibacterial, antiviral; reduces inflamed throat, mouth.
- Increases resistance to infections, colds and flus, similar to echinacea.

Tea Tree Oil***—Melaleuca alternifolia
- Internally, destroys fungi, viruses, bacteria (even antibiotic resistant).
- Externally, used for fungal or candida infections such as athlete's foot, toenail fungal infections, vaginitis and ring worm.

Usnea**—Lichen/Usnea species
- A lichen capable of destroying systemic candida and bacterial infection.
- Applied externally, also effective for ringworm, athlete's foot.
- Used for respiratory infections, colds or flus, or to enhance immunity.

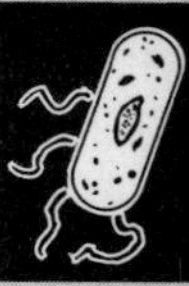

CHILDBIRTH

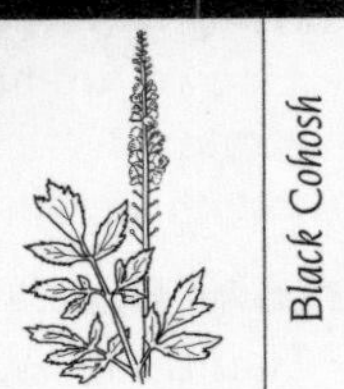

Select the herbs that are most suitable for your condition.

The Herbal Approach

The process of childbirth involves a coordinated action between the uterus and secretions from the pituitary that stimulate the onset of labor. There are many complications possible in childbirth. Yet the institutionalization of childbirth and soaring number of cesarean sections (accounting for about 25% of all births) may not be justified. Whether one opts for a home birth assisted by a qualified midwife, a conventional hospital birth, or something in between, herbs are an important aid. In fact, one of the oldest traditions of herbal medicine is the knowledge known and applied by the female elders who assisted at births in every time and culture throughout history. This same valuable information, refined and tested, is available and effective today.

Specific herbs can help when uterine contractions are either inadequate or too severe. When the opening of the uterus, the os, does not dilate adequately, other herbs are capable of promoting this phase of labor. Additionally, there are herbs that can help stop excess bleeding, both during and after childbirth. Recuperation after pregnancy is helped by herbs that tone the uterus, like *Mother's Cordial* (see page 96), while adaptogens and tonics can rebalance hormones and help overcome fatigue. The use of alcoholic tinctures should be avoided during pregnancy, and all herbs should first be checked for their suitability (i.e. see the Dosage section or consult with a health professional). See also ■ Bleeding ■ Colic/Cramps ■ Dysmenorrhea ■ Fatigue ■ Injury/Wounds.

Black Cohosh***—Cimicifuga racemosa
- Increases and normalizes irregular uterine contractions during labor.
- Used when os fails to dilate, with sharp pains and radiating cramps.
- Relieves after-pains and prevents postpartum hemorrhage.
- Relieves nervousness experienced during labor and prior to delivery.

Black Haw***—Viburnum prunifolium
- Relieves pain of labor and childbirth. Prevents premature contractions.
- Reduces bleeding during and after birth. Prevents miscarriage, morning sickness. Restores tone to the uterus after birth, prevents prolapse.

Blue Cohosh***—Caulophyllum thalictroides
- Strengthens labor when weak, too painful or not proceeding regularly.
- Regulates contractions when erratic, intermittent. Helps when cervix fails to dilate. Good for prolonged or difficult labor, with exhaustion.
- Indicated when pains are too low in the pelvis, with nervousness.

Chamomile—Matricaria recutita
- A tea prior to delivery is a gentle nerve/muscle relaxant, pain reliever.
- Antiseptic, speeds wound healing. A compress or salve applied over the perineum after birth relieves tenderness and lessens chance of infection.

Feverfew*—Tanacetum parthenium
- Traditionally given after birth to help expel the placenta.
- Used since the Roman times during birth and also to strengthen uterus.

Motherwort**—Leonarus cardiaca
- Encourages and eases uterine contractions during labor.
- A uterus stimulant, useful to relieve false contractions.
- Useful during labor to soothe nerves, anxiety, and heart symptoms.

Partridge Berry*—Mitchella repens
- Used in last weeks of pregnancy to prepare uterus and organism for childbirth. Used to decrease or prevent postpartum hemorrhage.
- Helps prevent hemorrhage, relieves excess cramps. Tonic and diuretic.
- Increases uterine tone and promotes easier childbirth.

Raspberry Leaf**—Rubus idaeus
- Taken throughout or during late pregnancy and childbirth. Effective as a uterine stimulant.
- The astringent action helps to prevent postpartum hemorrhaging.
- Do not take this herb with a history of intense labor or miscarriage.

Shepherd's Purse***—Thlaspi bursa pastoris
- Stimulates an atonic uterus to contract after childbirth to reduce postpartum bleeding. Stops both internal and external hemorrhage.
- Due to its stimulant properties, do not use during pregnancy.

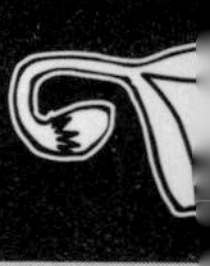

Trillium**—Birthroot/Trillium pendulatum or erectum
- Use prior to labor to decrease severity of possible hemorrhage and facilitate contractions, increasing their efficiency.
- Relieves intense cramping when hips and back feel as if broken.

Vervain**—Verbena officinalis
- Can be taken during labor for increasing contractions.
- A uterine stimulant; strengthens uterine contractions during labor.
- Nervine and tonic, relaxes the nervous system, eases tension, depression and exhaustion. Improves the flow of milk and assists in recovery.

CHOLESTEROL, HIGH

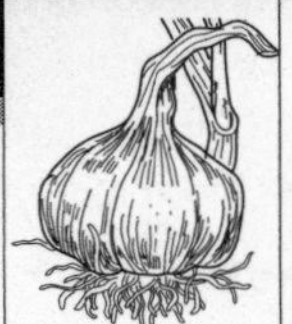

Select the herbs that are most suitable for your condition.

The Herbal Approach

Consumers are subject to a tremendous amount of misinformation regarding cholesterol. Simply, 80% of cholesterol is manufactured by the liver—only 20% is from the diet. From a food perspective, the greatest source of increased cholesterol is a high-sugar and refined-carbohydrate diet. The type of fats we consume is also generally at fault, since our diets are very deficient in essential fatty acids and high in trans-fatty acids. Further, a disordered liver metabolism is also responsible for disturbances in cholesterol. Vegetable fiber, as found in psyllium, oat bran and apple pectin, are all cholesterol-lowering agents. While cholesterol readings of 240 are high, those below 180 are considered too low for health.

Medicinally, several herbs have been shown to be far more effective than mainstream cholesterol-lowering drugs—and far safer. It is also a scientific fact that no cholesterol-lowering drug has ever been shown to lower overall mortality! They also create a deficiency in the heart's most important nutrient—CoQ10. Herbs also change the ratio of good (high density or HDL) to bad (low density or LDL) cholesterol. They can also work to correct a disordered liver and fat metabolism. Many of the plants listed below also provide antioxidant protection for blood vessel walls. See also ■ Arteriosclerosis ■ Heart Conditions ■ Liver Conditions.

Alfalfa**—Medicago sativa
- Blocks the absorption of cholesterol and prevents the formation of atherosclerotic plaques. Traditional tonic, improves digestion/absorption.
- Nourishing herb, rich in iron, protein, B6, K and detoxifying chlorophyll.

Artichoke**—Cynara scolymus
- Lowers LDL or "bad" cholesterol, increases HDL or "good" cholesterol.
- Reduces triglycerides, total serum cholesterol. A natural diuretic.
- Increases bile flow and liver function; used in treatment of cirrhosis.

Curcumin**—Turmeric/Curcumin longa
- Improves blood flow in arteries, while strengthening blood vessels.
- Reduces "bad" cholesterol, platelet stickiness and blood clot formation.
- Prevents free radical damage in arteries that leads to arteriosclerosis.

Fenugreek**—Trigonella foenumgraecum
- Inhibits cholesterol absorption and decreases its manufacture by liver.
- Contains a high amount of fiber; serving as a stool-softening agent.
- Lowers elevated triglycerides and lowers blood sugar in pre-diabetes.

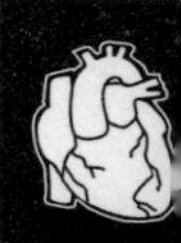

Fo-Ti**—Polygonum multiflorum
- Lowers cholesterol and reduces hardening of the arteries.
- Traditional longevity herb, heightens immunity, while energizing and tonifying the entire body. Improves impotence and infertility.

Garlic***—Allium sativum
- Shown to lower LDL cholesterol, while increasing HDL cholesterol.
- Studies show a reduction of 12% cholesterol and 15% triglycerides.
- Lowers high blood pressure, reduces blood platelet agglutination.
- Prevents oxidation of LDL cholesterol and build-up of arterial plaque.

Ginger***—Zingiber officinale
- Reduces cholesterol, lowers blood pressure, thins the blood.
- Strengthens the heart, reduces inflammation tendency, thus protecting the arteries and heart. antibacterial, antiviral, improves circulation.

Green Tea**—Camellia sinensis
- Inhibits cholesterol and increases excretion of this and other lipids
- Inhibits the enzyme that promotes blood vessel constriction.
- Polyphenols prevent arterial damage, fight cancer, regulate blood sugar.

Guggul***—Commiphora mukul
- Lowers cholesterol and triglycerides up to 30%, reduces LDL by 35% and increases HDL by 20% in 12 weeks. Prevents arteriosclerosis.
- Performs better than cholesterol-lowering drugs in several studies.
- Decreases platelet stickiness, reduces risk of heart disease and stroke.
- Stimulates thyroid, while removing excess uric acid. Reduces obesity.

Maitake**—Grifola frondosa
- Lowers cholesterol, regulates blood sugar, blood pressure and body weight. Powerful immune-strengthening and antiviral capabilities.
- A powerful adaptogen and tonic herb with overall anti-aging effects.

Olive Leaf**—Oleo europaea
- Prevents oxidation of cholesterol and formation of arteriosclerosis.
- Decreases high blood pressure, increases coronary blood flow.
- Effective against a wide range of viruses, bacteria, fungi, parasites.

Red Rice Yeast***—Monascus purpureus
- A traditional Asian medicine, lowers cholesterol, improves circulation, strengthens the heart. Inhibits liver enzymes that produce cholesterol.
- Contains chemicals found in the drugs Mevacor/Lovastatin, but safer.

Reishi***—Ganoderma lucidum
- Strengthens the heart; lowers total serum cholesterol and raises HDL, reduces platelet stickiness, prevents blood clots. Improves liver health.
- An adaptogen; relieves fatigue, enhances immunity; anti-inflammatory.
- Improves digestion, aids depression, insomnia and anxiety; antiviral.

COLDS & FLU

Yarrow

Select the herbs that are most suitable for your condition.

The Herbal Approach

The treatment of colds and flu provides a vivid contrast between different approaches to health and illness. During the time of Pasteur, the debate raged about the nature of infection. He maintained that the seed (bacteria) was the most important, while his adversary, Bechamp, insisted that the soil (the immune system and host resistance) was crucial. Today's medicine, based on Pasteur, has only half the answer.

Herbs work with both ends of the spectrum. Many have powerful antiviral and antibacterial effects, but mere suppression of symptoms can weaken the immune and nervous systems. Botanical medicines also stimulate, augment and strengthen disease resistance in dozens of ways. Traditionally, plant medicines have been relied upon to reduce fever (febrifuge herbs) and clear mucus (decongestant or expectorant herbs). Other herbs are used to treat specific sinus, throat or chest complaints. Of the many traditional cold formulas, the most famous is the trio of *peppermint, elderflower* and *yarrow*. From such plants, one can expect a shorter duration of a cold or flu, and less likelihood of recurrence or lingering symptoms. Using immune-strengthening herbs, one can naturally reduce the frequency of nasty colds or flu. See also ■ Cough ■ Ear Infections ■ Hay Fever/Allergy ■ Immune Weakness ■ Sinusitis ■ Sore Throat.

Andrographis***—Kalmegh/Andrographis paniculata
- Traditional Ayurvedic herb, rapidly relieves symptoms of nasal congestion, cough, sore throat, sinusitis, muscle soreness, cough and fever.
- Reduces recovery time by half, with five times less time lost from work.

Astragalus**—Milk Vetch/Astragalus membranaceous
- Boosts the immune system, increases T cells, protects against viruses.
- Protects the heart from viral infection (i.e. cocksackie-B virus).
- Reduces duration and frequency of colds if taken prior to the season.

Boneset**—Eupatorium perfoliatum
- Helps with colds, flu and fever. Loosens phlegm and encourages coughing, enhances immune resistance to viruses and bacterial infection.
- Promotes perspiration, alleviates nausea and deep muscle aching.

Cayenne**—Capsicum frutescens
- Taken at the first hint of a cold or fever to reduce the severity of illness.
- Promotes sweat in colds, flu, bronchitis. Increases warmth, circulation.
- A warming, stimulating, vasodilator herb for external or internal use.
- Also acts as a digestive stimulant, pain reliever and antiseptic.

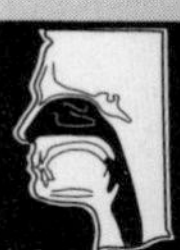

Catnip**—Nepeta cataria
- Soothing and relaxing herb for colds, flu, fevers; promotes sweating.
- A mild sedative, very useful for children. Antispasmodic in bronchitis.
- Helps intestinal flu with gas, indigestion, diarrhea, cramps and colic.

Chamomile**—Matricaria recutita
- Good for colds, flu and fever; promotes intense perspiration.
- Sedative that relieves pain, associated cramps, colic, calms irritability.
- Child needing it is hot, very thirsty, with alternate chills and fevers.

Echinacea***—Echinacea angustifolia
- Relieves acute colds, flu, fever and infection—over 350 studies done!
- Best taken in early stages; can be used as a preventive after exposure.
- Reduces duration of cold, risk of bronchitis; destroys infectious cells.
- Stimulates the immune system, increases interferon, T cells, white cells.

Elder***—Sambucus nigra
- Has antiviral properties; prevents viruses from invading healthy cells.
- Reduces fever, muscle ache, cough; speeds recovery, promotes sweats.
- Excellent gargle for sore throat. Contains antioxidant flavonoids.
- Part of a traditional cold formula: peppermint, yarrow, elderblossoms.

Eucalyptus**—Eucalyptus globulus
- Disinfects and decongests stuffy, blocked nasal passages and sinuses.
- Helps soothe throat irritation and coughs. Not for internal use.
- Used as an inhalation or rubbed topically for chest and lung ailments.

Eyebright**—Euphrasia officinalis
- Indicated for colds, flu or allergy with hot, acrid discharges from the eye, clear nasal discharge, light sensitivity and eye inflammation.
- Use sparingly with dry or blocked sinuses with no or little discharge.

Garlic**—Allium sativus
- Natural antibiotic properties: effective for many types of respiratory infections, including colds, flu, bronchitis as well as ear infections.
- Effective against a wide spectrum of bacteria, viruses, fungi, strep.

Ginger***—Zingiber officinale
- Active against a wide range of bacteria (staph, strep) and viruses.
- Produces sweating, lowers fever; cooling and anti-inflammatory.
- Powerful anti-cough effect, antihistamine; thins and expels mucus.
- Calms intestinal flu, effectively reducing nausea, inflammation.

Goldenseal**—Hydrastis canadensis
- In late stages, with development of yellow mucus, dries up secretions.
- Strong antibacterial and antiviral action; even effective against strep.
- Heals lining of the sinus, respiratory passages, throat; relieves cough.

Ground Ivy**—Glechoma hederacea
- Reduces fever in colds and flu. An astringent, decongestant herb for drying excess mucus in the throat, nose, ear, sinuses or bronchi.

Lomatium**—Lomatium dissectum
- Immune herb with antiviral, antibacterial and antifungal properties.
- Has a wide range of therapeutic action for various stages of cold or flu.
- Excellent for stubborn, chronic respiratory or urinary tract infections.

Meadowsweet**—Filipendula ulmaria
- Contains aspirin-like compounds that offer pain relief, fever reduction.
- Safe for children, soothes digestion, lowers stomach acidity.

Peppermint***—Mentha piperta
- Inhaling the essential oils, using tea or menthol relieves stuffed nose, sinus and chest congestion. Antispasmodic for coughs or easing colic.
- Induces sweating to "break a fever" in common cold or flu conditions.

Siberian Ginseng**—Eleuthrococcus senticosus
- Siberian Ginseng increases resistance to influenza. Helps increase resistance to physical stresses such as cold, heat, exhaustion, overwork.
- Excellent tonic for convalescence, weakness after illness.

St. John's Wort**—Hypericum perforatum
- Powerful broad spectrum antiviral activity for colds and influenza.
- Antibacterial, antifungal and anti-inflammatory. Contains potent immune-stimulating flavonoids. Relieves depression after flu or cold.

Wild Indigo**—Baptisia tinctoria
- An antiseptic, antibacterial herb, deeply stimulates immune function.
- Traditional use in sore throats, tonsillitis, flu and respiratory infections.
- Lowers fever, reduces swollen lymph glands in highly toxic, debilitated states. Indicated where there are foul secretions, exhaustion, aching.

Yarrow***—Achillea millefolium
- Reduces fever, promotes perspiration, often in conjunction with elderflower and peppermint. Also useful in allergies and hayfevers.
- Anti-inflammatory and a mild pain reliever for achiness of flus.

COLD & FLU HERBS

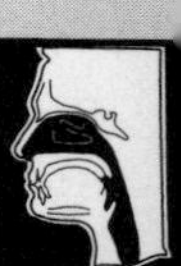

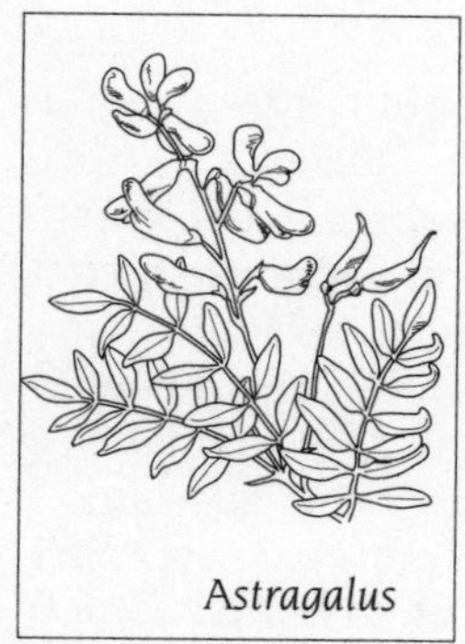
Astragalus

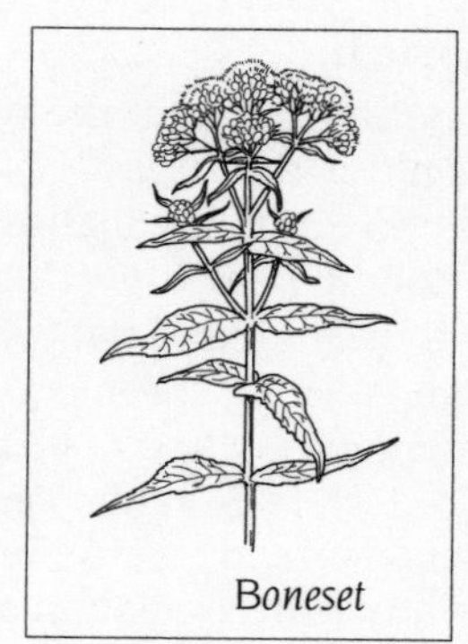
Boneset

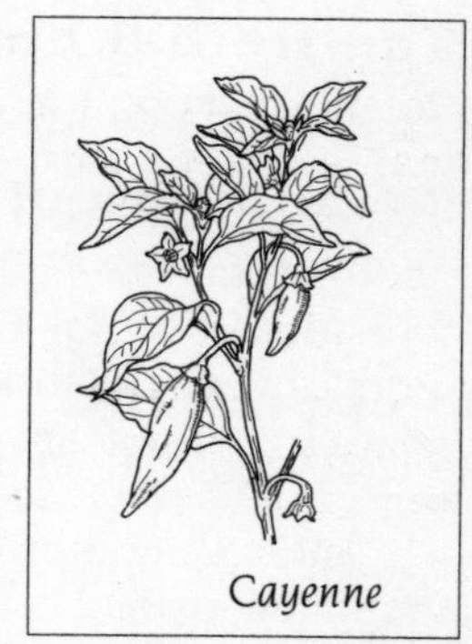
Cayenne

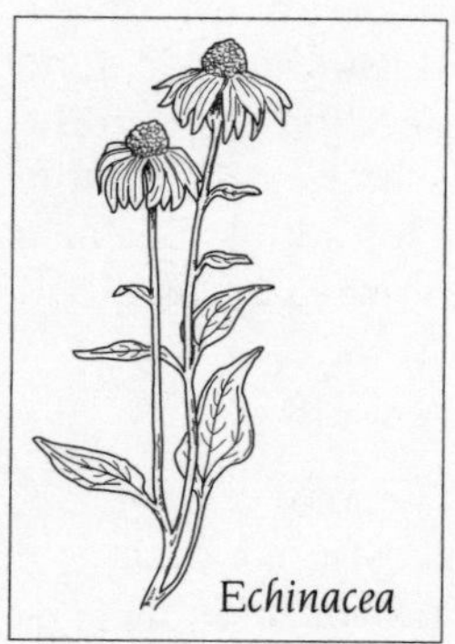
Echinacea

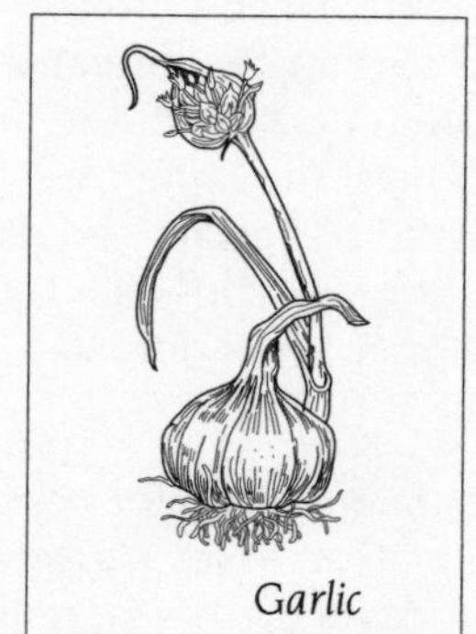
Garlic

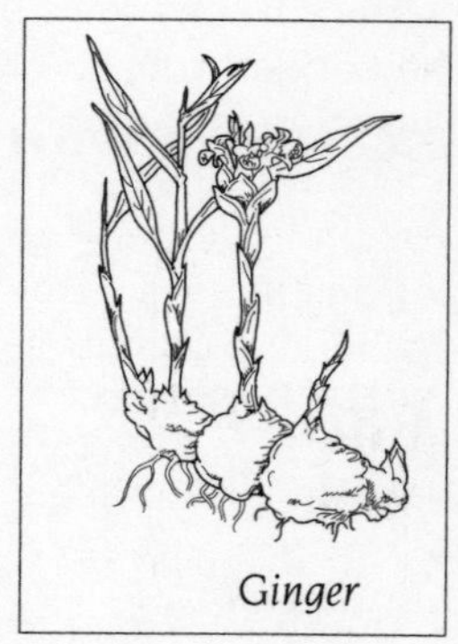
Ginger

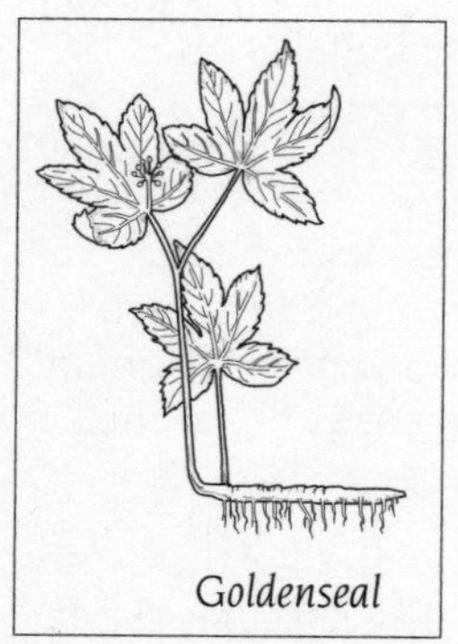
Goldenseal

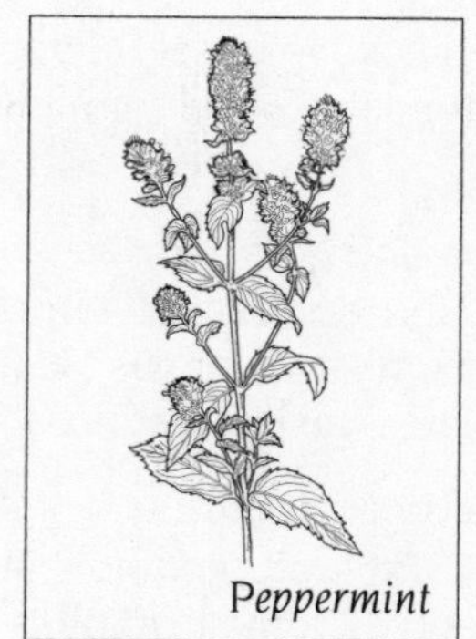
Peppermint

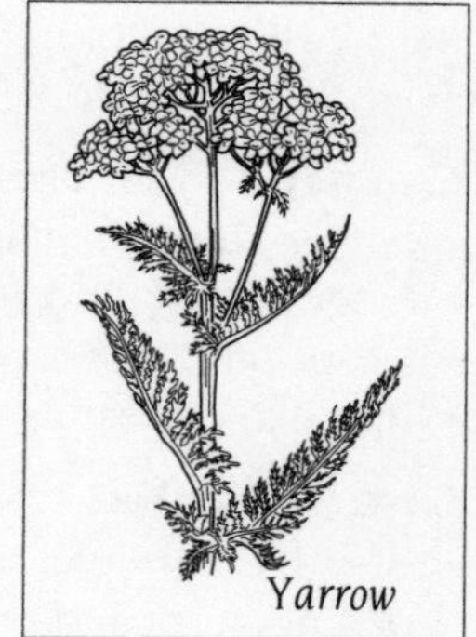
Yarrow

COLIC / CRAMPS

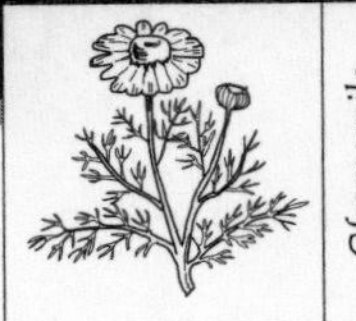

Select the herbs that are most suitable for your condition.

The Herbal Approach

Cramps can occur in any hollow organ of the body, but here we are primarily dealing with spasms in the digestive tract. Causes are many, including indigestion, infection or inflammation anywhere in the intestinal tract. Infantile colic, due to weak digestion, food allergies and gas formation, is a trial for both mother and baby. In adults, a variety of irritants can cause acute cramps, while chronic gut toxicity causes cramps relating to dysbiosis, irritable bowel and colitis. In all cases, underlying causes need to be addressed while painful spasms are being alleviated.

Antispasmodic herbs can provide a simple and non-toxic approach to calming painful cramps and colic. Such herbs are often *nervines* as well, providing sedative and calming effects for jangled nerves. Other needed herbs are also *carminatives*, helping expel excess gas, and *digestive tonics* with anti-inflammatory effects. Deeper problems can be improved with herbal detoxification programs for the intestines and liver. In colic, food allergies in the baby, or in a mother who is breastfeeding, need to be identified and eliminated, until the immune system can be re-regulated to eliminate these sensitivities. The same holds true for adults. See also ▪ Constipation ▪ Detoxification ▪ Diarrhea ▪ Dysmenorrhea ▪ Gas/Bloating ▪ Liver Conditions ▪ Stomach Conditions.

Anise***—Pimpinella anisum
- An important infant and child remedy for colic and general cramping.
- Antispasmodic and carminative, eases nausea, indigestion, bloating.
- Safe, gentle, tasty; can work via the breast milk. Improves appetite.

Caraway**—Carum carvi
- Similar to fennel and anise, relieves intestinal colic or cramps associated with gas, bloating, digestive upset, nausea and indigestion.
- Gentle enough for children, also good for menstrual cramping.

Catnip***—Nepeta cataria
- Relieves intestinal spasm and gas, diarrhea; mild relaxing effect.
- Relieves upset stomach, indigestion. Safe in children and the elderly.
- Is especially effective for intestinal or gastric upset of a nervous origin.
- Gentle and calming; sedates anxiety, reduces fever, eases headaches.

Chamomile***—Matricaria recutita
- Effective antispasmodic and colic remedy, soothes indigestion; anti-inflammatory and antiseptic. Calms irritability, restlessness, insomnia.
- Antidotes effects on nursing child of coffee or drug use by mother.

Cramp Bark***—Viburnum opulus

- Stronger antispasmodic than black haw; relieves painful cramping in abdomen, stomach, uterus or bladder. Relieves back pain, neuralgia.
- Effective for menstrual cramps, false labor pains. Helps with leg cramps.

Dill***—Anethum graveolens

- Relieves intestinal spasms, cramps, infantile colic and indigestion.
- Dispels gas and calms and improves the digestion; antibacterial action.
- Increases breast milk, which carries antispasmodic effects to the infant.

Fennel**—Foeniculum vulgare

- Stimulates digestion, relieves colic, flatulence, bloating and distension.
- Like anise and caraway, also used in coughs, as an antispasmodic and expectorant. Increases breast milk; has a reputation as a longevity herb.

Kava Kava**—Piper methysticum

- Muscle relaxant and antispasmodic for internal organs and muscle tension. Sedative pain and cramp reliever, reduces sensitivity to pain.
- Strongly reduces anxiety, relieves sleeplessness, is a mild antiseptic.

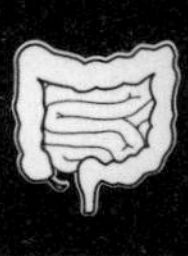

Lemon Balm**—Melissa officinalis

- Eases cramps and spasms, gas and bloating, indigestion and colic pains, gastric acidity. Useful for problems related to stress and anxiety.
- A good children's herb; soothes anxiety, irritability, restlessness.

Licorice**—Glycyrrhiza glabra

- Demulcent and anti-inflammatory, decreases the spasms of gastritis or intestinal distress, relieves stomach ulcers and body's stress response.
- Mild laxative, assists in the body's clearing of poorly digested foods.

Peppermint**—Mentha piperta

- Digestive antispasmodic; relieves colic, spasm, spastic constipation.
- Carminative, dispels gas and distention, with pain-relieving action.
- Stomachic, improves digestion, stimulates secretions and bile output.

Valerian**—Valeriana officinalis

- A sedative and antispasmodic, relaxing intestinal cramps, muscle tension. Relieves spasms and pain related to anxiety and emotional upset.
- For cramps with diarrhea, or after eating. Promotes restful sleep.

Wild Yam***—Dioscorea villosa

- Important antispasmodic for cramps in any hollow organ; intestines, stomach or gall bladder spasm. For colic that is relieved by stretching.
- Helps with gas and flatulence, belching, indigestion, upset from tea.

Yarrow*—Achillea millefolium

- A digestive antispasmodic, anti-inflammatory and pain reliever.
- For cramping pains or stomachache, distension, or gas pain.
- A sedative and tranquilizing herb that promotes tissue healing.

COLITIS/IBS

Select the herbs that are most suitable for your condition.

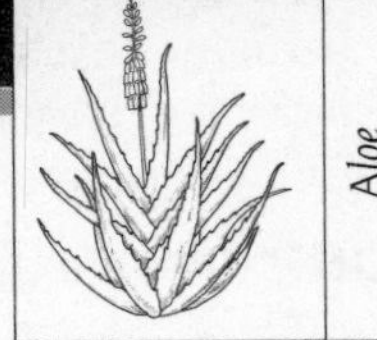

The Herbal Approach

The spectrum of intestinal illness ranges from spastic colitis or irritable bowel syndrome to far more serious inflammatory bowel disorders, such as Crohn's disease and ulcerative colitis. These chronic conditions affect over two million in the U.S., and can have an onset at an early age. The development of these illnesses begins with intestinal irritation from poorly digested and putrefying foods. The retention of toxic waste products, loss of normal intestinal flora and secondary infection forms a toxic soup called *dysbiosis*. As the intestines become inflamed, they allow toxic byproducts and partially digested foodstuffs to pass into the bloodstream, a condition known as "leaky gut syndrome." This sets the stage for the development of further food allergies, a toxic liver and a compromised immune system. The situation can progress into an autoimmune attack on one's own damaged intestinal cells. The vicious cycle continues.

For acute relief, anti-inflammatory, antispasmodic herbs often work far better than medical drugs, as referenced in the Bleeding and Inflammation section. Other plants treat underlying infection and dysbiosis. Herbs that improve the output of gastric and digestive enzymes are essential. As part of the healing process, the liver needs to be detoxified and the immune system strengthened. Using herbs and nutrients, removing food allergens and replacing bowel flora, these illnesses are actually curable. See also ■ Bleeding ■ Constipation ■ Diarrhea ■ Gas/Bloating ■ Immune Weakness ■ Inflammation ■ Infection ■ Liver Conditions.

Aloe***—Aloe vera/barbadensis
- Aloe gel soothes and promotes tissue healing in intestinal tract.
- Immune enhancing, antiviral, antibacterial and anti-inflammatory.
- Anti-inflammatory for Crohn's disease and irritable bowel syndrome.

Bayberry**—Myrica cerifera
- An astringent, deep-acting, antibacterial herb useful in treating colitis and irritable bowel syndrome. Effective for dysentery and bleeding.
- Astringent that tightens tissue and dries up excess mucus production.

Cat's Claw**—Uncaria tomentosa
- Effective for digestive inflammation and inflammatory bowel disease (IBS), including Crohn's disease, ulcerative colitis and diverticulitis.
- Helps ileocecal valve disorders, dysbiosis and leaky gut syndrome.
- Reduces diarrhea, chronic bleeding, stomach ulcers, hemorrhoids.

Chamomile**—Matricaria recutita
- For irritable bowel/colitis with alternating diarrhea and constipation.
- Reduces bloating, inflammation and spasm, while soothing the intestinal tract. Has antihistamine properties. Calms mental irritability.

Echinacea**—Echinacea angustifolia
- Antibacterial, antiviral, antifungal. Reduces intestinal dysbiosis.
- A strong immune stimulant for short-term, intense detoxification.

Goldenseal***—Hydrastis canadensis
- Anti-inflammatory, while healing lining tissue of the digestive system.
- Strong antimicrobial action against bacteria, parasites and candida.
- Aids digestion, promotes proper liver function, reduces bleeding.
- Useful in irritable bowel syndrome, colitis, gastritis, ulceration.

Myrrh**—Commiphora myrrha
- An astringent, antiseptic for intestinal disorders such as IBS, colitis and Crohn's disease. Useful to dry tissues with a excess mucus production.
- Ayurvedic medicine considered a blood cleanser and digestive remedy.

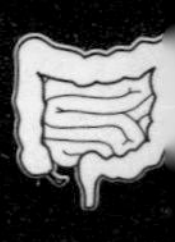

Olive Leaf***—Olea europaea
- Effective for dysbiosis; eliminates a wide range of organisms, including protozoa, viruses, fungi, bacteria, including antibiotic resistant ones.
- By clearing bacteria, reduces the immune burden. Antispasmodic.

Peppermint***—Mentha piperta
- Enteric-coated peppermint oil (preferable to tincture) reduces gas, relaxes cramping, gastroenteritis, soothes irritated intestinal linings.
- Antispasmodic, relieves nausea, irritable bowel. Not for use in infants.

Slippery Elm**—Ulmus fulva
- Soothing demulcent for irritation anywhere in the digestive tract.
- A highly absorbable, nutritional gruel that coats inflamed membranes.
- Use in IBS, Crohn's, constipation, diarrhea, hemorrhoids, diverticulitis.

Triphala***—Belleric, Chebulic and Emblic myrobalan
- Ayurvedic three-herb tonic that is anti-inflammatory and antiseptic.
- A soothing demulcent and gentle cleanser; regulates bowel, treats both constipation and diarrhea, tones the intestines, bowel and liver.

Valerian**—Valeriana officinalis
- Antispasmodic, eases intestinal cramps, bowel spasm, muscle tension.
- Relieves gas and bloating. Relaxes digestive upsets in nursing children caused by anger in the mother. Calms stress, anxiety, mood changes.
- Promotes relaxing sleep; helps with insomnia, twitching or tics.

CONSTIPATION

Select the herbs that are most suitable for your condition.

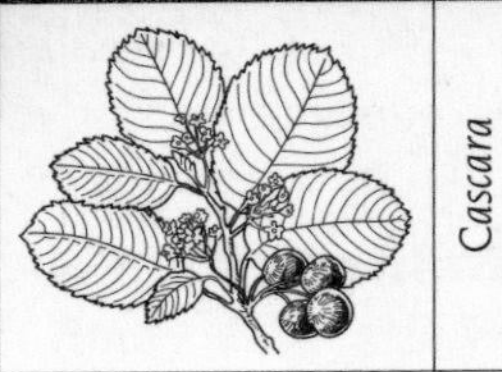
Cascara

The Herbal Approach

Atonic constipation is caused by weakness of the intestinal muscles or a lack of stimulating fiber, with no urge for days. *Spastic constipation* is produced by intestinal spasm, with a strong urging, but no result. The familiar symptoms, such as gas, bloating, cramps, headache, foggy thinking and bad breath, are produced by toxic by-products of intestinal fermentation. Hemorrhoids, from straining or hard stools, are a secondary effect. Of the many causes of constipation, stress, poor diet, inadequate enzymes, a sluggish liver and drug side effects are prominent. Aluminum absorbed from cooking pots or foil contributes to the problem, while adequate dietary fiber and water are essential to overcoming a sluggish bowel.

Herbal laxatives can be stimulating, bulking or lubricating. *Stimulating laxatives*, such as *cascara*, *buckthorn* and *senna* contain chemicals that promote contraction of the intestinal muscles. In fact, *cascara* is the most widely used laxative in the world and part of several over-the-counter medications. If overused, these herbs can weaken the intestinal muscles and nerves, resulting in a lazy bowel and increased constipation. Thus they should not be used for more than three or four weeks at a time. *Bulk laxatives* such as *psyllium*, *fenugreek* and *flax* provide fiber or intestinal mass that helps the colon to contract. These are better for long-term bowel management, as there are no weakening effects. Laxative herbal medicines are often combined with other digestive herbs, including *peppermint*, *ginger* and *chamomille*, that ease spasm, reduce inflammation and expel gas. *Lubricating laxatives*, like *slippery elm*, can help soften stool as well. See also ■ Colic/Cramps ■ Colitis/IBS ■ Detoxification ■ Diarrhea ■ Gas/ Bloating ■ Liver Conditions.

Aloe**—Aloe vera/barbadensis
- Aloe vera *gel* is a gentle and soothing cleanser, laxative and demulcent.
- Aloe *leaf extract* is a strong, cramping purgative and not recommended.
- Strong antibacterial action; promotes healing of intestinal linings.

Buckthorn*—Rhamnus catharticus/frangula
- Strong stimulating purgative, used only when gentler herbs fail.
- An ingredient in the over-the-counter laxative Movicol and also in the famous Hoxsey anti-cancer formula; may have anti-tumor effects.
- Avoid with chronic gastrointestinal complaints, ulcers, hemorrhoids.

Butternut**—Juglans cineria
- Gently relieves chronic constipation through its tonifying action.
- Like black walnut, a purgative, antimicrobial, antiparasitic and anti-tumor remedy with a wide range of applications. Valuable liver cleanser.

Cascara***—Rhamnus purshiana/Cascara sagrada
- Stimulates normal intestinal contractions by increasing water and salts in the bowels. Tones the intestinal muscles, with full effect in 8 hours.
- Stimulates pancreas, clears congestion of both liver and gall bladder.
- Not habit-forming and does *not* require progressively larger doses.

Chinese Rhubarb**—Rheum palmatum
- Stimulating laxative and purgative, with astringent, cleansing effects.
- Does not cause excessive cramping. Smaller doses effective in diarrhea.
- Reduces toxic bacteria, tones intestinal linings, improves appetite.

Dandelion**—Taraxacum officinale
- Gentle laxative action, stimulating bile production and liver function.
- Strengthens tone of digestive tract. Detoxifies and tones the gall bladder and liver. Strong diuretic effect, without potassium loss.

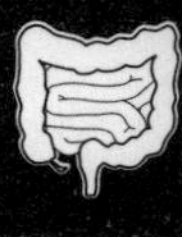

Flaxseed***—Linum usitatissimum
- High in mucilage, essential fatty acids and provides a bulking effect.
- Soothes and eases inflammation of the stomach and intestinal tract.
- May be taken as whole seeds or ground and ingested as a paste.

Peppermint**—Mentha piperita
- Antispasmodic, reduces spasm and colic, relieves spastic constipation.
- Soothes the irritated bowel and stimulates digestive secretions and bile. Relieves gas and bloating, antibacterial, useful in irritable bowel.

Psyllium Seed**—Plantago ovata or psyllium
- Bulk-forming laxative, forms a gelatinous mass that is easily expelled.
- Soothes intestinal lining and clears toxins from the large bowel.
- Both a laxative and anti-diarrhea herb, thus regulates bowel function.
- Very useful for irritable bowel, ulcerative colitis, Crohn's disease.

Senna**—Cassia senna
- A strong stimulating laxative, which also softens the stool; particularly useful in cases of fissure or hemorrhoids. Works within ten hours.
- Can cause cramping, so is best used in combination with other herbs.
- Should not be taken for more than two weeks to avoid weakening bowel.

Yellow Dock**—Rumex crispus
- Possesses mild laxative qualities, similar to Chinese rhubarb.
- Commonly used for constipation in the elderly and during pregnancy.
- Used in iron deficient anemia, for parasites or for general sluggishness.

COUGH

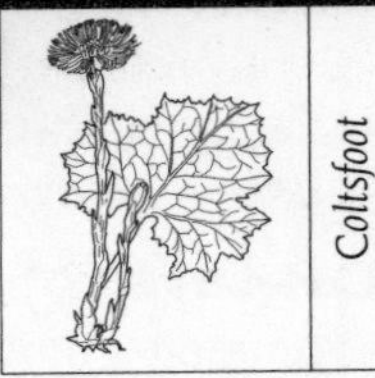

Select the herbs that are most suitable for your condition.

Herbal Approach

A cough is a natural reaction, designed to expel irritating, toxic material and mucus accumulations in the bronchial tubes. However, as everyone knows, even repeated coughing is sometimes ineffective at ridding the body of these irritants, and itself become fatiguing and debilitating.

For coughs, there are herbs that have a specific affinity to the chest and lung area (*pectorals*). Some herbs are true *antitussives* or cough suppressants (*coltsfoot, horehound, wild cherry bark, licorice*) or are just effective antispasmodics. Many are *demulcents*, soothing irritated bronchial tubes while others are *expectorants*, helping expel tough, adherent mucus. The powerful antibacterial and antiviral properties of many of these same plants makes them an excellent choice for getting at both symptoms and causes. Many herbal cough formulas are available that combine these various properties and are often superior to a single herb. The herbs below represent the best of literally hundreds of herbal cough medicines. Note that demulcent herbs are more applicable to dry coughs (*licorice, slippery elm, mullein, althea*), while astringent plants are more suitable to moist, rattly or congested coughs (*anise, eyebright, cowslip, thyme, eucalyptus*). See also ■ Asthma ■ Colds & Flu ■ Hayfever/Allergy ■ Infection ■ Sinusitis.

Anise***—Pimpinella anisum

- Helps expel mucus, while being anti-inflammatory, antispasmodic.
- For colds, coughs, bronchitis; also reduces nausea, gas, bloating.
- Safe for infants and children; a popular colic and indigestion remedy.
- Often mixed with other herbs for above effects and sweet licorice taste.

Coltsfoot**—Tussilago farfara

- Expels mucus, soothes irritated membranes and suppresses coughs.
- Coughs related to upper respiratory infections (colds), acute and chronic bronchitis, asthma, hoarseness, whooping cough and emphysema.
- See Dosage. Should not be used excessively or for prolonged periods.

Cowslip**—Primula veris

- Strong antispasmodic and expectorant for rattly coughs, chronic bronchitis with thick white mucus. Warming and sedative effects.

Elecampane***—Inula helenium

- For coughs and bronchitis, including chronic cough; gentle for children.
- Soothing expectorant; helps expel excess mucus, antibacterial effects.
- Relieves bronchial spasm in asthma, emphysema, bronchitis.

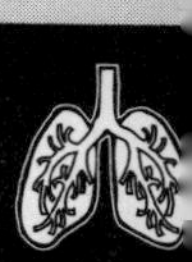

Eucalyptus**—Eucalyptus globulus
- Expectorant, natural decongestant, often used in rubs and liniments.
- Opens bronchial passages, clears mucus during colds, flu, bronchitis.
- Natural antiseptic. Use as an inhalant or lotion; high toxicity internally.

Grindelia**—Gumweed/Grindelia camporum
- For coughs of bronchitis and asthma, whooping cough or viral coughs.
- Clears tough mucus, improves breathing and smothering tendency on falling asleep. Slows rapid heart beat and reduces high blood pressure.

Horehound***—Marrubium vulgare
- Loosens mucus, soothes coughs; aids stuffy nose, sore throat and colds.
- For bronchitis, wheezing, congested chest, with inability to expel mucus.
- Treats asthma or chronic lung conditions with poor expectoration.

Hyssop***—Hyssopus officinalis
- Relieves coughs, bronchitis; loosens and expels mucus accumulations.
- Best in chronic coughs; a tonic, stimulating herb that speeds recovery.
- Asthmatic coughs in adults, children. Promotes sweat in colds and flu.

Irish Moss*—Chondrus crispus
- A mucilaginous, jelly-like seaweed used in many respiratory conditions.
- A soothing demulcent used for irritating coughs, inflamed membranes.
- An expectorant for phlegm and mucus, encourages a productive cough.

Licorice**—Glycyrrhiza glabra
- A powerful cough suppressant, soothing expectorant, demulcent and anti-inflammatory. Treats bronchitis, coughs, asthma, sore throats.

Lomatium**—Lomatium dissectum
- Powerful antiviral, antibacterial herb, kills at least ten bacterial strains.
- Eliminates a broad range of acute and chronic viruses.
- For flus, cold, chronic bronchitis, viral pneumonia. Expels hard mucus.

Lungwort* —Sticta pulmonaria
- For cough and bronchitis. For dry hacking night cough, preventing sleep.
- Treats lingering coughs after measles, flu, colds, whooping cough.
- Soothes tickling in throat, bronchi, where one cough incites another.

Maidenhair Fern*—Adiantum cappillus
- Used for coughs, bronchitis, asthma and general respiratory disorders.
- Soothes sore throats, expels mucus, helps chronic sinus congestion.

Mullein**—Verbascum thapsus
- Traditional cough remedy that soothes dry and inflamed throat and bronchi, clears mucus, allays bronchial spasms, shrinks swollen glands.
- Useful in colds, flu, bronchitis, asthma and even emphysema.

Osha**—Ligusticum porteri
- Antiviral, antibacterial herb, best taken at first sign of an infection.
- For sore throats and coughing, in colds, flu, or acute or chronic mucus conditions. Also useful when recuperating from digestive upsets.
- Dilates the bronchial passages and promotes expectoration.

Plantain**—Plantago officinalis
- Stops coughing, clears wheezing and chest pain in bronchitis and flu.
- Promotes expectoration of mucus from the entire respiratory tract.
- Antibacterial, demulcent, anti-inflammatory, promotes tissue healing.

Poplar**—Balm of Gilead/Populus canadensis
- A soothing, antiseptic demulcent for the linings of the respiratory tract.
- For dry and irritating coughs, bronchitis, colds, sore throats, laryngitis.
- Expectorant, antibacterial, pain-relieving and anti-inflammatory effects.

Slippery Elm**—Ulmus fulva
- A mucilaginous demulcent for coughs and respiratory tract irritation.
- Moistens a dry spasmodic cough, relieves pain and inflammation.
- May be eaten as a gruel in debilitated conditions and in the elderly.

Thyme**—Thymus vulgaris
- Powerfully antiseptic, useful for colds and flu, children's respiratory infections, asthma, bronchitis. Helps sore throat, headache, giddiness.
- Antispasmodic, dilates bronchi and clears mucus in coughs, asthma.

Usnea***—Lichen/Usnea species
- Inhibits strep, staph, pneumococcus, fungi and other organisms.
- Used in chronic coughs after colds or flu, and where fever accompanies the symptoms. Benefits chronic problems, pneumonia, pleurisy, TB.

Wild Cherry Bark***—Prunus serotina
- Astringent and antispasmodic; quiets coughs and dries up mucus.
- Relieves dry, irritating coughs in bronchitis, whooping cough, asthma.
- Eases indigestion and irritable bowel and other digestive complaints.

Yellow Dock**—Rumex crispus
- Soothes tickling in pit of throat and chest, not relieved by coughing.
- For long episodes of dry, teasing, hacking, fatiguing cough with little expectoration and tenacious mucus. For coughs that worsen outdoors.

Yerba Santa***—Eriodictyon californicum
- Native American herb used for asthma, chronic bronchitis and colds.
- Benefits dry coughs; an expectorant for difficult to expel mucus.
- Useful in urinary infections and as a poultice for bruises, arthritis.

Cough Herbs

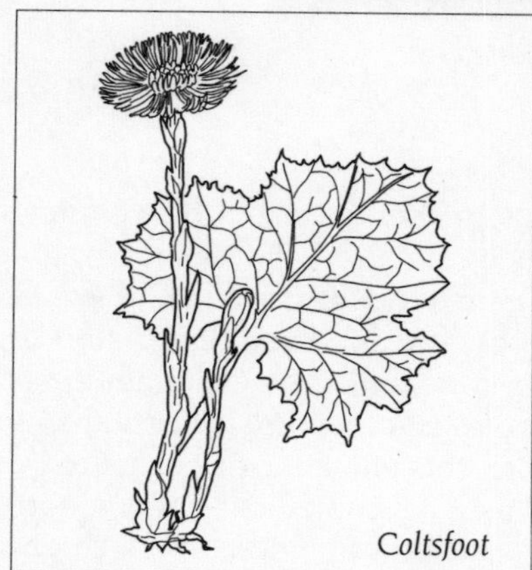
Coltsfoot

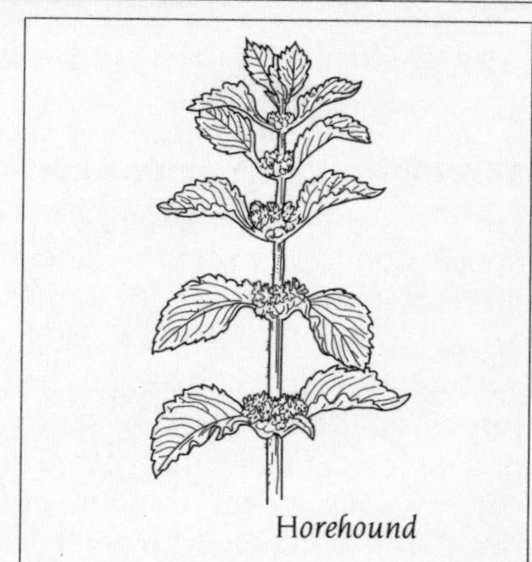
Horehound

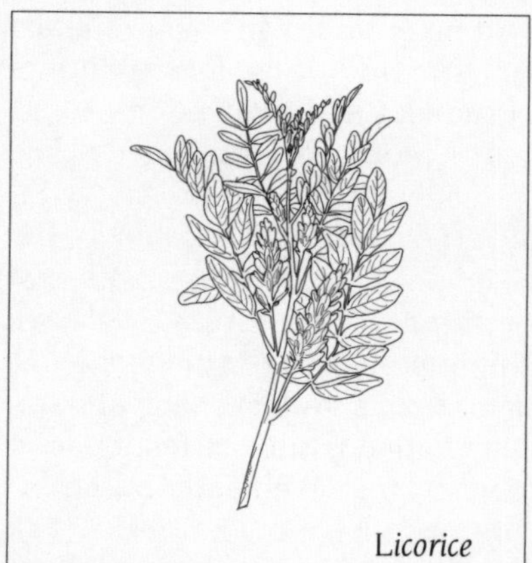
Licorice

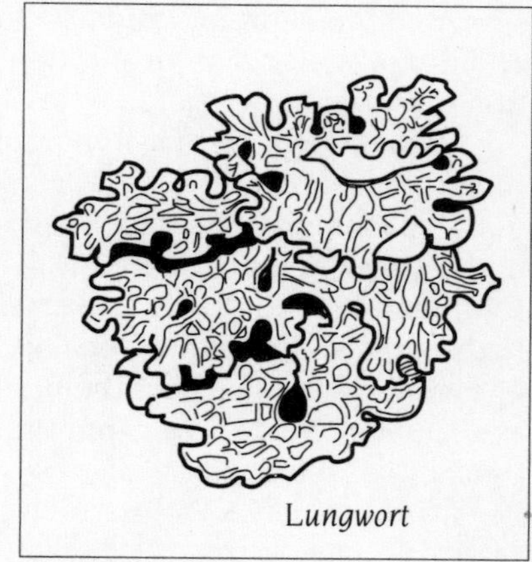
Lungwort

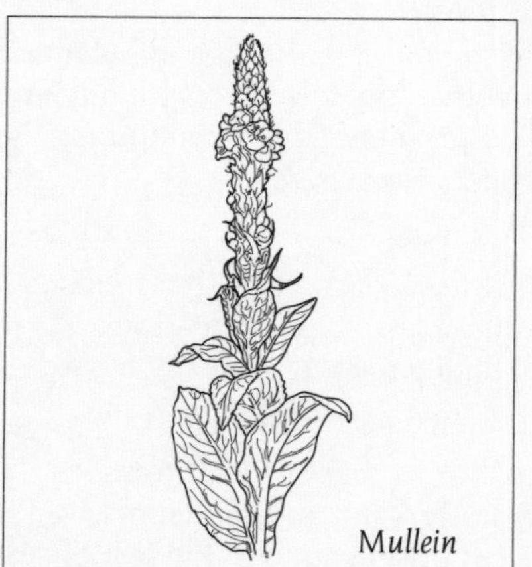
Mullein

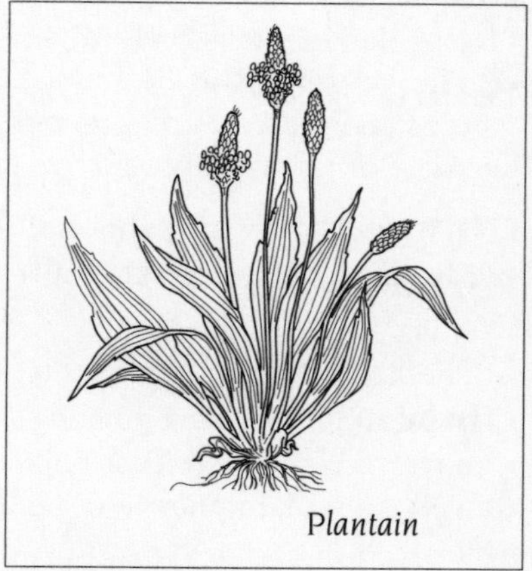
Plantain

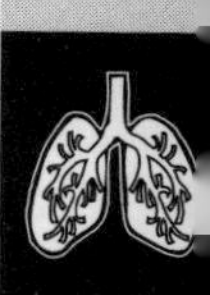

DEPRESSION

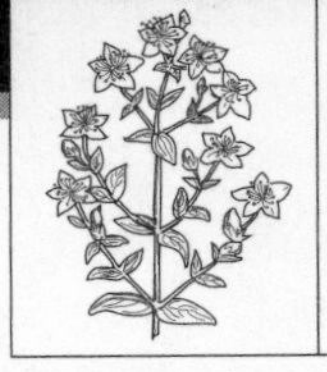
St. John's Work

Select the herbs that are most suitable for your condition.

The Herbal Approach

Feeling low or down is part of the human experience, but true clinical depression is described as a persistent combination of sadness, loss of interest, poor appetite, weight loss or gain, sleep disturbance, low sex drive, fatigue, low self-esteem, guilt, poor concentration, indecision or suicidal thoughts. Anxiety or irritability can be also be prominent features. The lifetime "risk" of such depression is about 15%, affecting 10% of people at any one time. More and more, this epidemic has come to be seen as a biological problem, as much as a psychological one. Indeed, two-thirds of people with depression also suffer from one or more chronic diseases. Deficiencies of folic acid, B12 and B6 are causes of depression, and the neurological impact of environmental toxins, heavy metals and drugs is also significant. In many holistic traditions, liver malfunction is known to be related to feelings of sadness and depression.

Herbal medicines have tranquilizing and mood-elevating effects, like their drug counterparts. However, they provide a gentler approach, without a deadening of emotions. Additionally they can address many of the underlying causes of depression. N*ervine* is the term given to plants that tonify, nourish, detoxify and strengthen the nervous system. A*daptogen* herbs are also important, rebalancing the immune and nervous systems. These plants also protect the brain against toxins and free radical damage. Our circumstances cannot always be changed, but our response to psychological and physical stress can be vastly improved and optimized. See also ▪ Anxiety ▪ Fatigue ▪ Liver Conditions ▪ Memory ▪ Stress.

Black Cohosh**—Cimicifuga racemosa
- Helps dark depression from emotional trauma or hormonal imbalance.
- Sedative properties, but also very effective for irritability and anxiety states centered around the menses, PMS or menopausal syndromes.
- A male or female reproductive tonifier and restorative.

Ginkgo***—Ginkgo biloba
- Relieves depression, especially in the elderly, or those with arteriosclerosis or heart disease, or after stroke. Improves brain circulation.
- Carries nutrients and oxygen to the brain, increases focus, memory.

Ginseng**—Panax ginseng
- An adaptogenic herb that balances the body's response to stress.
- Involved in maintenance of neurotransmitters involved in depression.
- Increases stamina, energy levels, concentration and immune response.

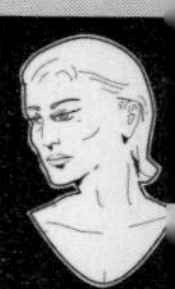

Gotu Kola**—Centella asiatica
- Adaptogen capable of tonifying, revitalizing and rejuvenating the body.
- Increases general mental functioning, memory and concentration.
- Useful in depression related to sub-clinical hypothyroid conditions.

Kava Kava***—Piper methysticum
- Best when anxiety is a component of the depressive syndrome.
- Relaxes and quiets the mind without producing hangover or sedation.
- Useful to decrease pain and muscle spasms; excellent for insomnia.

Lavender**—Lavandula officinalis (Tincture)
- Relaxes the entire nervous system, lifting depression and moodiness.
- Soothes and calms sleeplessness, irritability and tension headache.
- Helps digestion, relieves gas, bloating and cramping of nervous origin.

Lemon Balm**—Melissa officinalis
- Valued for its ability to raise the spirits in minor depression.
- Improves associated feelings of anxiety or panic, heart palpitations.
- Relieves restlessness, irritability, gastric acidity, spasms and bloating.

Rosemary**—Rosmarinus officinalis
- Used in mild to moderate depression, faintness, weakness.
- Helps vague feelings of poor health, undue fatigue or exhaustion.
- Assists recovery from long-term stress or illness, nourishes adrenals.

Schisandra**—Schisandra chinensis
- Provides nervous system rejuvenation, improves mental sharpness.
- Relieves depression, irritability and insomnia with disturbing dreams.
- Improves memory, concentration and sexual stamina.

Skullcap**—Scutellaria laterifolia
- Tones, nourishes and restores the nervous system. Used in serious mental exhaustion, depression, effects of overwork or prolonged sickness.
- Calms tension and stress, and is a help in insomnia, muscle spasms.

St. John's Wort***—Hypericum perfoliatum
- Improves mood, ability to function fully. Decreases feelings of sadness, hopelessness, worthlessness, exhaustion. Helps relieve insomnia.
- As effective as typical medical antidepressants, minus the side effects.

Valerian**—Valeriana officinalis
- Effective for depression with associated anxiety, panic attacks or pain.
- Relaxes spastic muscles, tremors, excitability and heart palpitations.
- Restores healthy sleep/wake cycle and decreases number of wakings.

Vervain**—Verbena officinalis
- Anti-depressive, valuable in PMS and menopausal mood alterations.
- For poor recovery after illness or viral infection, including Epstein-Barr.
- Lowers blood pressure, relieves headaches, treats spleen disorders.

DETOXIFICATION

Select the herbs that are most suitable for your condition.

Chickweed

The Herbal Approach

Detoxification is a cornerstone of natural systems of medicine. While the use of the term *toxin* may seem vague, it represents a major cause of chronic illness. *Extrinsic toxins* include heavy metals, pollutants, food additives, pesticides, viruses, bacteria and parasites. *Intrinsic toxins* are end-products generated by cells or organs, or from poorly eliminated wastes in the intestinal tract. These various poisons also act as free radicals, oxidizing and ultimately destroying living tissue. Accumulated free radical damage and toxicity spells aging, immune weakening and a host of illnesses with different names and a single cause.

The European-American tradition uses the term *alterative* or *blood purifier* for plants that cleanse and detoxify on the level of cells, tissues and organs. They are always important for the treatment and cure of chronic disease, stimulating immunity and clearing the lymphatic system. They also address underlying causes of many recurrent acute illnesses and can prevent the development of degenerative disease. Specific herbs have the ability to optimize the main detoxification channels of the body: the colon, skin, liver, kidneys and lungs. See also ■ Anti-aging ■ Constipation ■ Immune Weakness ■ Kidney Conditions ■ Liver Conditions.

Burdock***—Arctium lappa
- A potent alterative and detoxifier, antibacterial and antifungal.
- Useful in skin conditions (psoriasis, eczema, recurrent boils), rheumatism, dyspepsia, as well as in infections like colds, sore throats, coughs.
- Anti-inflammatory, liver and kidney cleanser. Helps clear heavy metals.

Chickweed**—Stellaria media
- An alterative and blood detoxifier, cooling and anti-inflammatory.
- Used in chronic skin disorders, vaginitis, boils, itching, rheumatism.
- Promotes healing, reduces enlarged glands, with cortisone-like effects.

Cleavers**—Galium aparine
- One of the most versatile lymphatic cleansers, restoratives and tonics.
- General detoxifier, helps eliminate waste products and build-up of excess fluid and swelling. Anti-inflammatory, reduces enlarged glands.

Dandelion***—Taraxacum officinale
- Very effective detoxifier of the liver, gall bladder and kidneys; eliminates toxins due to infection, pollutants. Useful in skin disorders, arthritis.
- Improves digestion, balances blood sugar during fasting programs.
- Gentle laxative effect; diuretic action without causing potassium loss.

Nettles**—Urtica dioica
- A restorative and nutritive tonic, high in detoxifying chlorophyll, rich in vitamins, protein, potassium and iron. Contains plant sterols.
- Clears toxins through the lungs, kidneys and stomach. Stimulates immunity, useful in anemia, neuralgia, arthritis, chronic skin conditions.

Poke Root***—Phytolacca decandra
- Lymphatic decongestant, stimulates waste removal, shrinks lymph glands; specific action on toxic or inflamed breast tissue, throat, joints.
- Fights chronic bacterial and fungal infection, especially with an inflammatory component: cellulitis, tonsillitis, arthritis, stomach ulcers.

Red Clover***—Trifolium pratense
- Immune-enhancing and blood-purifying herb, lymphatic cleanser.
- Specific for skin disorders, such as acne, eczema, rosacea, boils.
- Relieves congested, sluggish conditions. Safe for children and elderly.
- A remedy for ulceration, sores and part of traditional cancer formulas.

Red Root***—Ceanothus americanus
- A stimulating blood and spleen tonifier and detoxifying cleanser.
- Used internally to treat fevers and congested tissues of the body.
- Rids the body of excess heat and assists in tissue waste removal.

Queen's Delight***—Stillingia sylvatica
- Alterative and detoxifier that clears congestion of lymphatic vessels.
- Immune stimulant, anti-inflammatory, laxative, reduces swollen glands.
- Effective for chronic sore throat, bronchitis, chronic bone disorders, rheumatism. Helps clear mercury. Can be used as a local compress.

Triphala***—Belleric, Chebulic and Emblic myrobalan
- A combination of three Ayurvedic herbs, is a potent internal detoxifier, blood cleanser and bowel regulator. Promotes nutrient absorption.
- Detoxifies the liver, restores vitality, strengthens the nerves.

Wild Indigo**—Baptisia tinctoria
- An antiseptic, immune-stimulating Native American herb.
- For toxic states with chronic infections; for pustular tonsillitis, chronic intestinal toxicity, foul diarrhea, crops of boils, old ulcers.
- Indicated for systemic toxicity, with enlarged lymph nodes, exhaustion.
- Local use for chronic vaginitis, putrid sore throat, foul gum disease.

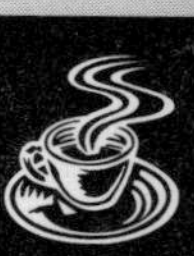

Yellow Dock**—Rumex crispus
- A blood purifier for people enfeebled by chronic toxicity and illness.
- For prolonged maldigestion with bloating and shortness of breath.
- Treats stubborn coughs, chronic skin disorders, old ulcers, toxic sore throats and enlarged glands. Liver and gall bladder tonic and laxative.
- Aids in treatment of anemia, eczema, acne, herpes, psoriasis.
- Used in both E*ssiac* and H*oxsey* detoxifying, anti-cancer formulas.

DIABETES

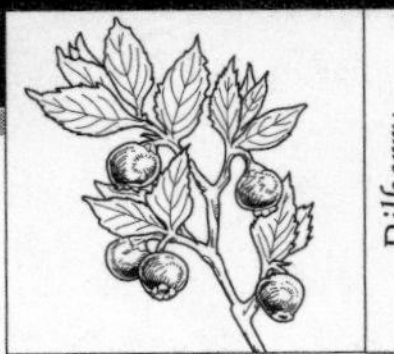
Bilberry

Select the herbs that are most suitable for your condition.

The Herbal Approach

Affecting 16 million Americans, diabetes is a national epidemic. For those in their thirties, its incidence has increased 70% in just ten years. While mainstream medicine seeks better kinds of insulin substitutes, the experience of holistic professionals is that adult (type II) diabetes can be greatly improved or even cured in many cases. Important, overlooked causes include chronic viral infections, autoimmune states, intestinal dysbiosis with absorption of endotoxins, and free radical damage from a wide variety of pollutants, drugs and chemicals. The adrenals are also critically involved, as is liver metabolism and the entire hormone system.

Results depend on how advanced the condition is, and medical management and monitoring is essential. Herbs are able to lower blood sugar levels, improve the body's ability to metabolize and respond to insulin, and regenerate the pancreas. Others reduce or eliminate the side effects of both diabetes and long-term insulin therapy, i.e. arteriosclerosis, obesity, poor circulation (including gangrene), neuropathy and retinal problems. Elimination of allergens and use of nutrients like chromium and zinc are essential. See also ▪ Heart Conditions ▪ Immune Weakness.

Bilberry***—Vaccinium myrtillus
- Reduces risk of diabetic complications: diabetic retinopathy, cataracts.
- Lowers and stabilizes blood sugar. Strengthens capillaries and arteries.
- Improves circulation in limbs. May help control blood sugar levels.

Bitter Melon***—Momordica charantia
- Traditional blood sugar lowering herb in China, India, Africa.
- Suppresses the neurological response to the stimuli of sweet taste.
- Improved glucose tolerance without increasing insulin levels in type II.
- Shown to stimulate the pancreatic beta cells that manufacture insulin.

Dandelion*—Taraxacum officinale
- Used for diabetes because it promotes healthy functioning of the liver.
- Helps to maintain stable blood sugar levels through liver metabolism.
- Promotes bile secretion and is a gentle laxative and diuretic.

Devil's Club***—Oplopanax horridum
- Normalizes blood sugar, balances fluctuations, regulates adrenals.
- Insulin-like activity in adult-onset diabetes; best suited for those who are slightly overweight. Reduces high blood pressure and blood lipids.
- An immune stimulant and adaptogen, similar to its relative, ginseng.

Fenugreek**—Trigonella foenumgraecum
- Lowers blood sugar and reduces need for insulin, improves glucose tolerance and excretion of glucose in the urine by up to 54%.
- Blood levels of insulin remain more stable; also lowers cholesterol.

Ginkgo**—Ginkgo biloba
- Prevents and treats common complications of diabetes: diabetic neuropathy and poor circulation to the limbs, and to the eyes and retina.
- A blood-thinning agent, improves brain blood flow, anti-inflammatory.

Ginseng**—Panax ginseng
- Enhances the release of insulin, increases insulin receptors in tissues.
- Adaptogen and tonic, improves mental concentration, co-ordination.
- In diabetics, shown to lower blood sugar levels, decrease weight, improve mood and motivation and assist in raising overall energy level.

Gymnema***—Gurmar/Gymnema sylvestre
- Regenerative effect on pancreas cells; raises insulin levels in the body.
- Decreases insulin needs by 45–75%. Lowers blood sugar, triglycerides.
- Reduces sugar craving and destroys ability to taste sweets for 3 hours.
- In type II diabetes, improves insulin's effects; may even substitute for oral sugar-lowering drugs. Use for 18–24 months for optimal effects.

Holy Basil**—Ocimum sanctum
- Shown to significantly lower blood sugar levels without side effects.
- An overall tonifying and invigorating herb that lowers stress levels.
- Has anti-inflammatory and analgesic properties, lowers blood pressure.

Jumbul***—Syzygium cumini/jambolanum
- Possesses the ability to lower blood sugar levels and reduce sugar in the urine; best for the beginning stages of type II, non-insulin diabetes.
- Also for type I diabetes with fatigue, increased urination, thirst.

Licorice**—Glycyrrhiza glabra
- Mediates body's stress and glucose response, maintaining even levels.
- Normalizes adrenal hormones (glucagon, corticosteroids), which control release of blood sugar from cells, or their absorption and storage.

Siberian Ginseng**—Eleuthrococcus senticosus
- An adaptogen that modulates the body's response to internal or external stressors, improving immune function, reducing overall exhaustion.
- Diabetes is very stressful to the body, and this herb helps the organism react to these blood sugar swings and imbalances more efficiently.

Stevia**—Stevia rebaudiana
- Stevia is 200–300 times sweeter than sugar, without affecting insulin.
- A natural, safe alternative sweetener for diabetics and hypoglycemics.
- A totally safe and effective sugar substitute, available in various forms.

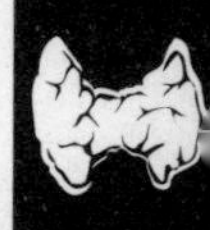

DIARRHEA

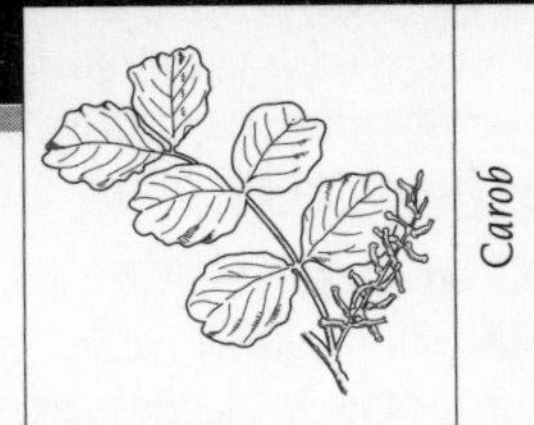

Select the herbs that are most suitable for your condition.

The Herbal Approach

Irritation or inflammation in the small or large intestines can be initiated by a wide variety of toxins. This includes food allergens, bacteria, fungi, additives and chemicals, and undigested or putrefying foodstuffs. Underlying this may be inadequate enzymes or digestive fluids, emotional upset or stress, hormonal imbalances, fluid shifts in the body, and so on. Treatment should address the causes, including eliminating dysbiosis and normalizing the flora of the colon.

Many anti-diarrhea herbs are simple astringents, which dry up secretions and tone the intestinal tract. Besides those listed below, other astringents commonly found in formulas include *bistort* and *agrimony*. The popular Kaopectate is herbal—apple pectin and clay. Demulcents soothe irritated linings, and plants with antimicrobial and tissue healing effects can detoxify the intestines. Antispasmodic herbs, like *chamomile*, reduce cramps, while carminatives reduce gas and fermentation. Fortunately, many herbs combine all these qualities as a synergistic whole. Additional treatment is advised to strengthen the liver and pancreas. Also consider stress-reducing remedies like *valerian*, *St. John's wort* and *kava*. See also ▪ Candida/Yeast ▪ Colic/Cramps ▪ Colitis/IBS ▪ Gas/Bloating.

Bayberry**—Myrica cerifera
- Digestive disinfectant for diarrhea, dysentery, gastritis, food poisoning.
- Astringent that tightens and dries out excess mucus in the intestines.
- Increases circulation, reduces colic through its antibacterial action.

Carob**—Ceratonia siliqua
- A nutritious chocolate substitute, with strong astringent effects, used to cure diarrhea; especially useful in infants and young children.
- Cleanses and calms intestinal inflammation. Contains tannins that bind toxins, reduce watery stools and stop bacterial overgrowth.

Chamomile**—Matricaria recutita
- Relieves inflammation and irritation of intestinal tract. Antispasmodic.
- Effective for both diarrhea and indigestion. Reduces gas, bloating.

Cinnamon***—Cinnamomum zeylandicum
- Powerful antibacterial, works against E. coli; best at onset of illness.
- Intestinal astringent; dries excess mucus, while warming and tonifying.
- Decreases diarrhea and symptoms of nausea and vomiting.

Geranium**—Cranesbill/Germanium maculatum

- Powerful astringent herb that helps cases of diarrhea, colitis, dysentery.
- Can relieve bleeding in colitis; helps painful or bleeding hemorrhoids.

Ginger***—Zingiber officinale

- Relieves diarrhea and associated gas, cramps and bloating, indigestion.
- Anti-inflammatory, inhibits bacteria; promotes protein breakdown.
- Soothes associated nausea or vomiting; warming for "cold" intestines.

Goldenseal***—Hydrastis canadensis

- Most effective for diarrhea due to infection or "traveller's diarrhea."
- Antibiotic against a wide variety of diarrhea-causing microbes, including E. coli, cholera, salmonella, shigella, giardia and amoeba.
- Blocks bacterial toxins, heals intestinal linings, strengthens the liver.

Meadowsweet**—Filipendula ulmaria

- Anti-inflammatory; contains aspirin-like substances but does not irritate, but heals the stomach, due to tannins. Reduces acid indigestion.
- Astringent that combats diarrhea, irritable bowel; safe for children.

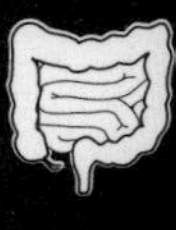

Oak***—Quercus rubor

- Used to stop acute and chronic diarrhea; also used for dysentery.
- Strong astringent, mild antiseptic; decreases parasitic infections.
- Also effective for hemorrhoids, mouth sores and vaginal discharges.

Peppermint**—Mentha piperita

- Antispasmodic, antibiotic, reduces spasm and colic, relieves diarrhea.
- Soothes irritated bowels and stimulates digestive secretions and bile.
- Relieves gas, bloating. Important for irritable bowel syndrome, colitis.

Potentilla*—Potentilla tormentilla

- More astringent than oak bark, stops diarrhea in colitis, irritable bowel, Crohn's disease and dysentery. Benefits hemorrhoids, rectal bleeding.
- May be used internally or applied externally to decrease bleeding.

Raspberry Leaf**—Rubus idaeus

- A superb remedy for diarrhea, high in tannins and very astringent.
- Relieves nausea, vomiting; antiviral, reducing herpes 2, coxsackie, influenza, polio virus, and retrovirus 1; also has antifungal properties.

Sangre de Grado**—Croton lechleri

- South American herb, effective against diarrhea and well tolerated.
- Effective in "traveller's diarrhea," as well as AIDS-related diarrhea.
- Can be used long term with no side effects or interaction with drugs.

Yarrow**—Achillea millefolium

- Anti-inflammatory and astringent, reduces diarrhea and dysentery.
- Relieves cramping, is anti-microbial and is strongly anti-hemorrhagic.

DRUG DETOX

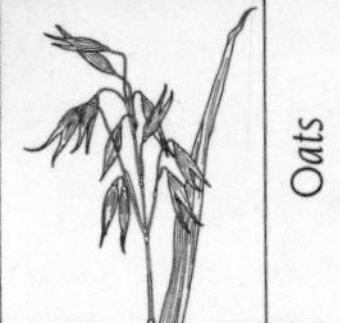

Select the herbs that are most suitable for your condition.

The Herbal Approach

One in four Americans has a substance abuse problem, with 3 million amphetamine users, 2 million cocaine addicts, 47 million smokers and 100 million caffeine addicts! At the same time, there are a million Prozac prescriptions written monthly, with 23,000 reports of adverse reactions and 1,300 deaths since 1985. There are over 110,000 deaths annually due to prescribed drugs in hospitals alone (and 8,000 from anti-inflammatories), making this the fourth leading cause of death. Undocumented cases could be 2 to 5 times as many. Yet the confusion around drug use and abuse is staggering. With recent changes in advertising rules, TV airways are filled with ads for sedatives and tranquilizers, side by side with spots to fight the war on drugs. One can go to jail for smoking an herb to relieve the nausea of anti-cancer drugs, yet giving speed (amphetamines and Ritalin) to children earns the prescriber a half million dollars a year!

Herbal medicines can be extremely useful in cessation and withdrawal from the use of medical or addictive drugs. These plants have calming effects and, moreover, nourish and promote healthy neurological functioning. Some have generalized tonic properties, while others are antidotes to a particular drug. Most also have a cleansing effect on the liver. All the tonic or adaptogen herbs have a role to play, augmenting nervous, hormonal and immune health and promoting adrenal function. See also ▪ Anxiety ▪ Depression ▪ Fatigue ▪ Liver Conditions ▪ Stress.

California Poppy**—Eschscholtzia californica
- Normalizes mental and emotional functioning in drug detoxification.
- Reduces anxiety, tension and nervousness during withdrawal.
- Related to the *opium poppy*, but not a narcotic herb and non-addictive.

Chaparral**—Larrea tridentata
- Antioxidant, anti-inflammatory and tissue healing. For the effects of and withdrawal from cocaine and speed, amphetamines and drugs like Ritalin. A tea can be sprayed directly into the nose via an atomizer.
- Excess or prolonged use purported to cause liver damage, hepatitis.

Chamomile**—Matricaria recutita
- A mild sedative and antispasmodic. Helps with sleep and nightmares.
- Excellent for high irritability, fits of rage, anxiety, restlessness, hypersensitivity associated with withdrawal. Specific antidote to coffee.

Ginger**—Zingiber officinale
- Helpful for weaning off medications. Binds to same brain receptors as

benzodiazepines (Valium, Xanax), relieves craving and withdrawal.
- Powerful antioxidant, reduces anxiety, improves digestion.

Ginseng/Siberian Ginseng***—Panax/Eleutherococcus
- Helps to regulate adrenal hormones, stress response, brain chemistry.
- Increases neurotransmitters and proteins. Improves strength and stamina; normalizes reactions to mental, physical, and emotional stress.

Goldenseal*—Hydrastis canadensis
- Has been used in the past to mask the detection of drugs in the urine, but in reality, has absolutely no effect on outcome of today's lab tests.
- May help reduce cravings, toning the liver and digestive system.

Gotu Kola***—Centella asiatica
- For effects of cocaine and other recreational drugs, or mixtures of drugs.
- Effectively combines with chaparral. Improves memory, intelligence.
- Energizes and strengthens nervous system, adrenals, immune system.

Holy Basil***—Ocimum sanctum
- Specific for withdrawal from pot or marijuana, as well as alcoholism.
- Increases immune function by up to 20%; broad action against bacteria, kills parasites and soothes a range of digestive disturbances.

Milk Thistle**—Silybum marianum
- Protects against damage to liver by alcohol, drugs and other toxins.
- Essential for cirrhosis; powerfully regenerates damaged liver tissue.

Oats***—Avena sativa
- Drug addiction: morphine, heroin, opium, cocaine, marijuana, tranquilizers, sedatives, alcohol, coffee, tobacco, anti-depressants (e.g. Prozac).
- Relieves chronic insomnia, impotency, amenorrhea, palpitations.
- Aids nervous exhaustion, fatigue, sexual weakness, poor concentration.
- For effects of anxiety, worry, over-study; relieves headache in occiput.
- Weans people off drugs while providing a healthful substitute "lift."

Passionflower**—Passiflora incarnata
- Relieves insomnia associated with drug withdrawal, without hangover effects. Combines well with kava, skullcap, valerian and hops.

Schisandra***—Schisandra chinensis
- Adaptogen; improves stress, irritability, depression, weak memory.
- Protects the liver, lessens alcohol damage, relieves night sweats, frequent urination, excess thirst. Tones the kidneys and adrenal glands.

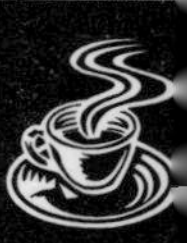

Skullcap**—Scutellaria laterifolia
- A nervine that helps ease drug withdrawal. Improves states of exhaustion, insomnia and headache. Sedative action, relieves anxiety, pain.
- Restorative for emotional and nervous system, for long-term balancing.

DYSMENORRHEA

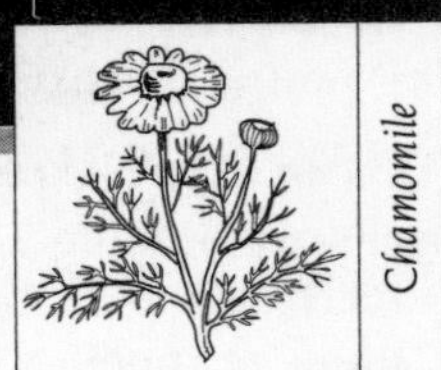

Select the herbs that are most suitable for your condition.

The Herbal Approach

Painful menstruation is a common problem, but in about 10% of women it is so severe that it significantly affects their ability to function. Dysmenorrhea is now considered a sub-type of PMS, as the causes are usually identical—an excess of estrogen in relation to progesterone. Dysmenorrhea can also be due to fibroids, ovarian cysts, endometriosis, infection or, rarely, more serious diseases. Contributing causes are food allergies or excess consumption of alcohol, spices, coffee, sugar or milk products. Deficiencies of omega 3 and 6 essential fatty acids, B6 (pyridoxine), magnesium, calcium and zinc are also significant factors.

Herbal treatment of menstrual cramps takes several forms. There are a variety of herbs that strongly relieve uterine spasms. They reduce inflammation by various pathways, such as decreasing inflammatory prostaglandins. A number of these healing plants, like *black cohosh* or *blue cohosh*, also have a tonifying and strengthening effect on the uterus. They also work to correct underlying hormonal imbalances, often reducing the estrogen to progesterone ratio. Besides their physical effects, many pain-relieving herbs also relieve anxiety, depression and erratic moods. In the case of menstrual cramps, several herbs are often combined for optimal effects. See also ■ Anxiety ■ Bleeding ■ Colic/Cramps ■ PMS.

Black Cohosh***—Cimicifuga racemosa

- Antispasmodic, relieves menstrual cramps, muscle tension, headache.
- Corrects imbalances in estrogen ratio; very effective at menopause.
- Also used to promote labor and ease labor pains and excess spasm.
- Relieves anxiety, depression. Benefits hypertension, rheumatism.

Black Haw***—Viburnum prunifolia

- Uterine antispasmodic, relieves menstrual cramps, tension headache.
- General pain reliever and sedative, with aspirin-like ingredients.
- Relaxes the intense spasms of the uterus before, during or after menses.
- Acts on the uterus variously as a stimulant, relaxant and tonifier.
- Regulates hormones; calming effects on the mood, relieving tension.

Blue Cohosh**—Caulophyllum thalictroides

- A uterine tonic that is antispasmodic; relaxes contracted uterine muscles. Helps in chronic uterine inflammation and associated arthritis.
- Relaxes congested uterine and back muscles during menses.
- Estrogen-balancing effects, promotes menses, regulates cycle.

Chamomile***—Matricaria recutita
- Antispasmodic for intense neuralgic pains, calms the nervous system.
- Calms and sedates irritability and anger, promotes relaxation, sleep.
- For menses that is too early, heavy, prolonged. Dark and clotted blood.
- Eases gas, distention, indigestion, diarrhea before or during menses.

Cramp Bark***—Viburnum opulus
- Relaxes menstrual cramps and uterine spasm before or during menses.
- Sedative and calming effects on mood, muscle tension, palpitations.
- Tonic effect on the uterus, regulates hormones, helps with PMS.

Dong Quai***—Angelica sinensis
- Antispasmodic, pain-relieving; lessens cramps, improves blood flow, reduces excess clotting. Mild sedative, helping insomnia, constipation.
- Helps in endometriosis, cramps, PMS, menopause, excess bleeding.
- A blood-builder in anemia, combats fatigue, strengthens immunity.

Ginger**—Zingiber officinale
- Analgesic and warming in nature; reduces cramps, lessens inflammation, increases blood flow and oxygen to the uterus.
- Increases the bioavailability of other herbs to maximize their effects.

Jamaican Dogwood**—Piscidia erythrina
- Antispasmodic, pain-relieving and sedative properties; calms tension.
- Relaxes menstrual cramping and muscular spasms, helps insomnia.
- Relieves anxiety, stress and heightened emotional sensitivity.

Kava Kava**—Piper methysticum
- Analgesic and antispasmodic; decreases pain and muscle tension.
- Quiets anxiety, relaxes the mood and reduces sensitivity to pain.
- May be taken anytime, without producing drowsiness or sedation.

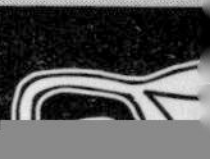

Meadowsweet**—Filipendula ulmaria
- Allays spasms, along with anti-inflammatory and pain-relieving effects.
- Contains salicylic acid, the herbal version of aspirin.
- Without gastric irritation, neutralizes stomach and general acidity.

Wild Yam***—Dioscorea villosa
- Powerful antispasmodic that combines well with other herbs for menstrual pain and cramping, PMS, ovary pain and menstrual irregularities.
- Regulates progesterone levels, supports the liver and uterus, and is used as a general anti-inflammatory.

Valerian*—Valeriana officinalis
- Antispasmodic that relaxes contracted uterus and eases menstrual pain and cramping. Calms the nervous system, anxiety and irritability.
- Promotes restful sleep, provides tension and stress relief. Good for PMS.

EAR INFECTION

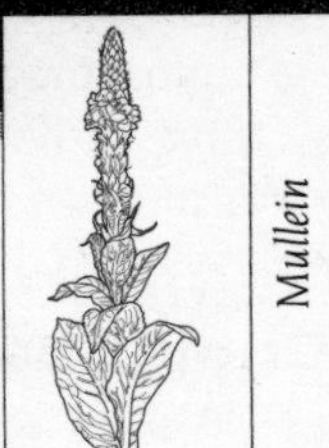

Select the herbs that are most suitable for your condition.

The Herbal Approach

Otitis media is the most common pediatric problem, affecting two-thirds of children, with a 50% increase in incidence over the last ten years. While 21% of *all* antibiotics are used for childhood ear infections, as many as 80% of these are due to antibiotic-resistant strains, viruses, fungi, or where no infective agent can be found. Children treated with antibiotics have recurrences two to six times more often than untreated children. Antibiotics cause injury to the immune system and set the stage for long-term systemic fungal infection. In fact, 90% of otitis cases are due to fluid accumulation in the middle ear from food allergies (especially dairy). Ear infections are often related to intestinal dysbiosis and are much commoner in children who are not breast-fed. Vaccines are another factor that can initiate chronic otitis.

Herbs are effective for ear infections, taken orally, placed directly in the ear, or, in the case of small infants, ingested through the mother's breast milk. A combination of internal and local medicines works best. Do not use eardrops if the ear drum is perforated or is draining. Avoid all herbs (and honey!) in young infants. Homeopathy is also an excellent treatment choice for permanently eliminating recurrent otitis. See also ■ Immune Weakness ■ Infection ■ Inflammation ■ Pain/Neuralgia.

Astragalus**—Milk Vetch/Astragalus membranaceous
- Antiviral, antibacterial herb for shortening duration of acute infection.
- Taken on a long-term basis to strengthen immune system, increases T cells to prevent recurring infection. Safe and effective for children.

Chamomile**—Matricaria recutita
- Gentle pain reliever, anti-inflammatory and antispasmodic. Especially effective for earache associated with teething, colic or diarrhea.
- Reduces fever and hot sweats. Calms irritability and crankiness.

Echinacea***—Echinacea purpurea
- Powerful, short-term immune stimulant and blood purifier; acts like interferon, rousing the body's overall response to acute infection.
- Antiviral and antibacterial against staph, strep. Can be used internally, as well as dropped into the ear along with other herbs or herbal oils.

Elder**—Sambucus nigra
- Internal use as an antiviral to prevent and treat infection, such as colds, fever; promotes perspiration. Astringent that dries mucus secretions.
- Relieves congestion, improves pain, helps stuffed ear, lost hearing.

Eucalyptus**—Eucalyptus globulus
- Pain-relieving properties, strong external antiseptic and disinfectant.
- Astringent and decongestant for mucousy colds, flu and chronic sinus.
- Anti-inflammatory for swollen membranes; use as local oil or tincture.

Garlic***—Allium sativa
- A wide-spectrum antibiotic for ear infections, otitis after cold, or flu.
- Effective against bacteria causing otitis, including antibiotic resistant strains. antiviral and antifungal, warm garlic oil can be put in the ear.

Goldenseal**—Hydrastis canadensis
- Internal or external antibacterial, effective against a wide spectrum of organisms, including staph, strep and antibiotic-resistance germs.
- Heals the mucus membranes and increases resistance to bacteria.
- Stimulates immune function and antibodies to prevent future infection.

Grapefruit Seed Extract**—Citrus paradisi
- A broad spectrum antibiotic, shown to be effective against almost 800 strains of bacteria and 500 types of fungus. A safe antiseptic agent.
- Several drops diluted in water can be placed in the ear, alone or combined with echinacea, licorice, mullein, plantain and garlic.

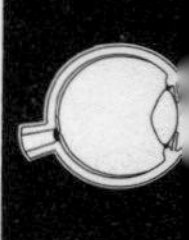

Larix**—Larix occidentalis
- Has antiviral action, highly effective against middle ear infections.
- Arabinogalactan extract has similar effects to echinacea, shiitake and astragalus. Enhances immunity, increases action of white cell activity.

Licorice—Glycyrrhiza glabra
- A soothing antiviral and antibacterial with anti-inflammatory effects.
- Increases the body's cortisol and immune-stimulating interferon.
- Take both internally and add to herbal ear drops with mullein, etc.
- Note: Deglycyrrhizinated licorice does not contain antiviral properties.

Mullein**—Verbascum thapsus
- Mullein oil put in the ear rapidly relieves pain, relieves blockage of swimmer's ear. Also treats facial pain radiating into the ear or vice versa.
- Inhibits viral replication. Internally, soothes coughs, expels mucus.

Plantain***—Plantago officinalis
- Plantain oil in the ear is pain-relieving, antibacterial, anti-inflammatory.
- Promotes tissue healing, dries up ear secretions, checks bleeding.
- Effective for ear pain during teething, after dental work or toothache.
- Use directly in ear, treats neuralgia of ear radiating into the face, teeth.

St. John's Wort**—Hypericum perforatum
- Used in eardrops to alleviate nerve sensitivity, pain and infection.
- Strong antiviral action, antibacterial and anti-inflammatory activity.
- Increases immune function, T cells, while treating irritability.

EYE CONDITIONS

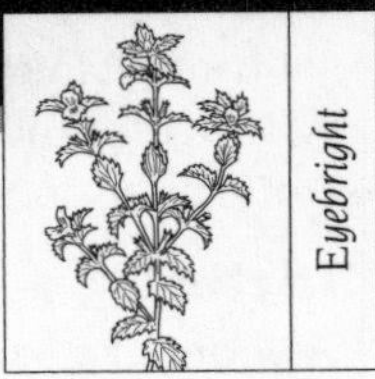

Select the herbs that are most suitable for your condition.

The Herbal Approach

The eye is subject to a variety of problems. The conjunctiva protects against the many irritants we encounter every day: smoke, pollution, dust, pollen or bright lights. Inflammation or infection results in conjunctivitis or "pink eye." Far more serious is cataract, mainly showing up by age sixty-five, the risk of this free radical induced condition is increased in smokers and users of steroids or tranquilizers. Cataract removal is now the most common surgery in the U.S., with over one million operations per year. Glaucoma affects as many as two million adults—2% of those over forty—causing 80,000 cases of blindness yearly. Meanwhile, the most common cause of blindness in people over sixty-five is macular degeneration, affecting between 20% and 40% of this age group. It is wholly preventable with antioxidants. Other important eye problems include retinal damage from diabetes, arteriosclerosis or retinitis pigmentosa.

For conjunctivitis or eye irritation, herbal remedies can provide lubricating, soothing and healing effects, while being antiseptic or antimicrobial. A number of powerful antioxidant herbs can improve the health of the tiny arteries supplying the retina and protect the various structures of the eye from free radical damage. Many can decrease the pressure inside the eye, associated with glaucoma, and stop the advance of cataracts. See also ■ Infection ■ Inflammation.

Bilberry***—Vaccinium myrtillus
- Strengthens and protects veins and arteries. Helps night vision, improves shortsightedness. Maximum effect in five hours; take before visual tasks.
- Protects retina against macular degeneration, retinitis pigmentosa, retinal damage in diabetes (also lowers blood sugar) and arteriosclerosis.
- Reduces pressure in glaucoma and can halt progression of cataracts.

Bupleurum*—Bupleurum chinense
- Chinese medicine considers eye problems to depend on liver weakness.
- A powerful liver tonic; simultaneously strengthens the eyes and vision.

Calendula***—Marigold/Calendula officinalis
- Heals and soothes, reduces inflammation and swelling, itching.
- Use in bacterial or viral conjunctivitis, irritation due to pollutants, allergies, and minor corneal injuries. Antiseptic and immune modulating.
- Apply as local compress and eyewash or in an eye drop formula.

Cayenne**—Capsicum frutescens
- Anti-inflammatory for irritated mucus membranes, conjunctivitis. Use in very small amounts, well diluted or in a compound eye drop formula.
- Initially causes redness, then pain relief, increases blood flow to eyes.

Coleus***—Coleus forskohlii
- Increases blood flow inside the eye and decreases intraocular pressure; dropped directly into the eye, effect lasts for several hours.
- Antihistamine, relaxes arteries, improves contraction of heart, increases thyroid function, insulin secretion. Useful in hypertension, diabetes.

Dusty Miller*—Cinerarea maritima
- For dissolving cataracts and corneal opacities, if taken in early stages.
- Effective after injury to the cornea (post-traumatic) or due to aging.
- Increase circulation to the eye for treating conjunctivitis.

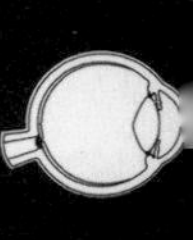

Eyebright***—Euphrasia officinalis
- For conjunctivitis or eye irritation/inflammation from pollutants, allergy, colds or flu, measles, etc. Relieves effects of eyestrain, bright lights.
- Soothes and heals bloodshot, burning, itching eyes, light sensitivity, sticky eye gum, or acrid yellow discharges. Use internally and as drops.
- Much safer and more effective long-term than commercial eye drops.

Ginkgo***—Ginkgo biloba
- Increases circulation and delivery of oxygen and nutrients to the eye.
- Prevents free radical damage, protects eye capillaries, clears toxins.
- Used in retinopathy, cataracts, macular degeneration, glaucoma.

Goldenseal***—Hydrastis canadensis
- Anti-inflammatory and antibiotic against a wide range of bacteria.
- Draws fluid from surrounding tissues and decreases swelling. Useful in conjunctivitis, irritation from pollutants, styes, infections of eye or lid.

Goldthread**—Coptis trifolia or chinensis
- Treats inflammation or infection of eyes, conjunctiva, mouth, throat.
- Antibacterial and antiviral, reduces inflammation; good pain-reliever.
- Use as both internally and, well diluted, as an external eyewash.

Grape Seed Extract***—Vitis vinifera
- Protects eyes from damage from exposure to sun and UV radiation.
- Procyanidins strengthen retinal capillaries, prevent clots or bleeding and provide vital nutrients; increases night vision and slows eye aging.
- Prevents and treats diabetic retinopathy, arteriosclerosis in the eye.

Lutein***—Spinach Extract/Spinacea oleoracea
- A carotenoid found in the eye and retina, capable of protecting and sometimes reversing macular degeneration, cataracts and blindness.
- Protects against aging effects of free radicals and UV radiation.

FATIGUE

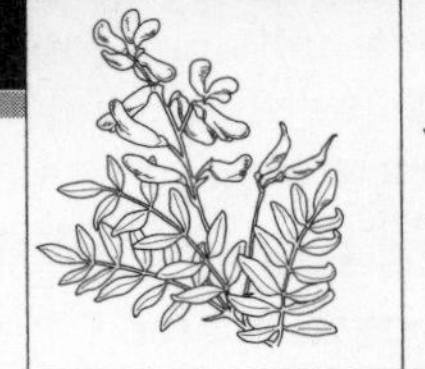

Select the herbs that are most suitable for your condition.

The Herbal Approach

Fatigue is the most common presenting complaint in doctor's offices, and can be part of scores of serious medical conditions, as much as from overwork or lack of sleep. Underlying causes need to be identified, and natural medicine recognizes many less obvious contributing factors. These include chronic intestinal dysbiosis, liver overload, adrenal exhaustion, hidden infections (yeast, viral or parasitic) and food allergies. Typical short-term solutions such as caffeine, tobacco, sugar and other stimulants are ultimately debilitating for the hormonal and nervous system.

Herbal medicines should be directed toward the underlying causes, but for simple fatigue, tonic and adaptogenic herbs can be relied upon. These have the ability to increase vitality and well-being, balancing and improving the function of the body's major control systems—immune, hormonal, cardiovascular and nervous. Thus they are particularly suitable for the effects of prolonged stress, both physical and psychological. This class of botanical medicines can help compensate for and overcome the effects of overwork, depression, prolonged illness and convalescence after illness. Optimal effects occur when tonics are taken long term (i.e. one to six months). They are best taken in chronic illness, rather than acutely and are typically used in a cycle of 3 weeks on and one week off.
See also ■ Anti-aging ■ Immune Weakness ■ Liver Conditions ■ Stress.

Alfalfa**—Medicago sativa

- Improves appetite, digestion; produces mental clarity and well-being.
- Increases stamina and strength, augments ability to respond to stress.
- For convalescence after long illness, extreme stress. Reduces toxicity.
- High in phytoestrogens, stimulates the body's hormone production.
- Note that alfalfa sprouts and especially seeds are potentially toxic.

Astragalus***—Milk Vetch/Astragalus membranaceous

- For general weakness, fatigue, loss of appetite, shortness of breath.
- Adaptogenic herb that stimulates immune function, improves stamina.
- Anti-inflammatory, antiviral, antibacterial effects; good for flu, cold.
- Strengthens people with cancer, after radiation or chemotherapy.

Cordyceps**—Cordyceps sinensis

- Builds strength, endurance, stamina and immunity. Reduces fatigue, promotes lung and kidney function. Increases blood flow to brain, heart.
- Increases male potency, female vitality. Improves appetite and sleep.

Ginseng***—Panax Ginseng
- Strengthens adrenals, improves vitality and ability to handles stress.
- Improves physical and mental performance, stamina; enhances mood.
- Increases visual and motor coordination, increases work capacity.
- Antioxidant, inhibits formation of free radicals, stimulates immunity.

Gotu Kola***—Centella asiatica
- Improves brain function, memory. Anti-stress, anti-anxiety, relaxant.
- Strengthens body's connective tissue and blood vessels, heals wounds.
- Tonic and rejuvenator, improves fertility, has anti-inflammatory effects.

Licorice**—Glycyrrhiza glabra
- Provides steroid-like factors for the the body's own production of adrenaline, cortisol; thus boosts adrenal function and adaptation to stress.
- Antiviral and immune-enhancing herb, valuable for weakened states.

Maitake**—Grifola frondosa
- Immune-stimulating effects; increases activity of immune cells (killer cells, etc.), as well as immune-modulating chemicals (interleukin 2).
- D-fraction has shown positive results in Epstein-Barr and chronic fatigue; inhibits virus production, protects cells from attack by toxins.

Oats***—Avena sativa
- Exhaustion from work, study, illness, drugs, alcohol, sexual excess.
- Nutritive effect on the brain, rather than temporary stimulatory effect.
- Greatly sharpens mental acuity, focus, memory before an exam etc..
- Eases heart palpitations, effective for insomnia due to overfatigue.

Schisandra***—Schisandra chinensis
- Improves adrenal and nervous system capacity. Counteracts effects of stimulants, coffee. Improves liver function and protects it from toxins.
- Increases work and efficiency level, improves mood, memory and sleep.
- Re-regulates immune system, helps skin problems, aphrodisiac effects.

Siberian Ginseng***—Eleutherococcus senticosus
- Adaptogenic herb, excellent for exhaustion, fatigue, immune weakness.
- For effects of long stress (physical, emotional, mental) or after illness.
- Increases mental alertness, work output and athletic performance.
- Enhances adrenals, increases immunity and protects against toxins.

St. John's Wort*—Hypericum perforatum
- Inhibits viral activity and replication of herpes virus and Epstein-Barr.
- Relieves depression that is a cause or effect of fatigue; improves sleep.

Yerba Mate*—Ilex paraguariensis
- Stimulates like caffeine, but without causing nervousness; calms, balances the nervous system. Improves sleep and mood, reduces allergy.
- Antioxidant, increases oxygen to the heart and brain.

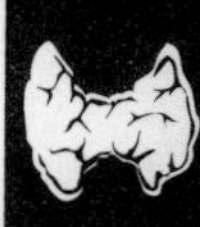

FIBROMYALGIA

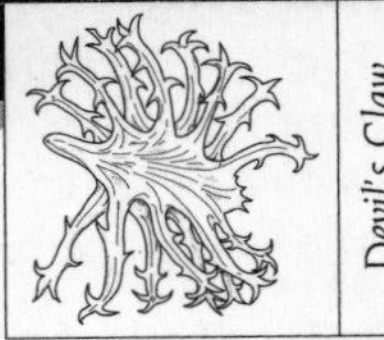
Devil's Claw

Choose the herbs that are most suitable for your condition.

The Herbal Approach

Fibromyalgia (FMS) is a systemic condition affecting up to 35% of women and 5% of men. The list of immune and connective tissue related symptoms includes fatigue, severe aching and tender muscular nodules with possible stiffness, insomnia, headache, cramps, irritable bowels, food allergies, weight gain, fevers, anxiety, irritability and poor concentration—but there are no definitive laboratory tests. FMS is linked to chronic fatigue syndrome, sleep disorders, phosphorus deposits in the tissue, chemical and environmental sensitivities, as well as chronic viral, bacterial or parasitic infections. A multi-faceted approach is needed for cure.

Herbal treatment includes a wide range of plants that influence the musculoskeletal system (joints, muscles, ligaments, etc.), as well as immune and hormonal modulators. Thus adaptogenic and general tonics are essential for building up and strengthening overall vitality. Anti-inflammatory plants play a major role, especially those with an affinity to fibrous tissues (*devil's claw, boswellia*). Apart from symptom control, antiviral and antiparasitic herbs are essential, as are both immune-stimulating and liver-enhancing herbs. Rounding out a program to include nutrition and homeopathy, this condition is curable. See also ▪ Arthritis ▪ Back Pain ▪ Detoxification ▪ Fatigue ▪ Immune Weakness ▪ Inflammation ▪ Liver Conditions ▪ Pain/Neuralgia ▪ Stress.

Astragalus***—Milk Vetch/Astragalus membranaceous
- Improves immune function of spleen and thymus, improves energy.
- Promotes the overall resistance to sickness, infection, tones liver.
- Resolves degenerative disease from chronic physical/emotional stress.

Black Cohosh***—Cimicifuga racemosa
- Relieves spasms of large muscles with stiffness, twitching and jerking.
- Anti-inflammatory for sore, heavy muscles, electric pains, numbness.
- Balances underlying hormonal problems related to menopause, PMS.

Bromelain**—Pineapple/Ananas comosus
- A proteolytic enzyme that inhibits swelling, pain in joints and muscles.
- Binds to partially digested proteins that initiate the antibody-antigen immune response, thus broadly decreasing inflammation.

Burdock**—Arctium lappa
- A liver herb tonifier and stimulating detoxifier, helps fibromyalgia.
- Drains lymphatics, promotes excretion of toxins and cellular wastes.
- Improves hormonal metabolism in the liver and acts as a mild laxative.

Cat's Claw**—Uncaria tormentosa
- Strengthens and stimulates a weakened or stressed immune system.
- Improves symptoms of muscle and joint pain, allergy and candida.
- Has anti-tumor, anti-inflammatory and antiviral properties.

Curcumin***—Turmeric/Curcuma longa
- Strong anti-inflammatory for pain and swelling in muscles, joints.
- Antioxidant properties bind free radicals and prevent cellular damage.
- Often combined in formulas with bromelain for increased effectiveness.

Devil's Claw**—Harpagophytum pubescens
- Anti-inflammatory and analgesic effects comparable to most NSAIDs.
- Helps muscle, back and joint pain, neuralgia and headaches.
- Improves poor digestion and absorption of nutrients.

Feverfew**—Tanacetum parthenium
- Decreases pain and inflammation symptoms of fibromyalgia.
- Reduces the incidence and frequency of migraine headaches.
- Anti-inflammatory action similar to COX-2 inhibitors, Vioxx, Celebrex.

Flax/Psyllium*—Linum usitatissimum/Plantago psyllium
- Important strategy in fibromyalgia for ongoing regulation of bowels.
- Patients report a greater sense of well-being and energy as the bowels become more active twice daily; relieves toxic burden in colon, liver.

Ginger***—Zingiber officinale
- Potent analgesic, anti-inflammatory with immune-stimulating qualities.
- Superior to NSAIDs in relieving muscle pain, swelling and stiffness.
- Helps with associated gastric ulcer, headache, nausea, weak digestion.

Kelp**—Bladderwrack/Fucus vesiculosis
- Provides organic iodine for strengthening the thyroid and various trace minerals for stimulating cell health. Reduces swollen lymph glands.
- Anti-inflammatory, traditionally used to relieve rheumatism.

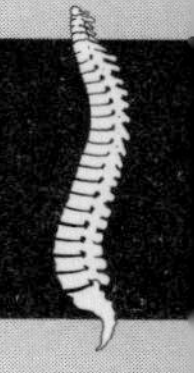

Licorice**—Glycyrrhiza glabra
- Improves adrenal function, energy levels and immune system function.
- Supports cortisol levels, the body's natural anti-inflammatory hormone.
- A healing demulcent to soothe irritated mucus membranes.

Milk Thistle***—Silybum marum
- Decreases chemical and environmental sensitivity in fibromyalgia.
- Potent antioxidant and free radical scavenger, protecting cells.
- Liver detoxification, regeneration and protection from toxic damage.

Olive Leaf***—Olea europaea
- An immune stimulant, effective for chronic viral and fungal infections.
- Effective against Epstein-Barr, herpes, resistant bacteria, yeasts, parasites and for fibromyalgia, chronic fatigue, CMV infection.

Pau D'Arco**—LaPacho/Tabebuia avellanedae
- Helps fibromyalgia symptoms, chronic infections, fatigue, inflammation. Folk cure in South American medicine for cancer and leukemia.
- Antibacterial, antiviral and antifungal, with a wide range of action.

Poke Root**—Phytolacca decandra
- A lymphatic drainer, clearing tissues of toxic load on an intercellular level, stimulates immune cells. Relieves swollen lymph nodes.
- Improves fibromyalgia, arthritic symptoms and local inflammations.

Prickly Ash***—Xanthoxylum americanum
- An antispasmodic herb, pain reliever for neuralgia and neuritis, with specific to electric-like shooting pains, tingling and muscle cramps.
- Effective for swollen glands, fevers, intestinal infection, diarrhea.

Shiitake**—Lentinus edodes
- The "ginseng of mushrooms" has adaptogenic, tonifying and especially immune-boosting power; antiviral and anti-tumor properties.
- Lowers cholesterol, regulates blood clotting and blood sugar.

Siberian Ginseng**—Eleuthrococcus senticosus
- Anti-fatigue and anti-stress; enhances stamina and mental performance.
- Improves immune function and resistance, sharpens memory, balances hormones. Protects the liver from metabolic and chemical toxins.

FIBROMYALGIA HERBS

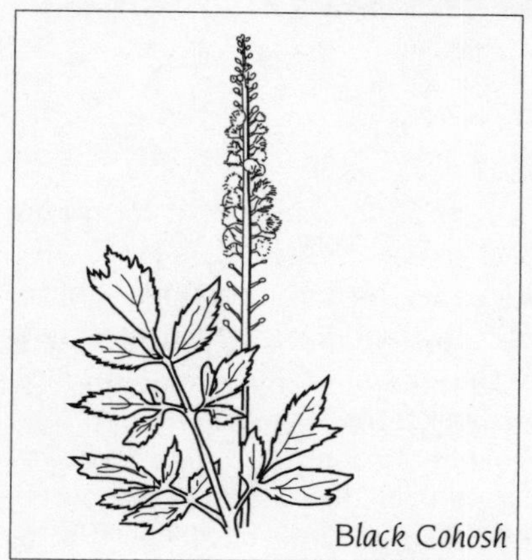
Black Cohosh

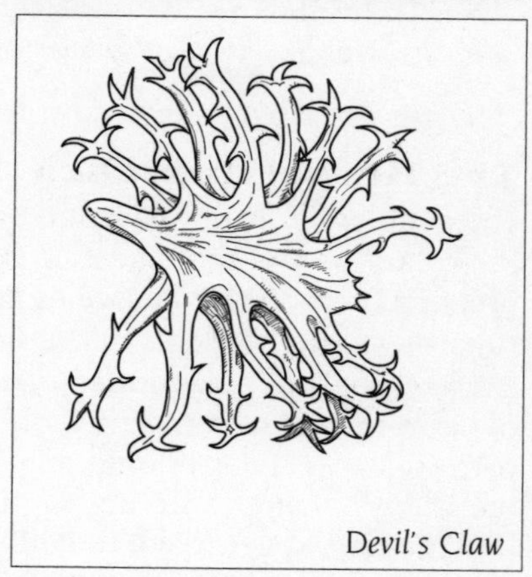
Devil's Claw

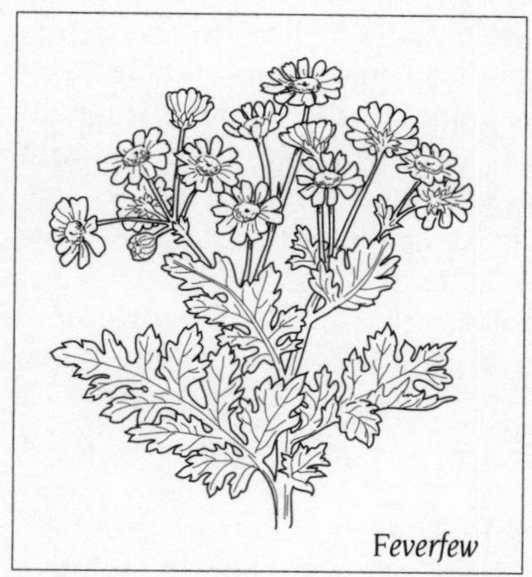
Feverfew

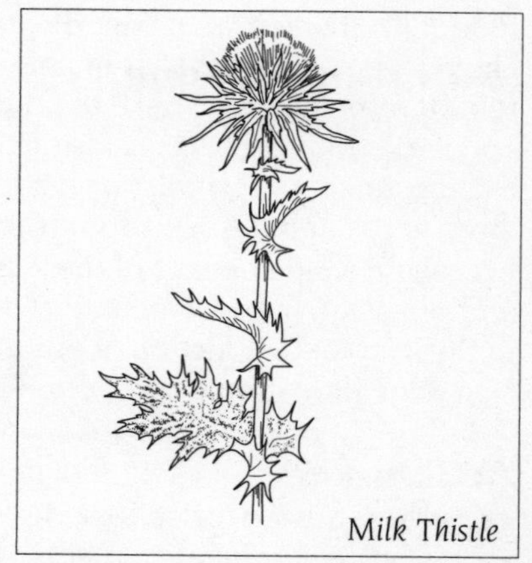
Milk Thistle

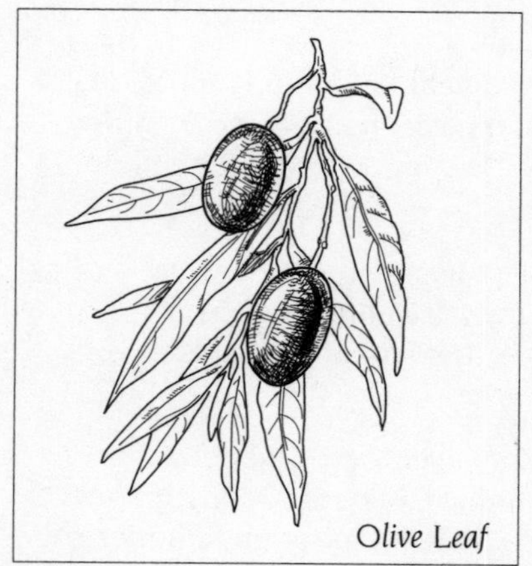
Olive Leaf

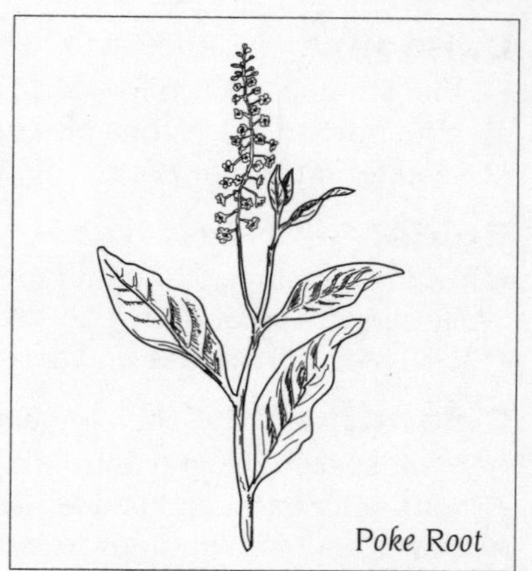
Poke Root

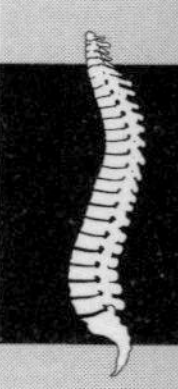

GALLBLADDER

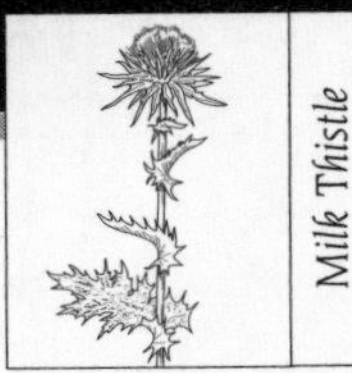

Select the herbs that are most suitable for your condition.

The Herbal Approach

The gallbladder is both a reservoir for bile produced by the liver and an important part of the digestive system. It makes fats soluble for digestion and breakdown by enzymes from the pancreas and intestines. Unfortunately, toxic overload of the liver, bacteria and various irritants can cause chronic or acute inflammation of this organ. In fact, the gallbladder is commonly a repository for chronic infections (bacteria, amoeba or parasites), which lay dormant until a weakened immune or digestive system allows them to flare-up, producing conditions like diarrhea or colitis.

The herbal approach to gallbladder inflammation (cholecystitis) is to use specific anti-inflammatories that help soothe and heal the gallbladder linings. Antispasmodic herbs are useful in acute attacks, while cholegogues (herbs that stimulate bile production) are important in long-term treatment. They make the bile more liquid and flush out a stagnant and toxic gallbladder. This also helps to prevent gallstones and deal with existing ones. Many holistic practitioners find that a combination of nutrients, herbs and detoxification therapy makes gallbladder surgery a rare necessity. A side benefit of these lipotropic herbs that stimulate the liver and bile is an improvement of blood cholesterol (which is manufactured in the liver) and reduction of obesity. See also ■ Cholesterol, High ■ Infection ■ Inflammation ■ Liver Conditions.

Artichoke**—Cynara scolymus

- Liver tonic, used for gallbladder, cirrhosis. Protects liver from toxins.
- A digestive stimulant that helps break down fats, stimulates bile flow.

Balmony**—Turtlehead/Chelone glabra

- A bile stimulant, used for gallstones and gallbladder inflammation.
- For jaundice due to stone obstruction, relieves nausea and vomiting.
- Useful for intestinal worms, mildly laxative. A good herb for children.

Boldo**—Peumus boldo

- Specific treatment for gallbladder; dissolves and removes gallstones, relieves inflammation (cholecystitis), liver or gallbladder pain.
- Stimulates bile release and detoxifies a stagnant and sluggish liver.

Celandine***—Chelidonium majus

- An antispasmodic and anti-inflammatory liver tonic and detoxifier.
- Treats gallstones, gallbladder pain, jaundice, hepatitis, constipation.
- Relaxes gallbladder, improves bile flow. Excellent for gallbladder colic

with pain in right upper abdomen, radiating to back or shoulder blade.

Culver's Root**—Leptandra virginica
- Anti-inflammatory, antispasmodic and strong bile stimulant.
- Relieves liver congestion. Useful in jaundice, chronic constipation.
- Treats gallbladder inflammation; not for use with gallstones.

Curcumin***—Turmeric/Curcuma longa
- Doubles the bile output and increases its solubility.
- Hepatoprotective: protects the liver from free radicals and toxicity.
- Effective against most bacteria associated with gallbladder inflammation.

Dandelion***—Taraxacum officinale
- May help dissolve existing gallstones, while preventing their formation.
- Important for gallbladder inflammation or jaundice, constipation.
- Powerful liver detoxifier, clearing pollutants and accumulated toxins.
- Strong diuretic action, clearing the kidneys, yet supplying potassium.

Fringe Tree***—Chionanthus virginiana
- A bile stimulant for preventing and dissolving cholesterol gallstones.
- Can be used for acute gallbladder attack or jaundice from gallbladder obstruction. Also therapeutic for hepatitis, cirrhosis, illness recovery.
- Effective tonic for the liver, pancreas and spleen; useful in pre-diabetes.

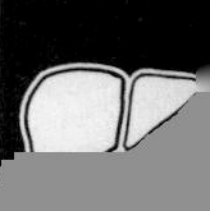

Garlic**—Allium sativa
- Suitable for eradicating many of the bacterial, viral and parasitic organisms that cause gallbladder inflammation; supports normal flora.
- Lowers cholesterol, anti-inflammatory. Protects the liver from damage.

Milk Thistle***—Silybum marianum
- Reduces the cholesterol levels in bile, helps treat and prevent stones.
- Detoxifies and regenerates the liver, protects against poisons, alcohol.
- Liver antioxidant that fights inflammation in bile ducts, gallbladder.

Oregon Grape***—Mahonia/Berberis aquifolia
- Similar to goldenseal, mahonia is a bitter bile stimulant that tonifies the gallbladder and improves liver functioning.
- Used for jaundice, skin disorders related to poor liver or gallbladder function (i.e. psoriasis, eczema). Improves digestion, regulates colon.

Peppermint*—Mentha piperta
- Reduces cholesterol level in bile, increases its flow and emulsifies it.
- Relieves the chronic belching common to gallbladder conditions.
- Digestive stimulant that is antispasmodic, relieves gas and bloating.

Wild Yam**—Dioscorea villosa
- Antispasmodic for relieving cramps and colic in the entire GI tract.
- Relieves the pain of gallbladder colic and spasm; acts rapidly.
- Stimulates bile flow and is anti-inflammatory; a good herb for children.

GAS / BLOATING

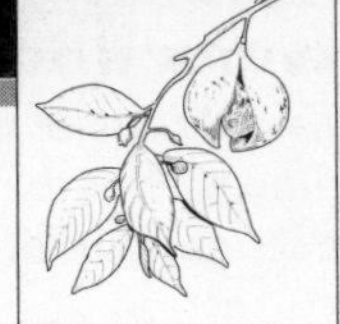

Select the herbs that are most suitable for your condition.

The Herbal Approach

Belching refers to gas "burped" or expelled from the upper stomach, while flatus indicates gas from the small intestines and colon. Besides its embarrassment and discomfort, the fermentation and maldigestion that underlies foul gas and bloating have far-reaching effects on overall health. As mentioned under the topics Colitis and Diarrhea, gas production indicates an imbalance of the bacterial colonies in the intestine, a state of dysbiosis. Toxins thus produced are absorbed into the liver and bloodstream, and act to gradually weaken the immune system and cause free radical damage in the farthest reaches of the organism. They also damage the intestinal linings, initiating the development of food allergies.

Carminatives is the term given to herbs that reduce the production of gas. Many members of the mint family act as carminatives, relieving stomach and intestinal gas, allaying spasms and soothing the digestive tract. These include *basil, lemon balm, marjoram, oregano, horsebalm, sage, thyme* and, of course, *peppermint*. Many seeds (actually tiny dry fruits) in the carrot family are traditional carminatives with similar properties, including *aniseed, dill, fennel, coriander* and *cumin*. There are many other herbs that both improve digestion and reduce gas production. The most effective of these are listed below. Many of these plants also address underlying intestinal or stomach imbalances, improving digestive secretions and reducing the colonies of pathogenic (toxin-producing) bacteria. See also ■ Colitis ■ Constipation ■ Diarrhea ■ Stomach Conditions.

Anise***—Pimpinella anisum
- Dispels gas and flatulence, eases colic; aids digestion, sweetens breath.
- Safe and gentle for children; also works through the breast milk.

Calamus***—Acorus calamus
- Specific herb for relieving gas and associated colic, cramping, distention. Soothes digestive tract and helps underlying gastritis, ulcers.
- Improves appetite, helps exhaustion and weakness due to gastritis.

Caraway**—Carum carvi
- Eases nausea, gas, indigestion, cramping and stimulates digestion. An antispasmodic herb, excellent for colic or bloating in children.

Cardamom**—Eletteria cardamomum
- A carminative and warming herb for digestive gas and cramping.
- Beneficial when gastric, urinary and respiratory symptoms coincide.

- Traditionally used to improve the flavor and taste of other herbs.

Chamomile***—Matricaria recutita
- Relieves bowel gas and distention, soothes indigestion, diarrhea.
- Relieves cramping; helps where gastritis causes insomnia.
- Gentle sedative and relaxant, safe for children and the elderly.

Cinnamon*—Cinnamomum zeylandicum
- Carminative for cramping, gas, bloating; combines well with other herbs.
- Intestinal astringent, dries excess mucus while warming and tonifying.
- Decreases nausea, vomiting and diarrhea; antimicrobial capability.

Fennel**—Foeniculum vulgare
- Traditional gas-reducing herb, relieves boating, distension and pain
- Relieves cramps, stimulates appetite, improves digestion.
- Safe for infantile colic. Anti-inflammatory herb, also lowers blood sugar.

Fenugreek***—Trigonella foenumgraecum
- Spice used for loss of appetite, indigestion, stomach acidity, bloating and distension. Acts as a stool softener and mild laxative.
- Lowers elevated cholesterol and triglycerides; balances blood sugar.

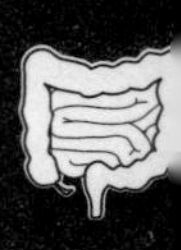

Ginger***—Zingiber officinale
- Relieves gas, heartburn, cramps, bloating, nausea and diarrhea.
- Strengthens overall digestion, especially of fats and protein.
- Safe for morning sickness in pregnancy; relieves motion sickness.

Nutmeg*—Myristica fragrans
- Powerfully reduces gas, nausea, as well as diarrhea and gastroenteritis.
- Stimulates the appetite, promotes better digestion, eliminates spasms.
- Use only small doses: hallucinogenic and toxic in large doses.

Parsley**—Petroselinum crispum
- Diuretic that reduces bloating caused by gas or water retention.
- Digestive and nutritive tonic, for indigestion, gas, cramps and bloating.
- Masks body and breath odors from foods such as garlic or onions.

Peppermint**—Mentha piperita
- Relieves gas, bloating and flatulence from both the stomach and bowel.
- Antispasmodic, reduces colic, soothes the irritated bowel and stimulates digestive secretions and bile. Helps in irritable bowel syndrome.

Sage*—Salvia officinalis
- Settles an upset stomach, relieves gas and bloating after meals.
- Calms inflammation of the digestive tract, soothes irritated membranes.
- Relieves excess sweating, night sweats, dries up congested mucus.

HAIR LOSS

Horsetail

Select the herbs that are most suitable for your condition.

The Herbal Approach

Skin problems with the hair often reflect the overall metabolism and health level of the individual. Stress, nutrient deficiency, free radical damage and lack of antioxidants all play a role. Hair loss also mirrors the hormonal balance of the body. Adrenal strength particularly influences hair loss in men and woman. Male pattern baldness, triggered by genetics, results from an accumulation of dihydrotestosterone (DHT) in the scalp. This breakdown product of testosterone blocks the follicle and prevents new hair growth. Toxins, fungal infection or dandruff contribute to hair thinning and loss exceeding growth.

Propeica, the first medical for hair loss, is none other than Finasteride, the main treatment for enlarged prostate. Since *saw palmetto* and other herbs have been shown to be 2 to 3 times more effective for diminishing prostate size, we can expect similar results in preventing hair loss—and without side effects. Herbal treatment may also be directed toward the adrenals and levels of estrogen/progesterone in women. Herbs that help the circulation, particularly *ginkgo* (internally) and *cayenne* (externally) are an additional help. *Gotu kola* and others can revitalize existing hair follicles. The earlier one begins, the better, and it will require some months to see evidence of slowed hair loss or regrowth. See also ■ Anti-aging ■ Infection ■ Prostate Problems ■ Menopause ■ Skin Conditions.

Amla**—Phyllanthus emblica
- Helps prevent gray hair, tonifies the blood. Promotes healthy and lustrous hair. Enhances cellular regeneration, nutritive and restorative.
- Bhringraja (*Eclipta alba*) may also reverse hair loss, 500 mg 3 times daily.

Arnica**—Arnica montana
- Stimulates circulation, strengthens connective tissue and hair follicle.
- Traditionally used as a local application to stimulate hair growth.
- Anti-inflammatory; helps regulates function of oil glands.

Bay Oil**—Pimenta racemosa (West Indies)
- Locally, essential oil of bay is used over time to encourage healthy hair growth and stimulate scalp circulation. Avoid use during pregnancy.

Fo-Ti***—Polygonum multiflorum
- Traditional Chinese herb used to restore color to gray hair. Hinders production of DHT. Available as internal capsules and in topical creams.
- Halts hair loss and thinning of hair and may encourage regrowth.

Gotu Kola**—Centella asiatica

- Stimulates hair and nail growth. Helps remove micro-scar tissue that blocks new hair growth. Strengthens connective tissue around follicles.

Horsetail**—Equisetum arvense

- Contains high amounts of silica; increases strength of connective tissue and follicles; strengthens keratin, promotes regrowth of hair.

Lavender Oil**——Lavandula officinalis

- Externally, helps reduce hair loss and is an effective dandruff treatment.
- Helps with psoriasis or eczema of the scalp, promotes skin healing.

Neem***—Azadirachta indica

- Used topically in Ayurveda for centuries to promote hair growth.
- Thickens hair, heals damaged hair follicles, cleanses scalp tissues.
- Increases scalp circulation, strengthens fine, thin hair, softens dry hair.

Nettles**—Urtica dioica

- Local and internal use to prevent baldness, stimulate hair growth.
- A traditional herb for darkening gray hair, added to many shampoos.
- High silica content, may be part of its effects by strengthening follicles.

Pygeum**—Pygeum africanum

- Works similarly to saw palmetto, reducing DHT in the scalp and thus promoting hair growth. Anti-inflammatory effects on the skin.

Rosemary***—Rosmarinus officinalis

- Used locally (rosemary oil), stimulates circulation and hair growth.
- Protects small capillaries that deliver oxygen and nutrients.
- Antioxidants help to promote healthy heart, circulation to the head.

Sage**—Salvia officinalis

- Contains thymol with antiseptic and astringent effects.
- A hair rinse that helps with dandruff and restores color to graying hair.

Saw Palmetto***—Sabal serrulata

- Works to unblock hair follicles, by same mechanism as it heals prostate, (i.e. decreasing residues of dihydrotestosterone in the scalp).
- Since it is three times as effective as Proscar in shrinking the prostate, it may be three times better than Rogaine (the same drug) for hair loss.

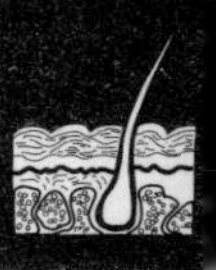

Tea Tree Oil**—Melaleuca alternifolia

- Massage scalp with a few drops before shampooing.
- Penetrates top layers of the scalp, kills bacteria and fungi that contribute to dandruff and scalp disorders; accelerates tissue healing.

Yarrow**—Achillea millefolium

- Traditionally used to cleanse hair follicles and improve scalp circulation. Darkens the hair. Anti-inflammatory that combats dandruff.

HAYFEVER / ALLERGY

Select the herbs that are most suitable for your condition.

Plantain

The Herbal Approach

Affecting 22 million Americans, allergies are the most common respiratory condition. The well-known symptoms of itchy eyes, nose, palate, sneezing and runny nose are due to release of histamines and other inflammatory substances by the sensitive mucus membranes of the allergy sufferer. The underlying causes are often food allergies or other long-term factors that undermine the immune system.

Herbs are effective antihistamines, without their many side effects and secondary toxicity. Specific herbs for short-term allergy symptom relief are also anti-inflammatory and antioxidant, protecting respiratory linings from damage. Many can help break up and expel mucus, while acting as astringents to dry up excess secretions. Adaptogenic, immune-balancing herbs like *astragalus* and *ginseng* are important parts of a long-term allergy strategy. Others are needed to correct underlying digestive disorders, food allergies and liver toxicity. Treatment should start weeks to months before the allergy season to prevent or minimize seasonal allergies. See also ■ Colitis ■ Immune Weakness ■ Liver Conditions.

Bromelain***—Pineapple/Ananas comosus

- Pineapple-based extract acts as an anti-inflammatory, stops the enzyme cascade that stimulates mast cells and histamine release.
- Proteolytic enzymes break up poorly digested proteins and polypeptides circulating in the blood that initiate an allergic immune response.

Chinese Skullcap***—Scutellaria baicalensis

- Contains anti-inflammatory, anti-allergy flavonoids.
- Effective for hayfever, respiratory and digestive allergy, asthma.
- A cooling herb, useful for feverish colds & flus with thick yellow phlegm.

Curcumin***—Turmeric/Curcuma longa

- As effective as anti-inflammatory drugs or cortisone in reducing allergy symptoms; stops release of histamine and other allergic chemicals.
- A powerful antioxidant; combine with bromelain for increased effect.

Dong Quai**—Angelica sinensis

- Inhibits production of allergic antibodies; increases interferon, stimulates white cells. Also antispasmodic, antibacterial and expectorant.

Echinacea**—Echinacea angustifolia

- Stabilizes cells that produce histamine and promote allergy symptoms.
- Dozens of immune-stimulating effects keep white blood cells within the

normal range. Useful for hayfever, asthma, food allergy reactions.
- Prevents secondary infection, including colds, sinusitis, bronchitis.

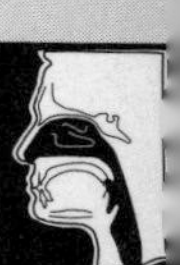

Elder**—Sambucus nigra
- Lowers mucus membrane sensitivity to allergens. Antiviral, strengthens resistance to colds, flu. Astringent, dries up excess mucus.
- Gentle for children and the elderly, taken as a pre-seasonal preventive.

Ephedra**—Ma Huang/Ephedra sinensis
- Reduces runny nose, watery eyes, sneezing, swelling of nose and eyes.
- Helps drain sinus cavities and passages, opens up breathing pathways.

Eyebright**—Euphrasia officinalis
- Anti-inflammatory, astringent, reduces swelling, soothes and dries up tearing and mucus secretions of eyes, nose, sinuses, mouth, throat.
- Due to strong astringency, do not use if nose is stuffy or too dry already.

Garlic**—Allium sativum
- High in bioflavonoids and sulphur-containing compounds, has powerful antihistamine and antioxidant effects. Natural anti-inflammatory.
- Has wide-ranging antibacterial, antiviral and antifungal effects.

Ginkgo**—Ginkgo biloba
- Reduces allergic wheezing by relaxing bronchial spasms.
- Protects and strengthens cell membranes, reduces inflammatory PAF.
- Strengthens blood vessels, making them less fragile to inflammation.

Goldenseal**—Hydrastis canadensis
- Heals the mucus membranes of the body; stops swelling and allergic hyper-sensitivity; antibacterial, antiparasitic; drys up membranes.

Horseradish**—Armoracia rusticana
- Eases watery, irritated eyes, membranes of the nose, sinuses, mouth.
- Stimulating herb, like cayenne, that encourages flow of discharges; may be applied externally as a poultice to clear congestion.

Licorice**—Glycyrrhiza glabra
- Adrenal tonic that helps maintain the body's own supply of cortisone.
- Anti-inflammatory, helps alleviate allergy, reduces hypersensitivity.

Nettles***—Urtica dioica
- Encapsulated freeze-dried form is an antihistamine, effective in 60% of sufferers, reduces itchy eyes, sneezing and nasal discharge.
- Stimulates immune function. Has diuretic, toxin-reducing effect.

Plantain*—Plantago lanceolatum
- Expels excess phlegm, soothes inflamed mucus membranes. Relieves coughs and bronchitis; dries mucus secretions in allergies.

HEADACHE

Feverfew

Select the herbs that are most suitable for your condition.

The Herbal Approach

It may be surprising to learn that 70% of people are headache sufferers. While muscle contraction or tension headaches account for about 90%, migraines affect some 25 million individuals. The diverse causes include eyestrain, sinusitis, hormonal imbalance, dental toxicity, digestive disturbances, psychological stress, fatigue and toxins. Yet the majority of migraines involve food allergies.

Herbs for headaches are variously anti-inflammatory, antispasmodic, anti-nausea and pain-relieving. Those that treat migraine also help rebalance the circulation. Still, underlying causes must be addressed, and herbs for the liver, such as *dandelion* and *milk thistle*, are often essential. Others that treat underlying infection or toxicity—especially within the digestive or respiratory tract—may be called for. For hormonal-based headache, or those with allergy syndromes, the herbs specific to those individual problems are required. It may take some detective work to pinpoint the group of factors that culminate in this eminently curable condition. See also ■ Anxiety ■ Depression ■ Immune Weakness ■ Liver Conditions ■ PMS ■ Sinusitis ■ Stress.

Chamomile*—Matricaria recutita
- Sedative and antispasmodic; best results in muscle tension headache.
- Effective where nervousness and irritability are part of the symptoms.
- Calms accompanying upset stomach, allergies and menstrual pain.

Feverfew***—Tanacetum parthenium
- Cures migraine totally in 25%, while 70% have improvement in severity, duration and frequency. Best results when taken as a daily preventive.
- Relieves nausea, vomiting. Improves sleep and relieves depression.
- Reduces histamines and serotonin, normalizes dilated blood vessels.
- Anti-inflammatory action similar to COX-2 inhibitors, Vioxx, Celebrex.

Ginger**—Zingiber officinale
- Relieves nausea, improves circulation, a potent anti-inflammatory.
- For tension headache or migraine, reduces pain-causing prostaglandins.
- May abort a migraine if taken at the onset. Can be used liberally in cooking or the fresh root can be juiced daily to prevent headaches.

Jamaican Dogwood**—Piscidia erythrina
- Relieves migraine, tension headache or facial neuralgia. Strong sedative and calming effects, reduces tension, relieves insomnia
- Powerful pain relief in facial neuralgia or from eye or ear inflammation.

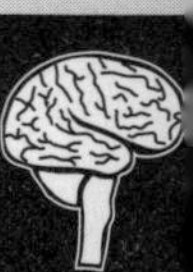

Kava Kava**—Piper methysticum
- Analgesic and antispasmodic, decreases pain and muscle tension.
- Quiets anxiety, relaxes mood and reduces sensitivity to headache pain.
- May be taken at anytime; will not cause drowsiness or sedation.

Lavender**—Lavandula officinalis
- Eases painful headaches and migraines, relaxes muscle tension, spasm.
- A relaxant and mood elevator. Use oil externally, tincture internally.
- Helps in insomnia and irritability, relieves neuralgia, stomach upset.

Linden**—Tilia europaea
- Relieves migraines related to nerves or high degree of stress. Relieves tension and sinus headache. Promotes sleep, lowers blood pressure.

Meadowsweet**—Filipendula ulmaria
- Anti-inflammatory that relieves headaches; herbal forerunner of aspirin, contains salicylic acid but, unlike aspirin, doesn't cause gastric upset.
- Actually neutralizes stomach acid and overacidity of the whole system.

Petasites**—Butterbur/Petasites hybridus
- Powerful analgesic, for acute pain of migraine and other headaches.
- Reduces spasms or cramps in muscles, urinary tract, bronchi, stomach.

Skullcap**—Scutellaria laterifolia
- Effective for headaches associated with muscular tension.
- Restorative, provides long-term balancing for emotions and nervous system. Helps relieve effects of excess worry or thinking, sleep loss.

Valerian**—Valeriana officinalis
- Sedative action, pain-relieving, calms nervous tension and anxiety.
- Relieves tension headache, calming muscle spasms of neck, shoulders.
- Relieves stress, insomnia; sedative effect without causing drowsiness.

Verbena**—Vervain officinalis
- For migraine connected to premenstrual or menopausal syndromes.
- Nervine and tonic for exhaustion following long-term stress or illness.
- Has anti-depressant and anti-anxiety effects; improves digestion.

Willow**—Salix nigra
- Salicylic acid and other co-factors are anti-inflammatory ingredients that inhibit pro-inflammatory substances (prostaglandins, etc.).
- Decreases pain of headache, as well as arthritis and muscle pain.

Wood Betony**—Stachys officinalis
- Relieves headaches caused by nervous tension and anxiety.
- Nutritive and soothing during a crisis or nerve-induced illness.
- Supports the proper functioning of the central nervous system.

HEART CONDITIONS

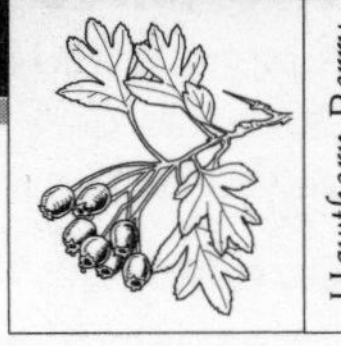

Select the herbs below that are most suitable for your condition.

The Herbal Approach

Though it is America's number one killer, claiming a quarter of a million lives annually, heart disease is both preventable and reversible in most cases. Apart from dietary change and exercise, nutrition and herbs play a crucial role in heart health. Botanical medicines can both prevent and treat illness in the cardiovascular system and are an important part of rehabilitation and recovery after heart attack or stroke. Obviously medical diagnosis, treatment and often hospitalization are needed for serious or acute heart problems. Care also must be taken to avoid those herbs that interact negatively with cardiac drugs (see Dosage section). That being said, the following botanical medicines have unique properties for actually *healing* the heart and arteries—unlike *any* medical drug—and are widely used in Europe, India and China.

Plant medicines provide antioxidant protection and detoxifying capabilities for the heart, strengthening the heart muscle and improving the metabolism and the function of heart cells. Many of the same herbs lower cholesterol significantly and can prevent and reverse arteriosclerotic changes in the blood vessels. Other herbs target associated problems, correcting the liver's cholesterol metabolism or the kidney's ability to clear fluids and toxins. See also ■ Arteriosclerosis ■ Cholesterol, High ■ High Blood Pressure ■ Kidney Conditions ■ Veins/Circulation.

Arjuna***—Terminalia arjuna
- Main Ayurvedic heart herb; regulates blood pressure, heart rate.
- Increases circulation to coronary arteries. Lowers cholesterol levels.
- Used in angina, congestive heart failure, arrhythmia, as well as asthma.

Bromelain***—Pineapple/Ananas comosus
- Natural blood thinner: prevents platelet stickiness and clot formation, while having anti-inflammatory and immune-modulating effects.

Coleus**—Coleus forskohlii
- Lowers blood pressure. Increases heart contractility, relaxes arteries, regulates rhythm, increases blood flow to coronary arteries and brain.
- Used in congestive heart failure, angina, after stroke, arteriosclerosis.

Curcumin**—Turmeric/Curcumin longa
- Improves blood flow in the arteries, while strengthening blood vessels.
- Reduces "bad" cholesterol, platelet stickiness and blood clot formation.
- Prevents free radical damage in arteries, leading to arteriosclerosis.

Dong Quai**—Angelica sinensis
- Strengthens the heart's force and volume, smooths irregular rhythms.
- Increases blood flow to coronary arteries, reduces blood pressure.
- Helps poor circulation, combats blood clots, rebuilds blood in anemia.

Ginkgo**—Ginkgo biloba
- Improves circulation, blood flow to the heart and coronary arteries.
- Protects against lack of oxygen to the heart (ischemia) and blood clots.

Green Tea**—Camellia sinensis
- Improves circulation, assists the liver in clearing high cholesterol.
- Powerful antioxidant that protects heart and arteries; diuretic effects.
- Reduces risk of heart disease and stroke, prevents arteriosclerosis.

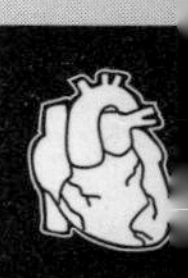

Hawthorn***—Crataegus oxycantha
- Essential heart tonic, strengthens heart muscle, protects from damage.
- Reduces cholesterol, prevents and reverses deposits on arterial walls.
- Increases strength and regularity of heart, slows rate, lowers pressure.
- Dilates coronary arteries, increasing blood supply and oxygen to heart.
- Slows advance of heart disease, helps in rehabilitation after heart attack.
- Use in mild arrhythmias, mild hypertension, angina, shortness of breath.

Motherwort**—Leonarus cardiaca
- Lowers blood pressure, if excessive. Calms and steadies heart rhythm.
- Balances electrolytes within heart cells. Improves blood flow to heart.
- Strengthens heart, calms cardiac problems related to anxiety, tension.
- Reduces excessive heart rate, calms palpitations of nervous origin.

Olive Leaf*—Olea europaea
- Lowers blood pressure, relieves arrhythmias, prevents spasms.
- Combats infection anywhere, including heart. Reduces LDL cholesterol.

Red Sage**—Dan Shen/Salvia miltiorrhiza
- Chinese herb used to assist patients recovering from heart attack.
- Dilates coronary arteries and increases blood flow to the heart.
- Stimulates circulation, lowers cholesterol; reduces angina, palpitations.

Reishi***—Ganoderma lucidum
- Benefits coronary heart disease, improves palpitations, angina, edema.
- Tonifies the heart; lowers total serum cholesterol and raises HDL, reduces platelet stickiness, prevents blood clots. Improves liver health.
- An adaptogen; relieves fatigue, enhances immunity; anti-inflammatory.

Shiitake**—Lentinus edodes
- Lowers cholesterol, prevents clot formation, regulates blood sugar.
- Prevents heart attack, stroke and diabetes. Powerful immune stimulant.
- Antioxidant protection, inhibits the formation of arteriosclerotic plaque.

HEMORRHOIDS

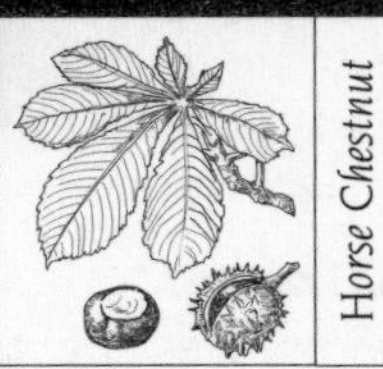

Select the herbs that are most suitable for your condition.

The Herbal Approach

Hemorrhoids occur when the rectal veins become swollen and engorged, because of collapsed back-flow valves within the veins and because of excessive pressure—similar to varicose veins. Hemorrhoids can occur in more superficial veins, with protruding external piles, or in deep veins, where only bleeding and pain signals their presence. Underlying factors are constipation and congestion of the venous system in inner organs—most commonly the liver or uterus. Weakness of the valves and vein walls often indicates overall damage to the body's connective tissue.

Herbs for hemorrhoids are often astringents that tighten and shrink swollen, inflamed tissue. Apart from those listed below, other traditional astringents used for hemorrhoids include *bistort, cranesbill, oak, pilewort, silverweed* and *tormentil.* Other effective herbs for the veins are strong antioxidants, with the ability to strengthen and heal the blood vessels. Still others act as local demulcents or emollients, soothing the area, like *aloe,* helping heal the tissues. Other plants that can be used for tissue healing include herbs for healing wounds, including *marigold* and St. *John's wort.* Herbs recommended for hemorrhoids may work by regulating the bowels, to prevent the straining or pressure that damages veins. Ultimately, other congested organs that contribute to the problem, particularly the liver, uterus and colon must be corrected. See also ■ Bleeding ■ Bruises ■ Colitis ■ Constipation ■ Diarrhea ■ Liver Conditions ■ Veins/Circulation.

Aloe**—Aloe vera/barbadensis
- Internally, taken as a commercial preparation, aloe vera gel relieves constipation, reduces liver congestion and heals hemorrhoids.
- Externally, the gel or fresh aloe is used directly on the hemorrhoid itself.

Butcher's Broom**—Ruscus aculeatus
- Internal use for hemorrhoids and varicose veins, reduces inflammation, Helps poor circulation. External use to reduce hemorrhoidal swelling.

Comfrey*—Symphytum officinale
- Anti-inflammatory, soothes irritation and promotes healing of tissues.
- Use locally as ointment, powdered root, or tea from the leaf or powder.
- Astringent contracts swollen, dilated tissue and decreases recurrence.

Horse Chestnut**—Aesculus hippocastanum
- Strengthens blood vessels, tones the veins; anti-inflammatory effects.
- Shrinks hemorrhoids, reduces swelling, pain, itching, blood clots.
- Can be taken internally or can be used as a local ointment or gel.

Mullein*—Verbascum thapsus
- A soothing emollient for hemorrhoids that are dry, sore and irritated.
- Mullein flower oil or infusion is applied locally to speed tissue healing.

Peony**—Paeonia officinalis
- Helps with burning, itching or irritated hemorrhoids or pain after stool.
- For fissures, ulcerations and fistula, with oozing of offensive moisture.

Plantain**—Plantago major
- An astringent that shrinks swollen veins, decreases related bleeding.
- Apply the ointment directly for relief of irritation and swelling.

Psyllium Seed**—Plantago psyllium
- Taken orally, relieves itching, bleeding and pain by correcting bowels.
- Benefits hemorrhoids by decreasing irritation from frequent loose stools or from overstraining due to constipation or hardened stool.
- Soothing to the digestive tract, draws toxins, metals from the body.

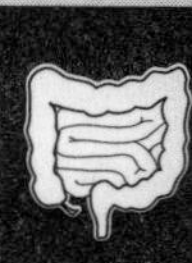

Slippery Elm***—Ulmus fulva
- Demulcent with a gel-like mucilage, used orally and locally.
- Externally, used to coat and soothe hemorrhoids, tighten up tissues.
- Internally, used in both constipation and diarrhea, or in irritable bowel and other colon disorders (e.g. diverticulitis, bowel inflammation).

Stone Root**—Collinsonia canadensis
- Relieves pain, itching, burning of chronic protruding or internal piles.
- Reduces bleeding; helps with chronic atonic constipation or diarrhea.
- Aids congested or toxic liver, anal prolapse. Use before rectal surgery.

Witch Hazel**—Hamamelis virginiana
- A soothing astringent that relieves pain and swelling, contracts and shrinks veins, heals bleeding hemorrhoids and helps with anal prolapse.
- Apply locally as an ointment, lotion or in a compress; used in most commercial hemorrhoid preparations or available full strength.

HERPES

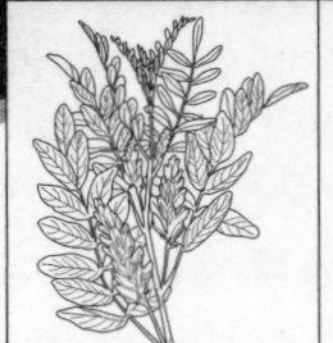

Select the herbs that are most appropriate for your condition.

The Herbal Approach

Herpes virus 1, related to the smallpox/chickenpox and Epstein-Barr virus group, is the cause of facial herpes, also known as cold sores or fever blisters. Once one is infected, this virus stays dormant in the nerves and skin, erupting when resistance is weakened by factors such as exposure to the sun, colds, fever, emotional stress, drugs or fatigue. Genital herpes is causes by herpes virus 2, and is usually sexually transmitted. Again, this virus stays latent in the lower nerve ganglia, and flare-ups occur around the vulva, penis, anus or on the thighs or buttocks. In both types, there may be itching, burning, tingling or numbness before an outbreak, extreme tenderness and sometimes overall fatigue or mild fever and swollen glands. Herpes zoster or shingles occurs along the course of the nerve of the chest wall or face (where it can dangerously affect the eye). Medical treatment requires constant or occasional use of Acyclovir, which only suppresses and has many toxic side effects.

There are a variety of herbs that can actually destroy herpes and other related viruses. Some work by stimulating specific immune-response factors, like interferon, while others slow or stop replication of the virus itself. In addition to the herbs below, *aloe* and *calendula* tincture (not cream), diluted in water (1–5 ratio) is an excellent and non-suppressive treatment for accelerating healing, used several times daily. See also ▪ Infection ▪ Inflammation ▪ Pain/Neuralgia ▪ Skin Conditions.

Cayenne**—Capsicum frutescens
- Internally has antiviral properties, helps prevent outbreaks.
- Use externally for pain relief during acute stages; apply for lingering pain or neuralgia after herpes or shingles.

Chaparral**—Larrea tridentata
- An antioxidant, antiseptic, antiviral and blood-purifier; can be applied directly to affected area. Fights associated colds, flu or digestive upset.

Echinacea**—Echinacea angustifolia
- Antiviral and antibacterial, a strong short-term immune stimulant.
- Take internally and apply as a wash or lotion to the infected area.

Goldenseal/Bearberry/Goldthread***—Berberis spp.
- A related group of herbs containing berberine. Antiseptic and anti-inflammatory, lessen duration of outbreak, support liver and digestion.
- Dries up fluid-filled blisters and cools the heat symptoms typical of herpes (facial or anal). Also benefit sores, abscesses, hives and burns.

Grapefruit Seed Extract***—Citrus paradisi
- Broad antibiotic action against bacteria, fungus, parasites and viruses.
- Effective when used externally, well-diluted, for facial or genital herpes.

Lavender Oil***—Lavandula angustifolia
- Antiviral, anti-inflammatory and antiseptic for sores, protects skin.
- Reduces pain and tissue sensitivity both before and during outbreak.
- Externally, useful for pain or neuralgia after herpes.

Lemon Balm***—Melissa officinalis
- Potent antiviral effects; combats herpes simplex, prevents its spread.
- Reduces symptoms of itching, burning, tingling, swelling and pain.
- Cuts healing time by half, while doubling the time between outbreaks.
- Use internally, as well as an external ointment several times daily.

Licorice**—Glycyrrhiza glabra
- An immune stimulant and adrenal booster with powerful antiviral and anti-inflammatory effects, used internally and as an external ointment.
- Reduces pain and speeds healing of herpes; inactivates the virus.

Lomatium**—Lomatium dissectum
- Antiviral activity against both DNA and RNA viruses, herpes 1 and 2, shingles and Epstein-Barr; also has broad antibacterial properties.
- Provides symptom relief; best taken at the beginning of an outbreak.

Olive Leaf**—Olea europaea
- Effective against a wide spectrum of viruses, including herpes simplex and genitalia, shingles. Can be taken as a preventive after exposure.
- Immune booster that also fights Lyme disease, candida, parasites.
- Interferes with amino acids needed for growth and life cycle of viruses.

Passionflower**—Passiflora incarnata
- A pain reliever and nervine that strengthens nerves, relieves anxiety.
- Effective for neuralgia after viral infections such as shingles or herpes.
- Used long term, may prevent attacks brought on by excess stress.

Pau D'Arco**—LaPacho/Tabebuia avellanedae
- Effective for herpes and many other viruses, bacteria and fungi.
- An antioxidant that relieves pain, reduces inflammation and allergy.

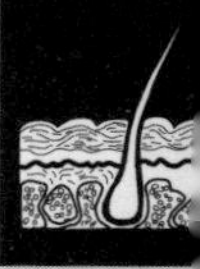

St. John's Wort***—Hypericum perforatum
- Potent antiviral for a wide range of viruses, including herpes 1 and 2.
- Useful internally during all phases, helps with post-herpes neuralgia.
- Use external cream to heal tissue, decrease pain and inflammation.

Tea Tree Oil***—Melaleuca alternifolia
- Antiviral, antiseptic and immune stimulant; relieves dryness, itching and irritation during prodrome and outbreak period. Prevents scarring.

High Blood Pressure

Select the herbs that are most suitable for your condition.

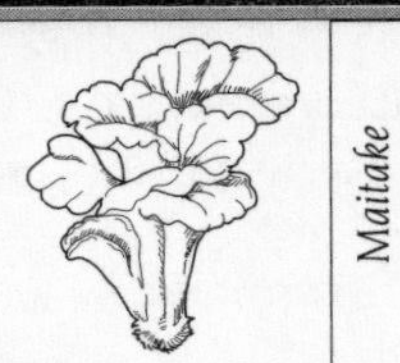

The Herbal Approach

Blood pressure reflects the tension within arterial walls, fluctuating according to the body's need for oxygen and nutrients. Elevated blood pressure is a disease of modern culture affecting over 40 million. This predisposes to heart attack and stroke, weakens the heart and can damage the eyes, brain and kidneys. Over 90% of cases are due to arterial constriction related to an overactive sympathetic nervous system. More serious is hypertension due to hardening of the arteries, preventing dilation of the vessels. Other underlying causes are kidney problems, increased levels of stress hormones, obesity, diet, and toxins such as heavy metals and alcohol.

Diet, herbs and natural therapeutics have been shown to both prevent and reduce blood pressure significantly, aided by stress-reducing methods like meditation and yoga. If medications are being used, herbs should be used, as an addition or substitution, only under professional supervision. Some of the best anti-hypertensive herbs are antispasmodic and nervine, while others are cardiac tonics. Most also lower cholesterol, combat arteriosclerosis and thin the blood. Diuretics like *cornsilk*, *parsley* and *chickweed* may also be useful, and liver herbs may be needed to correct cholesterol metabolism. See also ■ Arteriosclerosis ■ Cholesterol, High ■ Heart Conditions ■ Liver Disorders ■ Stress.

Cayenne**—Capsicum frutescens
- Improves elasticity of the blood vessels regulating blood pressure.
- Stimulates blood flow, lowers cholesterol; may aid arteriosclerosis.
- Reduces risk of clotting, increases heart output, strengthens vessels.

Curcumin**—Turmeric/Curcuma longa
- Reduces cholesterol and blood lipids, prevents blood clot formation.
- Powerful antioxidant that prevents arteriosclerosis, improves arterial blood flow, strengthens blood vessels. Corrects liver metabolism.

Garlic***—Allium sativa
- Lowers blood pressure, reduces blood stickiness, lowers cholesterol, triglycerides, increases ratio of HDL. Prevents cholesterol oxidation.
- Keeps plaque from adhering to artery walls, promotes clot dissolution.

Ginger**—Zingiber officinale
- Improves and stimulates circulation; relaxes the small muscles surrounding peripheral blood vessels, dilates blood vessels.

- Strengthens and tones heart; improves its contractions and efficiency.
- Lowers blood lipid levels, prevents clots; prevents arterial damage.

Ginkgo**—Ginkgo biloba
- Dilates blood vessels, improves flow through arteries, reduces pressure.
- Helps with vertigo, memory loss, cognition and peripheral circulation.

Hawthorn***—Crataegus officinalis
- Excellent heart tonic with anti-hypertensive effects. Dilates blood vessels, especially coronary arteries. Gradually reduces arteriosclerosis.
- Long-term treatment for elderly, rehabilitation after heart attack.
- Useful for weak valves or heart muscle, aneurism, angina, heart failure.

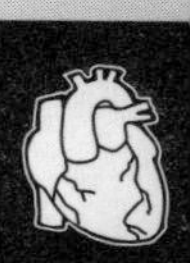

Linden***—Tilia europaea
- Valuable for arteriosclerosis and reducing high blood pressure.
- A sedative and antispasmodic; relieves anxiety, insomnia, stress effects.
- Combines well with heart tonics: hawthorn, motherwort or ginkgo.

Maitake***—Grifola frondosa
- Anti-hypertensive, lowers plasma LDL and HDL cholesterol levels.
- Produces a decrease in both systolic and diastolic blood pressure; one study showed a mean of 14 mm Hg systolic and 8 mm Hg diastolic.

Mistletoe*—Viscum album
- Used for hypertension, enlarged heart, weak valves, angina, palpitations. Lowers blood pressure, promotes sleep, relieves anxiety.

Motherwort**—Leonarus cardiaca
- Lowers blood pressure, normalizes heart rhythm and slows rate.
- A heart tonic that improves blood flow to the coronary arteries.
- Sedative properties, helping calm anxiety, tension, relieve palpitations.

Olive Leaf*—Olea europaea
- Lowers blood pressure, relieves arrhythmias, prevents spasms.
- Reduces LDL cholesterol. Combats viral, bacterial and fungal infection.

Rosemary**—Rosmarinus officinalis
- Normalizes blood pressure. Protects blood vessels and is a warming circulatory stimulant. Promotes healthy heart, enhances the adrenals.
- Improves circulation to head, increases mental acuity, benefits moods.

Siberian Ginseng—Eleutherococcus senticosus
- Helps equalize blood pressure, lowering or raising it to normal levels.
- An adaptogenic herb that influences the adrenals and nervous system.
- Improves circulation, increases stamina and vitality.

Valerian**—Valeriana officinalis
- Lowers blood pressure, increases levels of GABA, while acting as a mild tranquilizer and sedative. Reduces tension and anxiety, aids sleep.

HIV/AIDS

Select the herbs that are most suitable for your condition.

The Herbal Approach

It is difficult to do justice to this complex condition here, except to state that there are many herbs that have an essential role to play in slowing the progression of HIV, prolonging life and helping create remissions. Herbal use in these infections has been the topic of intense research, with very promising results. Useful herbs for HIV and AIDS are as diverse as the conditions themselves. There are those that have been shown to slow or stop viral replication, or prevent infection from progressing to various AIDS syndromes. Other herbs are essential for their unique ability to enhance immunity, while infection fighting plants take stress off an already over-burdened system. A coordinated program is necessary to integrate the many botanical medicines referred to here and in the cross-references. See also ■ Anti-aging ■ Cancer ■ Depression ■ Diarrhea ■ Immune Weakness ■ Infection ■ Liver Conditions.

Astragalus***—Milk Vetch/Astragalus membranaceous

- Antiviral, immune stimulant; improves white cells, infection resistance.
- Adaptogen that increases the body's energy reserves, relieves night sweats, reduces thirst, protects the liver against toxic chemicals.

Cat's Claw*—Una de Gato/Uncaria tormentosa

- A number of reports indicate that this herb improves various symptoms and overall well-being, as well as blood counts in AIDS patients.
- A commercial extract, Krallendorn, may halt HIV progression to AIDS.

Curcumin***—Turmeric/Curcuma longa

- Inhibits specific proteins (HIV integrase) necessary for viral replication.
- Anti-inflammatory; reduces chemical cascades prompting HIV multiplication; viral load is greatly decreased using 3 gm daily for eight weeks.

Garlic***—Allium sativa

- Antiviral effects; inhibits the chemical cell signals that stimulate inflammation and subsequent HIV replication.
- Antioxidant effect, decreases the toxicity of cell-damaging compounds.

Ginseng***—Panax ginseng

- Tones the adrenals, pituitary, thyroid, thymus, liver and spleen.
- Increases interferon production, number of cytotoxic and natural killer cells. Stimulates liver detoxification, increases resistance to colds, flu.

Isatis**—Isatis tinctoria

- Used for viral, fungal and bacterial infections; shown to be effective for

common viral conditions, as well as hepatitis and HIV.
- Works against strep and a variety of secondary HIV-related sequelae.

Licorice***—Glycyrrhiza glabra
- Elevates T cells, improves liver, tones adrenals, stimulates interferon.
- Inhibits HIV replication and the progression from HIV to AIDS.
- Antiviral for Epstein-Barr, herpes, HIV; fights allergies & inflammation.

Maitake***—Grifola frondosa
- Strongly stimulates immune function (e.g. interleukins, lymphokines).
- As effective as AZT to prevent HIV destruction of helper and killer T cells.
- Promotes survival of infected cells, improves many AIDS symptoms.
- Reduces cancers; used topically with DMSO to clear Kaposi's sarcoma.

Milk Thistle—Silybum marum
- Increases overall immune response, protects the liver against toxins and poisons, regenerates liver cells even after damage has occurred.
- Increases the vital antioxidants glutathione and superoxide dismutase.
- Inhibits HIV replication through its anti-inflammatory properties.

Olive Leaf**—Olea europaea
- Interferes with virus's ability to make enzymes necessary for replication.
- Provides defense against protozoa, bacteria and fungi, including drug resistant bacteria. Decreases enteritis, bronchitis, sinusitis, herpes.

Pau D'Arco**—LaPacho/Tabebuia avellanedae
- Combats bacteria, viruses, parasites and fungi in the intestines, vagina, in immunosuppressed conditions like HIV/AIDS and cancer.
- Anti-inflammatory, antioxidant, pain-relieving and anti-allergy.

Reishi***—Ganoderma lucidum
- Enhances immunity; stimulates macrophages, TNF, interleukins.
- Prevents HIV progression to AIDS by protecting the body's T cells.
- An adaptogen that improves liver health; can markedly relieve fatigue.

Shiitake***—Lentinus edodes
- Stimulates immunity; increasing interferon, T cells, macrophages.
- Antiviral effects; may be more effective than AZT at blocking initial stages of HIV infection. Antioxidant, inhibits various cancers, tumors.

Siberian Ginseng**—Eleuthrococcus senticosus
- Immune stimulant, restores vigor, regulates insomnia, depression.
- Improves poor memory, resistance to infection and speeds recovery.
- Provides fortification in times of overwork or conditions of fatigue.

St. John's Wort**—Hypericum perforatum
- An antiviral herb, hypericin extract has effects against the HIV virus.
- Greatly extended the life span of people with AIDS in one study.
- Hypericin is in the second stage of a clinical AIDS research study.

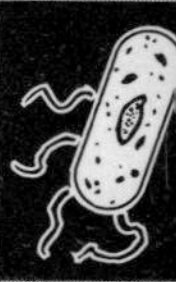

HIVES

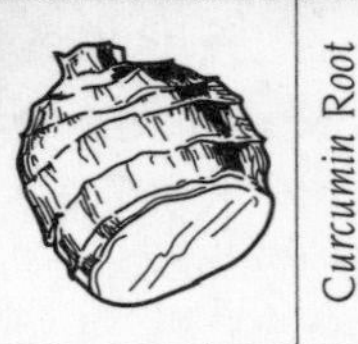

Select the herbs that are most suitable for your condition.

The Herbal Approach

Hives or urticaria are an allergic reaction that manifest as extremely itchy welts of varying size. The most common cause is food or airborne allergens, or direct contact with dyes, chemicals, clothing or other materials. However, side effects from prescription or over-the-counter medications are another frequent and easily overlooked cause. Often the tendency toward hives is due to intestinal parasites or fungi, and part of a larger picture of disordered intestinal bacteria (dysbiosis), liver toxicity, and immune system weakness. Flare-ups can also occur with exposure to cold air or exercise. Hives are often acute allergic reactions, but chronic hives are becoming much more common, where the cause of the problem is obscure and medical treatment is strictly symptomatic.

There are many extremely effective antihistamine herbs, outshining their drug counterparts, without side effects such as drowsiness and fatigue. They also prevent tissue damage and remove debris left by the inflammatory process. Detoxifying herbs and a program of liver and immune system rehabilitation can go a long way toward eradicating hypersensitivity reactions to foods, chemicals and environmental toxins. See ■ Detoxification ■ Hayfever ■ Immune Weakness ■ Skin Conditions.

Aloe**—Aloe vera

- Applied topically, reduces inflammation, provides protective coating.
- Cooling to the tissues, relieves itching, redness, stinging and pain.
- Internally, stimulates immunity and elimination of inflammatory toxins.

Bromelain***—Pineapple/Ananas comosus

- More effective anti-inflammatory than most drugs, decreases the allergic response, alleviating hives, skin irritations. Accelerates healing.
- Non-toxic in large internal doses; may be applied directly to the hives.

Burdock**—Arctium lappa

- A liver and blood detoxifier, diuretic, digestive stimulant; assists in clearance of cellular and lymphatic debris, reduces tissue swelling.
- Purifies skin problems such as hives, acne, boils, eczema and psoriasis.
- Stimulates the immune system; antibacterial, antiviral, antifungal.

Chinese Skullcap**—Scutellaria baicalensis

- Contains potent flavonoids that are anti-allergic and anti-inflammatory.
- Stabilizes body during increased immune stress or allergen overload.
- Cools conditions of "damp heat" such as hives, fever, infections.

Curcumin***—Turmeric/Curcuma longa

- Stimulates the body's natural anti-inflammatory corticosteroids.
- Very effective natural antihistamine and antioxidant for hives and a variety of inflammatory skin ailments. Protects liver against toxins.

Echinacea***—Echinacea angustifolia

- Anti-inflammatory; reduces sensitivity to allergens, stings or bites.
- Encourages blood and lymph drainage, modulates and balances a hyper-reactive immune system. antiviral and antibacterial effects.

Ginger***—Zingiber officinale

- Rapidly quells the onset of hives, itching or other allergic responses.
- A potent anti-inflammatory and antihistamine, improves skin circulation, relieves swelling and carries away inflammatory waste products.

Goldenseal/Coptis/Oregon Grape**—Berberis spp

- Soothing herbs for swelling, itching; ideal for hives and skin disorders such as boils, sores, abscesses and fluid-filled or pustular eruptions.
- Tonic and detoxifying to the liver, gall bladder, stomach and intestines.

Green Tea***—Camellia sinensis

- Strong antihistamine, reducing hives and other allergic inflammations.
- High in antioxidant polyphenols and flavonoids that protects against oxidative, toxic damage to the tissues. Enhances the immune system.

Licorice**—Glycyrrhiza glabra

- Antihistamine and anti-inflammatory, increases levels of cortisone.
- Immune stimulating, improves stress response, antiviral activity.
- DGL form is not effective for allergy. Also use locally as a tea or lotion.

Nettles***—Urtica dioica

- Freeze-dried form provides fast-acting antihistamine, symptom relief.
- Anti-inflammatory and astringent to relieve swelling or edema of hives.
- Detoxifying and diuretic, encourages excretion of inflammatory wastes.

Quercetin***—Quercetin

- A non-toxic, potent antihistamine bioflavonoid, decreases inflammation of allergic skin and hay fever conditions. Strengthens capillaries
- May be taken acutely during hive outbreak or as a preventive measure.

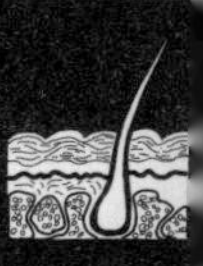

Schisandra**—Schisandra chinensis

- Chinese herb that alleviates hives, eczema and swollen tissues.
- A tonic for the adrenals, increases ability to deal with chemical stress.
- Improves sluggish or deficient liver and protects it from various toxins.

Yarrow***—Achillea millefolium

- Pain-relieving astringent, antiseptic and anti-inflammatory action.
- Take internally or apply directly to hives to quell inflammation and pain associated with swollen tissues. Detoxifies tissues of cellular waste.

IMMUNE WEAKNESS

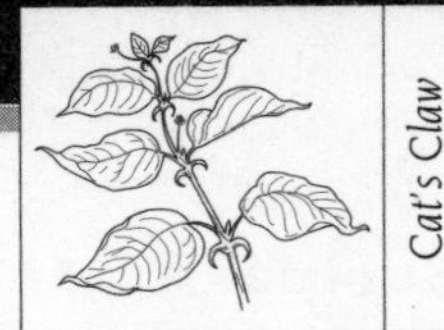

Select the herbs that are most suitable for your condition.

The Herbal Approach

Less than 25 years ago, the "greater defense system" was not recognized as a separate body system and the tonsils and appendix were considered to be a vestigial—the body's unwanted leftovers. Today we know the immune system as the central command post that provides continual surveillance and monitoring of the body's farthest frontiers. With the thymus as the immune "brain" and the spleen as the workhorse, specialized chemicals and a variety of cells seek out and neutralize toxins, microorganisms, allergens and cellular wastes. A vast system of lymphatic channels and lymph nodes filter out and destroy debris. Understandably, this overworked system can become weakened or damaged. Various drugs, viruses and heavy metals can be immunosuppressive. Chronic allergy and immune imbalance can also result in autoimmunity, implicated in thyroid disease, arthritis, diabetes and a whole host of chronic conditions.

Herbs are the most potent agents known for improving immune function. Many are immune modulators, either boosting or calming a disordered immune system. Many specific effects have been demonstrated, but these tonic and adaptogenic herbs have the global result of re-organizing and revitalizing this most crucial system, with its subtle and intelligent functioning. See also ■ Hayfever/Allergies ■ HIV/AIDS ■ Hives ■ Infection.

Astragalus***—Milk Vetch/Astragalus membranaceous

- Powerful tonic and immune strengthener, increases T cells, killer cells, interferon. Increases resistance to infection, flu; speeds recovery time.
- Excellent in hepatitis, AIDS, colds, viral disease, fevers, chronic fatigue, repeated infections, bronchitis; improves circulation, heart health.

Cat's Claw**—Una de Gato/Uncaria tormentosa

- Boosts immune function, increases circulation, reduces heart rate and cholesterol and improves response to viral and respiratory infections.
- Has been used in chronic fatigue syndrome, lupus, diabetes, arthritis.

Cordyceps***—Cordyceps sinensis

- Enhances immunity, increasing helper T cells and killer cells, speeds up spleen regeneration. Improves uptake of oxygen by brain and heart.
- Hormone enhancement, greatly increasing endurance and performance.

Echinacea***—Echinacea angustifolia

- Short-term immune booster; increases interferon, T cells, number and activity of white cells, chemical barriers and lymphatic drainage.
- Protects against viral and bacterial infection; destroys infected cells.

Ginseng***—Panax ginseng
- Adaptogenic and tonic for the adrenal, pituitary, thyroid, liver, spleen.
- Enhances immune-modulating interferon and interleukin-2, increases numerous immune cells including killer T cells. Strong vitality booster.

Larix**—Larix occidentalis
- Arabinogalactan extract has similar effects to echinacea, shiitake and astragalus. Enhances immunity, increases action of macrophages.
- Useful against various viruses and in the treatment of cancer, colds, flu, allergy, middle ear infections, asthma.

Licorice**—Glycyrrhiza glabra
- An adaptogen, stimulating or calming the immune system's activity.
- Stimulates interferon production, inhibits atrophy of thymus, improves adrenal health and cortisol production. antiviral and antibacterial.

Maitake**—Grifola frondosa
- Stimulates immune system, increases natural killer cells, macrophages, interleukin 1 & 2, white cells. Inhibits cancers, protects healthy cells.
- Most powerful and best absorbed of the medicinal mushrooms.

Pau D'Arco**—LaPacho/Tabebuia avellanedae
- Treats cancer and other severe immune deficiencies. Combats bacteria, viruses, parasites, fungi. Anti-inflammatory, antioxidant and pain killing.

Reishi**—Ganoderma lucidum
- Adaptogen, relieving fatigue, enhancing immunity in numerous ways; increases T cells, interleukin 2 production, protects against radiation.
- Antiviral, anti-inflammatory; improves depression, insomnia and anxiety. Protects and enhances the liver, balances blood sugar. Heart tonic.

Schisandra***—Schisandra chinensis
- Tonic to the immune system, circulation, nerves and digestion.
- Protects and heals the liver. Protects against toxins and viral infection.
- Improves mood, memory and sleep; increases work and efficiency.
- Counters effects of stimulants, coffee. Helps skin, has aphrodisiac effects.

Shiitake***—Lentinus edodes
- Stimulates immunity; increasing interferon, T cells, macrophages.
- Inhibits various cancers; used for stomach cancer in Japan. The extract Lentinan is used as injectable anti-tumor drug. Has antiviral capacity.

Siberian Ginseng**—Eleuthrococcus senticosus
- Adaptogenic herb, improves response to stress and fatigue, increases resistance. Decreases incidence of colds and flu by 40%.
- Immune stimulant that increases T cells, counteracts environmental toxins and effects of toxic drugs. Tonic for weakness and convalescence.

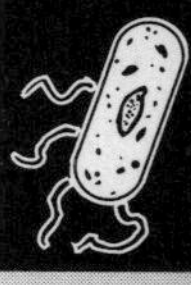

IMPOTENCE/MALE INFERTILITY

Select the herbs that are most suitable for your condition.

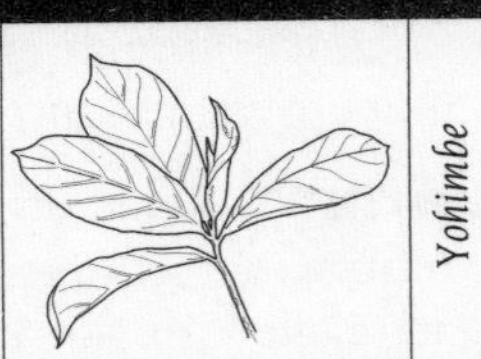

The Herbal Approach

Erectile dysfunction (ED) is increasingly common, affecting 30 million Americans between ages of 30 and 70. Most cases—some 80% are due to circulatory problems, drug side effects, hormonal imbalance, prostate problems or injury. Smoking, high blood pressure, diabetes, obesity and depression are also definite causes. Additionally, a reduction in male hormones, rise in male infertility and a global decrease in sperm count is mainly due to the estrogen-like effects of pesticides and other environmental toxins. Thus infertility in couples is due to the male in 35% of cases. "Male menopause" is also a fact of life, expressed as a decrease of testosterone and related functions.

Some herbs work like Viagra, increasing circulation to the pelvic area and penis. Others act through mental relaxation or by stimulating specific brain areas. Importantly, tonic and adaptogenic herbs have long-term androgen/testosterone–building effects, rejuvenating the pituitary, adrenals and gonads to balance hormones and increase sex drive. Viagra does none of these. The result can be a permanent improvement in both sexual function and total health. See also ■ Fatigue ■ Infertility ■ Prostate Problems ■ Stress.

Ashwaganda**—Withania somnifera
- Ancient tonic for promoting longevity, vitality. Increases sperm count.
- Normalizes reproductive hormones. Improves endurance and fatigue.

Astragalus**—Milk Vetch/Astragalus membranaceous
- Increases sperm count, vitality, energy, sexual function and endurance.
- Normalizes reproductive glands, improves nervous and immune function.

Chaste Tree**—Agnus castus
- Treats impotence, infertility and emissions, especially in old age, from sexual overindulgence, excess masturbation or after venereal disease.
- Regulates the pituitary, increases sperm count, increases testosterone.

Cordyceps**—Cordyceps sinensis
- Helps impotence, improves sexual function and release of reproductive hormones, increases sperm activity and is used in states of exhaustion.

Damiana***—Turneria aphrodisiaca
- Stimulates circulation in the penis and clitoris, increases sensitivity.
- Enhances pleasure, stimulates sexual performance, relieves anxiety.
- Strengthens hormonal and nervous systems; testosterone-like effects.

Ginkgo**—Ginkgo biloba
- Improves circulation to the penis to help erectile function. Helps with impotence due to antidepressant drugs; effective for depression.

Ginseng**—Panax ginseng
- Stimulating tonic and adaptogen. Impotent men show a 60% increase in sex drive and ability to achieve erection. Increases interest, function.
- Increases sperm production, growth of testes, testosterone levels.

Maca***—Lepidium meyenii
- Traditional Peruvian aphrodisiac and cure for impotence, infertility.
- Increases sex drive, sexual stamina and strength; improves erectile dysfunction, male impotence, increases sperm count, counters fatigue.
- Improves physical strength; helps maintain activity in geriatric men.

Muira Puama***—Ptychopetalum olacoides
- Increases sexual desire, helps in impotency or maintaining erection.
- May work through nervous system or increase sex hormone production.
- Studies show it increases libido in 62% and improves impotence in 51%.

Oats**—Avena sativa
- For impotence due to nervous exhaustion, overwork, mental stress.
- Helps with substance withdrawal. Neurological tonic, improves libido.

Sarsaparilla**—Smilax officinalis
- Contains precursors to synthesis of male sex hormones. Used traditionally in Central and South America, as well as China and Caribbean.
- A tonic and aphrodisiac, increases muscle mass, treats impotence.

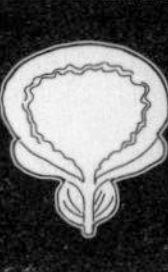

Schisandra***—Schisandra chinensis
- Sexual tonic and aphrodisiac, stimulates libido, sexual secretions.
- Enhances overall stamina and longevity. Improves stress response.
- Improves mood, sleep, efficiency. Counteracts effects of stimulants.

Siberian Ginseng**—Eleuthrococcus senticosus
- Heightens sexual performance, increases sperm count, reproductive vigor and vitality; balances hormones. Helps impotence due to stress.
- Promotes sound sleep, increases endurance, well-being, mental acuity.

Tribulus**—Tribulus terrestris
- Helps low sex drive, impotence, infertility; improves heart, liver, kidney.
- Markedly stimulates libido, fertility in both sexes; increases testosterone and estriol levels significantly (30% in 5 days). Helps menopause.

Yohimbe*—Pausinystalia yohimbe
- Increases ability to achieve and maintain erection, working on circulation to the penis. Has adrenaline-like activity and potential toxicity.
- FDA approved for impotence, requires 6 to 8 weeks for maximum effect.

Infection

Goldenseal

Select the herbs that are most suitable for your condition.

The Herbal Approach

In the 1940s, medicine promised a cure for bacterial infection, stating outright that this ancient scourge of humankind would be a thing of the past. This was also the time when some 60% of the herbs that were in the U.S. Pharmacopoeia disappeared, to be replaced by hugely profitable, patented pharmaceutical drugs. Yet the antibiotics of yesterday and today have not lived up to their promise, but have produced generations of increasingly resistant bacteria. Antibiotics have been so overused that they themselves are a major health hazard, with side-effects that damage the liver, kidney, nervous and immune systems.

Herbs have been used safely for thousands of years to treat infections of every kind, be they viral, bacterial or fungal. There are enough of these to write several books, but below are some of the most powerful and often used infection-fighters. Others are cross-referenced below. Additionally, detoxifying and immune-building herbs are needed to increase resistance and eliminate underlying tendencies to infection. See also ■ Candida/Yeast ■ Detoxification ■ Immune Weakness ■ Parasites.

Bayberry**—Myrica cerifera
- Widespread antibiotic effects for gum disease, sore throats, coughs, colds, flu; used as a vaginal douche and externally for ulcers, abscess.
- Digestive disinfectant for diarrhea, gastritis, colitis, food poisoning.

Echinacea***—Echinacea angustifolia
- Stops viral and bacterial infection, colds, bronchitis, sinusitis, strep throat, abnormal pap smears; externally for wounds, stings, boils.
- Intensifies immunity, interferon production, T cells, macrophages.

Garlic***—Allium sativa
- Effective against at least 30 types of bacteria, viruses, fungi, amoeba and parasites. Used for intestinal or respiratory infection, otitis.
- Activates immune system, stimulates it to attack invading organisms.

Goldenseal***—Hydrastis canadensis
- Wide-spectrum antibiotic against staph, strep, E. coli, giardia, amoeba.
- Anti-inflammatory and astringent; useful for every lining tissue: eyes, mouth, intestines, throat, bronchi, stomach, intestines, vagina, skin.

Grapefruit Seed Extract***—Citrus paradisi
- Along with garlic, the most effective agent against over 1,000 bacteria, yeasts, fungi. Safe and non-toxic for both internal and external use.

Lemon Grass**—Cymbopogan citratus
- Antibiotic for flu, coughs, fevers and pain, colic, gas, stomach problems.
- Essential oil is antifungal and antibacterial, used locally on ringworm.

Lomatium***—Lomatium dissectum
- Immune herb with antiviral, antibacterial and antifungal properties.
- Best for stubborn, chronic respiratory or urinary tract infections.

Myrrh***—Commiphora myrrha
- Antiseptic, antimicrobial, anti-inflammatory and astringent herb.
- A rinse or gargle for mouth, gums, throat. Internally for infections of the lungs, colitis; use externally for boils, abscesses, wounds, vaginitis.

Neem**—Azadirachta indica
- Blood purifier and detoxifier, stimulates immune system to respond to infections. Broad effects against parasites, fungus, malaria and TB.
- External use for ringworm, lice, skin fungus, eczema, ulcers, wounds.

Olive Leaf***—Olea europaea
- Powerful action against many viruses, bacteria, yeast and fungi, including HIV, Epstein-Barr, retrovirus, malaria, parasites, colds and flu.
- Treats fevers, sore throat, respiratory or sinus infections, herpes, yeast or fungal infections, toothaches, chronic fatigue and allergy symptoms.

Oregano Oil***—Origanum vulgare
- Volatile oil exits via the lungs, loosens phlegm, kills most organisms.
- Effective for intestinal infection, parasites, worms. Antispasmodic effect.
- Expectorant and antibiotic for colds, flu, coughs, chest congestion.

Osha**—Ligusticum porteri
- Antiviral and antibacterial, works best during initial stages of infection.
- Treats respiratory infections, sore throats, coughs, colds, flu and digestive upsets. Good for fevers related to measles. Also antispasmodic.

Pau D'Arco**—LaPacho/Tabebuia avellanedae
- Fights viruses, bacteria, fungi, including herpes, candida, HIV.
- Used for nose and throat infections, intestinal dysbiosis, cystitis, prostatitis. An immune stimulant, blood purifier and pain reliever.

Tea Tree Oil***—Melaleuca alternifolia
- External use for bacteria, virus and fungi, even drug-resistant germs.
- Effective in acne, candida, ringworm, bites, athlete's foot, shingles, nail infections, wounds, bronchitis, colds, sinusitis. Use as wash, vaporizer.

Usnea***—Lichen/Usnea species
- Destroys staph, strep and many other bacteria, TB, fungus infections, ringworm, athlete's foot, candida. Good for respiratory infections, colds.
- Anti-parasitic against vaginal infections: trichomonas, chlamydia.

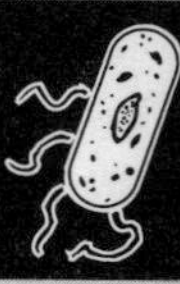

INFERTILITY

False Unicorn

Select the herbs that are most suitable for your condition.

The Herbal Approach

By 1995 there were over 6 million women between ages 15 and 40 who had difficulty in having children, with some 10 million women using infertility services. Two million married couples have such problems, affecting one in five couples between ages 35 and 40. In fact infertility—defined as the inability to conceive after one year of trying—is the most common disorder of men and women of reproductive age. The greatest single cause of this epidemic is, without doubt, environmental estrogen-disruptors, in the form of pesticides, PCBs, DDT and even estrogen via municipal water supplies—residues of women on the pill. Yet, even in the aging population, natural therapies have been shown to produce excellent results in a majority of cases. Of course infertility also results from hormonal imbalances, with ovarian cysts leading the way. Undiagnosed and asymptomatic infections are also present in up to half of all infertile couples. Fertility drugs should be a last resort when underlying causes cannot be found and natural therapeutics are ineffective. However, half of all pregnancies from the fertility drug Clomiphene are miscarried. Herbs are *extremely* effective in promoting fertility and preventing miscarriage. Check the Dosage section, and once pregnant, take herbs only under the direction of an herbal expert. A phytoestrogen-rich and pesticide-free diet will go a long way toward promoting fertility, naturally. See also ■ Amenorrhea ■ Detoxification ■ Impotence/Male Infertility ■ Liver Conditions ■ Menopause ■ Miscarriage ■ PMS.

Black Cohosh***—Cimicifuga racemosa
- Optimizes use of estrogen in the body, balancing excess or deficiency.
- Re-regulates and normalizes cycles, helps delayed or missed periods.
- Promotes pituitary hormones that stimulate release of egg from ovary.

Chasteberry***—Vitex agnus castus
- Working via the pituitary, increases progesterone formation in the body.
- Normalizes menstrual cycle, increasing fertility (take for 12–18 months).
- In human studies, Vitex led to pregnancy in approximately 15% of cases.
- Regulates menses after the pill, emotional upset, exercise, illness.

Dong Quai***—Angelica sinensis
- Traditional Chinese herb to promote fertility, reestablish normal menstrual cycle after discontinuing the pill. Often used in combination.
- Increases progesterone and balances estrogen/progesterone ratio.
- Promotes blood flow, so do not use once pregnant or during menses.

False Unicorn***—Helonias/Chamaelirium luteum
- Excellent tonic for weak, prolapsed uterus and tendency to miscarriage.
- Hormonal and ovarian regulator, brings on absent or delayed menses.
- Prevents miscarriage, relieves pelvic congestion, improves libido.

Fo-Ti***—Polygonum multiflora
- Ancient Chinese longevity herb, increases fertility in men and women.
- Strengthens the reproductive organs, liver, kidney and blood.
- Promotes vitality, sexual vigor. Good for older women trying to conceive.

Licorice***—Glycyrrhiza glabra
- Balances estrogen, progesterone and testosterone ratio, regulates infrequent periods or amenorrhea. Helps to correct ovarian cysts.
- Helps with stress response, improving health of adrenals, immunity.

Maca***—Lepidium meyenii
- Peruvian aphrodisiac, increases hormone levels, energy and stamina.
- Enhances fertility. In animal tests, increases number of pregnancies and birth weights. Regulates and balances menstrual cycle or amenorrhea.

Motherwort**—Leonarus cardiaca
- Improves fertility and frigidity. Helps to regulate the menstrual cycle after stopping the pill; brings on delayed menses. Helps tone the uterus.
- Calms anxiety and tension; a heart tonic that lowers blood pressure.

Partridgeberry**—Mitchella repens
- A Native American fertility and pregnancy herb; helps with amenorrhea and menstrual irregularities, relieves exhaustion and irritability.
- Improves uterine circulation, reduces congestion, improves its tone.

Red Clover***—Trifolium pratense
- Provides 4 phytoestrogen compounds; balances hormones, correcting deficient or excess pituitary or ovary output. Protects against pesticides.
- Improves uterine tone, general detoxifier; promotes lymphatic drainage.

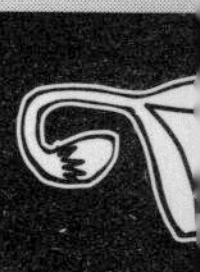

Shativari***—Asparagus racemosa
- Main Ayurvedic female tonic, promotes fertility and estrogen production.
- Prime female rejuvenator, sexual tonic; strengthens reproductive organs.
- Regulates menstrual cycle, helps loss of libido, threatened miscarriage.

Siberian Ginseng**—Eleuthrococcus senticosus
- Improves overall energy, vitality, well-being and stress adaptation.
- Acts on endocrine glands, including pituitary, to regulate hormones and reproductive function. Strengthens sexual organs and their function.

Wild Yam**—Dioscorea villosa
- Helps correct low progesterone and high estrogen ratio. Best taken from ovulation to menstruation. A muscle relaxant and antispasmodic.
- Strengthens and stabilizes uterus blood vessels, maintains its lining.

INFLAMMATION

Select the herbs that are most suitable for your condition.

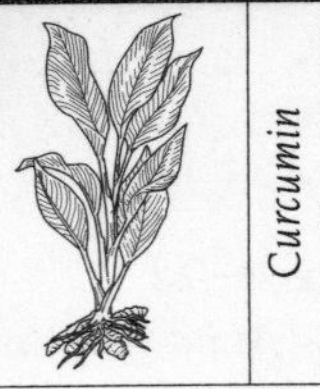

The Herbal Approach

Inflammation is a natural reaction of the body and one of its primary mechanisms for combatting infection, toxins, irritations and injuries. It plays a part in a majority of illnesses and in literally any area of the body. Inflammation can be acute (intense and short lived) or long standing. However, imbalances in the inflammation pathway can occur. Nutritional deficiencies, allergy, pro-inflammatory substances such as refined fatty acids, a disturbed digestive system, liver malfunction or immune weakness can result in unregulated and chronic inflammatory reactions.

In numerous studies, herbs have been shown to be both more effective and safer than medical anti-inflammatory drugs (NSAIDs) or even cortisone. In fact, NSAIDs inhibit a number of our positive chemical pathways that fight inflammation naturally. The newest NSAIDs, the Cox-2 inhibitors (Vioxx and Celebrex), are designed to be more specific, since they do not inhibit these pathways. But they have their own side effects. Natural Cox-2 inhibitors like *ginger*, *skullcap* and *curcumin* are more effective, without harmful side effects. See also ■ Burns ■ Injury/Wounds.

Boswellia—Boswellia serrata
- Reduces pain and swelling after injury; as effective as Ibuprofen.
- Effective anti-inflammatory for arthritis and may be taken preventively to stop the cascade of inflammatory and pain chemicals in the tissues.
- Does not produce stomach irritation or ulcers, even with long-term use.

Bromelain***—Pineapple/Ananas comosus
- Cuts healing time in half after injury, breaks down cellular wastes, which contribute to inflammation and swelling, improves local circulation.
- Most potent action compared to nine common anti-inflammatory drugs.
- Decreases the duration of swelling and pain after surgery.

Chamomile**—Matricaria recutita
- Anti-inflammatory and antihistamine, prevents redness, irritation, itching and swelling. Reduces digestive bloating, inflammation and spasm.
- Antioxidant, antibacterial, antifungal for cleansing wounds, ulcers.

Curcumin***—Turmeric/Curcuma longa
- Powerful anti-inflammatory, more effective than NSAIDs (Ibuprofen).
- Particularly useful for inflammation of the joints or digestive system.
- Prevents free radical damage, provides strong antioxidant protection.

Ginger***—Zingiber officinale
- Potent analgesic, anti-inflammatory and immune stimulant.
- Superior to NSAIDs in relieving muscle pain, swelling and stiffness.
- Reduces arthritic inflammation, used both internally and topically.
- Has protein-digesting enzymes 80 times more potent than pineapple.

Flaxseed***—Linum usitatissimum
- Ground seeds or flax oil contains anti-inflammatory omega 3 fatty acids.
- Promotes healthy cell membranes, reduces excess permeability.
- Maintains healthy prostaglandin pathway; long-term preventive.

Hawthorn***—Crataegus oxycantha
- Has flavonoids that prevent tissue destruction during inflammation.
- Inhibits production and release of inflammatory compounds.
- Protects connective tissue from damage, reinforces protein linkage.
- Inhibits the destruction of tissues caused by inflammatory enzymes.

Licorice***—Glycyrrhiza glabra
- Potent anti-inflammatory, promotes the body's own corticosteroids.
- Demulcent properties soothe and protect the body's membranes.
- Strengthens adrenals and inhibits inflammatory chemical pathways.
- Effective for inflammation anywhere: fibromyalgia, arthritis, colitis.

Meadowsweet**—Filipendula ulmaria
- Original source of salicylates (aspirin), a natural anti-inflammatory.
- Ironically, cures stomach inflammation/acidity, which aspirin causes.
- For joint and muscle inflammation, hyperacidity, bladder inflammation.

Quercetin***—Quercetin
- Potent bioflavonoid and systemic anti-inflammatory and antihistamine.
- Strengthens capillaries and blood vessels to reduce inflammatory tendency. Strong antioxidant action that neutralizes inflammatory toxins.
- Excellent for injury, joint inflammation, allergic reactions, colitis.

Willow Bark*—Salix nigra
- Contains salycic acid, active ingredient of aspirin, and many co-factors.
- Blocks body's pro-inflammatory chemicals, such as prostaglandins.
- Relieves headache, arthritis pain, menstrual cramps, muscle pain.

Yarrow**—Achillea millefolium
- Contains anti-inflammatory compounds and has antispasmodic action.
- Reduces allergy, such as hay fever, hives. Helps menstrual pain.
- Improves tone of circulation, lowers blood pressure, improves digestion, decreases excess bleeding in wounds and internally, lowers fevers.

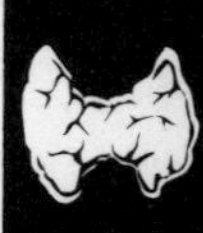

INJURY / WOUNDS

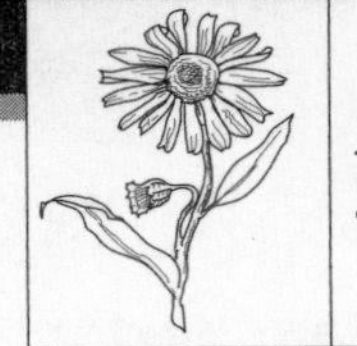

Select the herbs that are most suitable for your condition.

The Herbal Approach

From simple scratches to devastating accidents, trauma is the single most common medical condition. The herbs described here are for the entire range of injuries, including falls, muscular strains, joint sprains, cuts, fractures, wounds and bruising. A concentrated group of trauma-related plant medicines does duty for all these conditions, offering unique effects that are unavailable with drugs. Herbs that help with the healing of wounds are termed *vulneraries*. Many such plants offer anti-inflammatory and anti-infective effects, rapidly relieving pain, swelling and typical injury symptoms. But the unique physiological effect is the promotion and acceleration of tissue repair. Some, like *gotu kola*, even help prevent or correct the formation of scars and adhesions. Also included are herbs that have a specific effect on absorbing bruises. Note that many herbs can be used both externally and internally. *Arnica* is an extraordinary healer for trauma, but in herbal form is strictly for external application. *Calendula* is to wounds what *arnica* is to trauma, since it has the amazing effects of pulling the edges of cuts together. Another bonus is that timely use of healing plants greatly reduces the possibility of long-term effects of injury and the incidence of "sequelae," such as arthritis. See also ■ Bleeding ■ Burns ■ Infection ■ Inflammation ■ Pain/Neuralgia.

Aloe***—Aloe vera/barbadensis
- Externally apply to cuts, scrapes, burns. Protects and soothes the skin.
- Accelerates wound healing, stimulates growth of new tissues.

Arnica***—Leopards Bane/Arnica montana
- Use for any injury, blow, fall, surgery; to prevent or heal bruises.
- Effective for muscular strains, joint sprains, charley horse, overexertion.
- Prevents bruising, reduces swelling, pain, tenderness, inflammation.
- For continued after-effects of sprain or other injuries.
- *Not for internal use*, nor to be used on open wounds or broken skin.

Boswellia—Boswellia serrata
- Natural anti-inflammatory, stimulates tissue immunity.
- Reduces pain, swelling, stiffness after injury; as effective as Ibuprofen.
- Promotes repair of damaged tissues with improved circulation.

Bromelain**—Pineapple/Ananas comosus
- Natural protein-digesting enzyme that is anti-inflammatory; reduces pain, swelling, speeds healing. Heals bruises rapidly, relaxes muscles.

- Extracted from pineapple, reduces inflammation, helps absorb fluids.

Calendula***—Marigold/Calendula officinalis
- External use in wounds, scrapes, cuts, bleeding, inflammation.
- Stops bleeding from wounds, especially from the scalp and mouth.
- Rapid healing of wounds, seals the edges, prevents scarring.
- Prevents and treats infected wounds, abscess, ulceration, gangrene.

Cayenne**—Capsicum frutescens
- Capsaicin cream has been shown to markedly speed skin regrowth.
- Reduces pain, reduces substance P in the nerve cells.
- Applied as an external ointment, improves circulation locally.

Chamomile***—Matricaria recutita
- Anti-inflammatory, eases spasms; relieves pain, reduces swelling.
- Promotes the body's own cortisone and stress response mechanisms.
- Relieves mental stress, tension and irritability, promotes rest and sleep.

Comfrey***—Symphytum officinale
- In fracture; pain relief and cuts bone healing time by half. Use in non-union of fractures, after amputation. For bone inflammation, osteitis.
- Excellent for bone bruising, puncture, blows to eye socket, skull or face.
- External: as a root paste or leaf tea, stops bleeding, promotes healing.

Curcumin***—Turmeric/Curcuma longa
- Anti-inflammatory; may be used on minor wounds and cuts, sprinkling some powder on the cleansed area, or made into a dilute paste.
- Powerful anti-inflammatory effects, reducing pain, swelling, tenderness.
- Shown to be as effective as medical drugs, including cortisone.
- Use both as an internal herb and as a topical cream for pain relief.

Echinacea**—Echinacea angustifolia
- Antimicrobial and immune-boosting effects to prevent infection from wounds, bites and stings, blood poisoning; speeds removal of debris.
- Use internally and externally as a poultice to accelerate wound healing.

Eucalyptus Oil*—Eucalyptus globulus
- External application only. Reduces pain and inflammation of sprains.
- Promotes wound healing. Relaxes muscular spasms.

Ginger***—Zingiber officinale
- Reduces inflammation, pain, swelling in bursitis, arthritis, tendonitis.
- Blocks the body's formation of inflammatory chemicals (prostaglandins, leukotrienes). Can be used as an external application simultaneously.

Gotu Kola***—Centella asiatica
- Promotes skin and wound healing, repair of ulcers. Prevents scarring.
- Stimulates collagen synthesis for healing tendons, ligaments, etc.

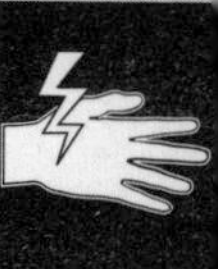

- Wounds from childbirth, surgery, abrasions, after radiation therapy.
- Use after surgery (tonsils, ears, etc.). Reduces skin inflammation.

Horse Chestnut***—Aesculus hippocastanum
- Reduces bruising, swelling and pain quickly after injury, sprains.
- Used in pre- and post-operative swelling and bruising, lymphedema after mastectomy, head injury, even brain edema. Strengthens blood vessels.
- Use internally (capsules) and as an external ointment.

Kava Kava*—Piper methysticum
- Anti-inflammatory and antispasmodic, reducing pain and cramps.
- Does not lose effectiveness in long-term use. Relieves stress, anxiety.

Lavender Oil**—Lavandula officinalis
- External use for pain relief, reduction of spasm and muscle tension.
- Antiseptic; enhances healing of wounds, sores, insect bites and burns.

Myrrh**—Commiphora myrrha
- External antiseptic for wounds, prevents infection; immune stimulant.
- Anti-inflammatory and astringent, promotes tissue healing, cleansing.

Plantain**—Plantago officinalis
- Taken internally and as a poultice is anti-inflammatory, antiseptic and pain-relieving. Stops bleeding, tightens tissues, promotes healing.

St. John's Wort**—Hypericum
- Anti-inflammatory and wound-healing effect, promotes nerve healing.
- Externally, stops bleeding, prevents infection, heals bruises, burns.
- Relieves muscle aches and pains. Protects against effects of radiation.

Witch Hazel**—Hamamelis virginiana
- External application to prevent infection, promote healing.
- Helps bruising, damaged blood vessels. Best on unbroken skin.
- Applied externally for all bruises, black eye, injury to veins, to testes.
- Quickly prevents or reduces bruising. Improves pain and tenderness.
- Stops bleeding and helps varicose veins, phlebitis, hemorrhoids.

Yarrow**—Achillea millefolium
- A traditional wound remedy; staunches internal and external bleeding.
- Anti-inflammatory and antispasmodic, promotes healing with astringent properties. Antiseptic effects, soothing irritation and pain.

HERBAL MAN

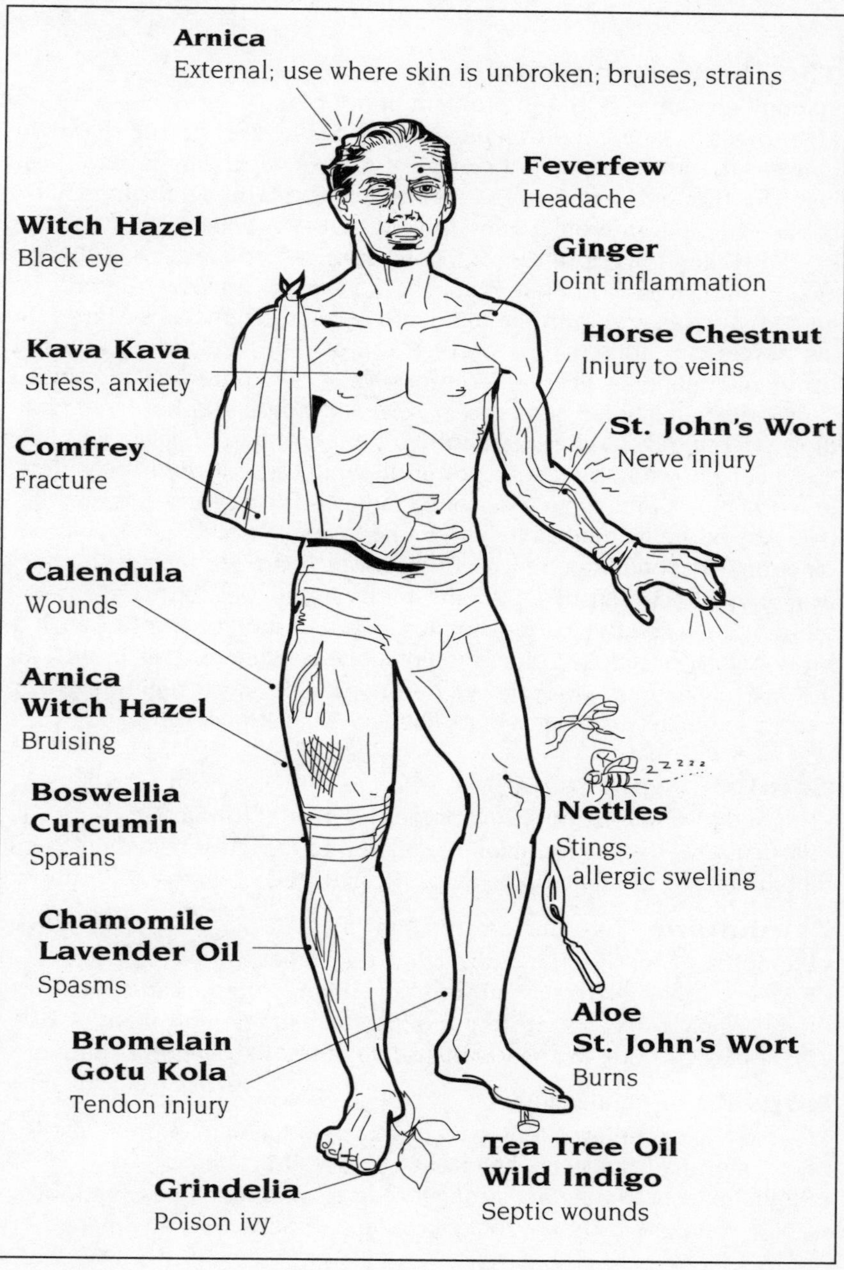
Arnica
External; use where skin is unbroken; bruises, strains
Feverfew
Headache
Witch Hazel
Black eye
Ginger
Joint inflammation
Horse Chestnut
Injury to veins
Kava Kava
Stress, anxiety
St. John's Wort
Nerve injury
Comfrey
Fracture
Calendula
Wounds
Arnica
Witch Hazel
Bruising
Boswellia
Curcumin
Sprains
Nettles
Stings,
allergic swelling
Chamomile
Lavender Oil
Spasms
Aloe
St. John's Wort
Burns
Bromelain
Gotu Kola
Tendon injury
Tea Tree Oil
Wild Indigo
Septic wounds
Grindelia
Poison ivy

INSOMNIA

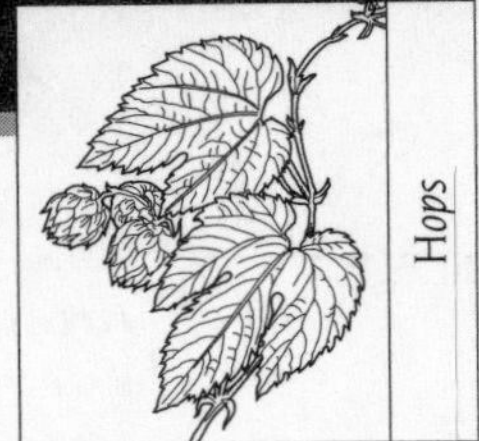
Hops

Select the herbs that are most suitable for your condition.

The Herbal Approach

Insomnia includes both the problem of not being able to get to sleep and waking (and staying awake) during the night. Causes are numerous, including lack of oxygen (sleep apnea), overheating, irritation in the digestive or respiratory systems or stirrings in the bladder or other internal organs. Waking at 1–3 a.m. is often a symptom of liver stagnation. Yet much of insomnia arises from everyday tension, anxiety and stress. The herbal approach is to use *nervines*, tranquilizing herbs that relax and calm the mind and sooth the nervous system without narcotic or addictive properties. The overall result is an improved depth and quality of sleep, with fewer wakings and refreshed mornings.

Of the herbs listed here, *valerian*, *hops* and *passionflower* have a long tradition of effectiveness and reliability. *Kava kava* and St. *John's wort* have now been shown to be just as powerful. While *passionflower* is considered less potent than the others, it is often indicated as a gentle nerve restorative. Any of the medicines below can be taken singly or in various combinations. Personal experience will show which is more effective for one's own unique metabolism. Optimally, herbs should be alternated to avoid building up a tolerance. Additionally, avoid stimulating herbs, such as *ginger*, *cayenne* or *ginseng*. Coffee should not be consumed at all, as its "half-life" is a full 24 hours, so that even morning coffee affects nighttime sleep. See also ▪ Anxiety ▪ Depression ▪ Fatigue/Exhaustion ▪ Stress.

Catnip*—Nepeta cateria
- Has sedative and tranquilizing properties similar to valerian.
- Particularly effective for insomnia related to digestive complaints, gas, infantile colic or menstrual cramps. Relaxing effect during colds, flu.

Chamomile**—Matricaria recutita
- Promotes sleep, with tranquilizing action similar to Halcion, Valium.
- Reduces stress-related chemicals in the brain, promotes adrenal health.
- Reduces pain, spasms, anxiety and insomnia in teething, menses, PMS, menopause or due to anger or digestive upset. Excellent for children.

Hops***—Humulus lupulus
- Calms nerves, relieves tension. For stress-induced insomnia, restlessness, starting from sleep, headaches, indigestion, alcohol.
- Similar effects to valerian; stronger than chamomile or passionflower.
- Good when one is drowsy, but can't sleep. Produces no a.m. hangover.

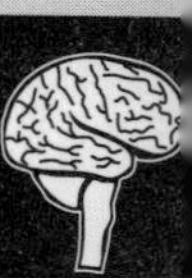

Kava Kava***—Piper methysticum

- Relieves anxiety, stress; reduces tension, with muscle-relaxing effects.
- Sleep is deeper, more restful, feel more refreshed on waking. Larger doses are sedative. Does not suppress dreaming phase of sleep.
- Comparable to medical benzodiazepines, but without their side effects.
- Best taken several hours before bed; smaller doses may be stimulating.

Lavender*—Lavandula officinalis

- Relieves restlessness, insomnia, especially due to intestinal or stomach disorders, exhaustion, neuralgia, hysteria, irritability or headache.
- A calming antidepressant, improves digestion and relieves gas, colic.

Lemon Balm*—Melissa officinalis

- For insomnia due to tension, digestive upset or nervous palpitations.
- Relieves anxiety, irritability, restlessness and nervous stomach.
- Sedative effects, relieving spasms. Also helps with overactive thyroid.

Passionflower**—Passiflora incarnata

- Insomnia from exhaustion, overwork, anxiety, stress, drugs, alcohol, asthma, teething, epilepsy, cough, pain; insomnia in infants or the aged.
- Tranquilizing, relaxes muscles, soothes the stomach, reduces anxiety.
- Acts as a mild MAO inhibitor, but no sedative hangover on waking.
- Suitable for nervous children or people with heart disease or asthma.

Skullcap**—Scutellaria lateriflora

- Relieves insomnia, especially due to anxiety, worry, emotional excitement or neuralgic pains, after effects of influenza, sinusitis, antibiotics.
- A mild sedative as well as nerve tonic. Reduces high blood pressure.

St. John's Wort**—Hypericum perforatum

- Acts as a mild MAO inhibitor, improving serotonin in the brain.
- Relieves anxiety, stress and depression and improves quality of sleep.
- Especially helps insomnia during menopause or hormonal imbalance.
- Improves mental clarity, energy. Well researched; no drug hangover.

Valerian***—Valeriana officinalis

- Nervous and muscle relaxant, improves falling asleep and sleep quality, reduces wakings; in some people has a late night energizing effect.
- Insomnia from mind activity, excitement, fright, fatigue, long journeys, menopause, after pregnancy, wine, emotional upset or palpitations.
- As effective as barbiturates, yet no side effects, grogginess or addiction.

Wild Lettuce*—Lactuca virosa

- Calms overactivity and overstimulation, promoting restful sleep.
- Sedative action is particularly recommended for excitable children.
- Formerly used as a substitute for opium, though non-addictive.

KIDNEY CONDITIONS

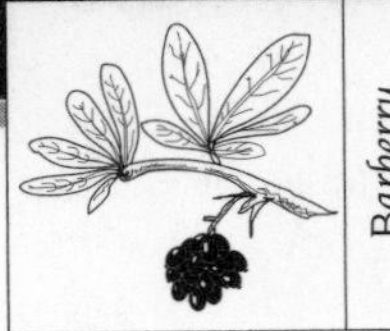

Select the herbs that are most suitable for your condition.

The Herbal Approach

With its miles of microscopic tubules, the kidney is the chief system for the filtration of toxins from the blood. Thus it easily becomes overwhelmed or weakened. Yet it is much overlooked in Western medicine, unless there is major pathology, such as an infection, kidney stones (calculi) or kidney failure. The kidneys are, however, subject to toxic damage from antibiotics, pain relievers, solvents, herbicides, heavy metals and endotoxins secreted by bacteria. Infection of the kidney can occur when bacteria migrate upward from the bladder, especially if there is blocked urine flow from prostate disease, stones or tumors. Autoimmune syndromes like lupus and cystic fibrosis can devastate the kidney tissue. Kidney stones, usually of calcium oxalate, occur in 1% of the population.

Herbs for kidney disorders are often *diuretic*, increasing the flow of urine to wash out toxins, bacteria and deposits. Many are *demulcents*, with mucilaginous properties that coat the urinary linings and promote tissue healing. *Antiseptics* effectively clear the infection from the urinary tract. Additionally, kidney herbs are used as diuretics in heart disorders, obesity and osteoarthritis. Such botanical medicines are also crucial for general detoxification programs for the skin, immune system and so on. See also ■ Bladder Infection ■ Infection ■ Liver Conditions.

Barberry***—Berberis vulgaris

- Disinfectant, pain relieving, healing for kidney or urinary infections.
- Antispasmodic, relieves pains from kidney stones, radiating down into thighs or whole body. Clears urine with thick mucus or red sediment.

Buchu**—Barosma betulina

- Only a mild diuretic, but a urinary antiseptic for chronic infections or inflammation with the formation of much mucus and acidic urine.
- A warming renal tonic for pyelitis, gravel, urethritis, prostatitis.
- Usually combined with other kidney herbs for maximum diuretic action.

Corn silk**—Zea mays

- Soothing diuretic for chronic cystitis, irritation of the bladder, urethra, prostate. Dissolves and reduces kidney stones. High in potassium.
- Effective for urinary difficulties in prostate disorders, bedwetting in kids.

Couchgrass*—Agropyron repens

- Diuretic, demulcent and kidney tonic, for dissolving kidney gravel or stones, cystitis, urethritis, prostatitis, pyelitis, first stages of nephritis.
- Lessens frequency and pain of urination with anti-inflammatory effects.

Dandelion**—Taraxacum officinale
- Diuretic agent, without causing potassium loss; reduces kidney inflammation or infection, prevents kidney stone formation. A gentle laxative.
- Effective liver detoxifier, bile stimulant. Helps regulate immune system.

Goldenrod***—Solidago virgaurea
- A gentle diuretic for such conditions as cystitis and especially nephritis or nephritic syndromes; flushes out kidneys, dissolves kidney stones.
- A useful urinary antiseptic, used in nephritis, prostate disorders.

Gravel Root**—Joe-Pye Weed/Eupatorium purpureum
- Specific for kidney stones and gravel, as well as bladder stone or infection. Diuretic, helps relax the pelvic area so stones can pass.
- Used for chronic cystitis, irritable bladder, enlarged prostate, sterility.

Hydrangea**—Seven Barks/Hydrangea arborescens
- Useful for bladder or kidney stones or gravel; helps to dissolve existing stones and aids in their expulsion; preventive for tendency to stones.
- Also for cystitis, nephritis and other kidney diseases, enlarged prostate.
- Diuretic, antispasmodic, antiseptic. Combine with althea, uva ursi.

Marshmallow**—Althea officinalis
- Soothing demulcent for cystitis; eases irritation and helps heal tissue.
- For stones of kidneys or bladder, coats the linings and eases passage.
- Decreases pain, irritation of urinary organs and is anti-inflammatory.

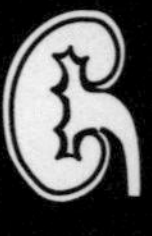

Parsley**—Petroselinum crispum
- A diuretic and urinary antiseptic, anti-inflammatory and detoxifier.
- For kidney irritation, urinary infections, kidney stones or gravel.
- Traditional use in water retention, edema. Use the root, not the seeds.

Pellitory**—Parietaria diffusa
- Useful diuretic to prevent and dissolve kidney stone and gravel; soothes urinary lining and has a restorative action on the kidney.
- For inflammation or infection of kidney/bladder, nephritis, renal colic.

Uva ursi**—Arctostaphylos uva ursi
- Antiseptic and disinfectant to the urinary tract. For acute nephritis.
- Helps inflammation or infection of the kidney and bladder.
- Useful for sand and small stones in the bladder or kidney.
- As a normal reaction, may turn the urine dark or greenish-brown.

Wild Yam**—Dioscorea villosa
- Antispasmodic for kidney colic, with pains shooting up into the back and down the legs; helps during passing of small kidney stones.
- Does not dissolve stones or act as a pain reliever to any extent, but works through relaxing muscles of the ureter, bladder, back, etc.

LIVER CONDITIONS

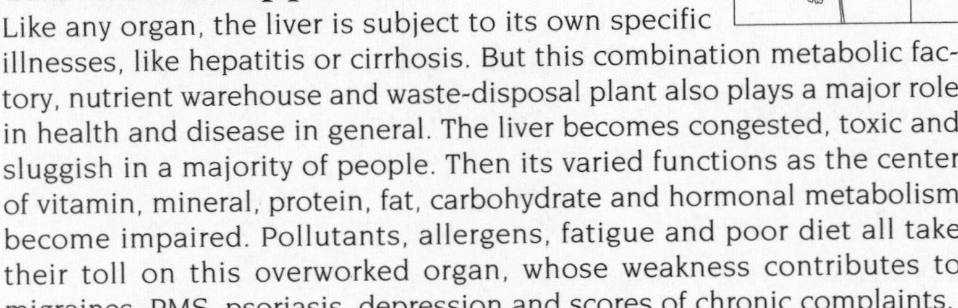
Celandine

Select the herbs that are most suitable for your condition.

The Herbal Approach

Like any organ, the liver is subject to its own specific illnesses, like hepatitis or cirrhosis. But this combination metabolic factory, nutrient warehouse and waste-disposal plant also plays a major role in health and disease in general. The liver becomes congested, toxic and sluggish in a majority of people. Then its varied functions as the center of vitamin, mineral, protein, fat, carbohydrate and hormonal metabolism become impaired. Pollutants, allergens, fatigue and poor diet all take their toll on this overworked organ, whose weakness contributes to migraines, PMS, psoriasis, depression and scores of chronic complaints.

Herbal *cholegogues* stimulate bile production and detoxification. Some also promote regeneration of liver tissue. Liver herbs or *hepatics* are integral to the treatment of any chronic illness and should be used as part of an annual or semiannual detoxification and preventive program. See also ■ Colitis ■ Gallbladder ■ Immune Weakness.

Artichoke**—Cynara scolymus
- Protects the liver from damage from toxins, chemicals and carcinogens.
- Increases bile flow; used for chronic liver disease, cirrhosis and gall bladder problems; relieves nausea, indigestion, bloating.
- Lowers cholesterol and blood sugar. Diuretic, useful in kidney disease.

Astragalus**—Milk Vetch/Astragalus membranaceous
- Protects liver against damage by various toxins, improves endurance.
- Improves degenerative conditions, including cirrhosis. Used for viral hepatitis, immune weakness, fluid retention. Highly energizing tonic.

Barberry***—Berberis vulgaris
- Useful for many liver and gallbladder problems, hepatitis, cirrhosis.
- Assists detoxification from effects of poor diet, medications or drugs.
- Stimulates the immune system, tonifies kidney and spleen.

Beet Leaf**—Beta vulgaris
- Tones the liver, gallbladder and bile ducts; promotes regeneration of liver cells, enhances immunity and increases metabolism of fat cells.
- Also known to affect headaches and hair loss; assists in weight loss.

Black Radish*—Raphanus sativus
- Stimulates bile flow, while aiding gas, bloating and indigestion.
- Stimulates appetite and tones intestines with a laxative effect.
- Avoid if ulcers or gastritis are present; use no longer than one month.

Bupleurum**—Bupleurum chinese.
- Anti-inflammatory, good for hepatitis; strengthens, protects the liver.
- Tones the digestion and spleen; for associated liver/spleen symptoms of bloating, nausea, indigestion, abdominal pain, dizziness, irritability.

Celandine***—Chelidonium majus
- For general liver detoxification or for skin diseases, arthritis, colitis.
- Treats liver or gallbladder inflammation, jaundice, gallstones.
- Relaxes gallbladder and improves bile flow. For liver problems or gall bladder colic with pains in right abdomen, radiating to shoulder blade.

Culver's Root*—Leptandra virginica
- Liver and gallbladder tonic with strong laxative effects; use small doses.
- Relieves gas and bloating; helps hemorrhoids and rectal prolapse.
- For skin problems where liver is a factor; not for use during pregnancy.

Curcumin***—Curcuma longa
- Shown to reduce liver inflammation and hepatitis; makes the liver cells more sensitive to the body's own cortisone. Rich antioxidant activity.
- Protects the liver from toxic damage, increases bile flow and solubility.

Dandelion****—Taraxacum officinalis
- Important liver detoxifier, clearing wastes, pollutants; stimulates bile.
- Treats gallstones, gallbladder inflammation, jaundice, as well as liver-related conditions, including constipation, acne, psoriasis, arthritis.
- Strong diuretic effects, while supplying adequate potassium salts.

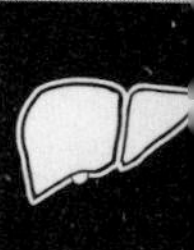

Fringe Tree***—Chionanthus virginiana
- Bile stimulant used in hepatitis, cirrhosis, enlarged liver and jaundice, as well as gallstones or inflammation. Liver detox in chronic illness.
- A tonic to aid recovery from illness; strengthens the spleen, pancreas.

Milk Thistle****—Silybum marianum
- Potent liver detoxifier, protects against damage by toxins, alcohol, etc.
- Promotes regeneration and repair, reversing liver damage and cirrhosis, good for chronic and acute hepatitis, fatty degeneration of the liver.
- Anti-inflammatory and free radical fighter, increases liver glutathione.

Rehmannia*—Rehmannia glutinosa
- Hepatoprotective, preventing liver damage and poisoning. Reduces blood pressure and serum cholesterol, improves blood flow to the brain.
- Treats impaired liver function and shown to be effective in hepatitis.

Schisandra**—Schisandra chinensis
- Improves liver function and protects it from damage by various toxins.
- Treats hepatitis with a 75% success rate, with no known side effects.
- Calming, reduces irritability and forgetfulness, improves sleep.
- An adaptogenic herb, tonic to the sexual organs; good for skin rashes.

MEMORY LOSS

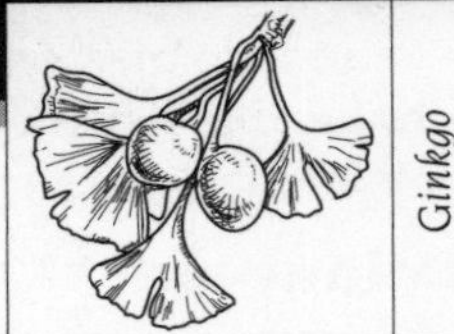

Select the herbs that are most suitable for your condition.

The Herbal Approach

With all its complexity and subtlety, the brain is highly sensitive to toxic impacts over time. Free radicals from dietary toxins, pollutants, dental mercury, pesticides, vaccine residues, drugs, artificial sweeteners, tobacco (the list goes on) add to the burden of toxic damage. As circulation becomes diminished, the brain receives less of its vital nutrients and antioxidants. While the epidemic of senility and Alzheimer's is expected to escalate to 14 million Americans by the year 2020, milder changes in memory and cognition are affecting every age group.

Specific herbs are known to enhance the levels of neurotransmitters, particularly acetylcholine, and improve blood flow to the brain, thereby increasing its oxygen and nutrient supply. More than this, such herbs augment the metabolism, detoxification and healthy functioning of brain cells. As free radical fighters, they can neutralize damaging toxins, as well as help prevent and reduce arteriosclerosis. Both scientific and clinical experience show definite and worthwhile results in using these safe and easily obtained herbal medicines. Any of the herbs below—used singly or in combination—must be used long term for optimal results. Additionally, a variety of herbs should be alternated over time to obtain maximal, full-spectrum results. See also ■ ADD/ADHD ■ Anti-aging ■ Arteriosclerosis ■ Depression ■ Fatigue ■ Immune Weakness ■ Veins/Circulation.

Bacopa**—Brahmi/Bacopa monnieri
- Improves intellectual capacity, acuity, clarity of thought, concentration.
- Improves memory, especially in the elderly; shortens learning time.
- Calming and sedative. Improves anxiety, important for hyperactivity.

Ginkgo***—Ginkgo biloba
- Improves brain circulation, increasing oxygen and nutrient delivery.
- Protects from free radical damage to brain, as well as effects of injury.
- Improves memory, alertness, clarity, depression and apathy.
- Also helps symptoms of tinnitus, dizziness, headache and anxiety.
- Effective in first stages of Alzheimer's disease, minimal effectiveness in later stages. Excellent results for senility from brain arteriosclerosis.

Ginseng**—Panax ginseng
- Improves mental sharpness, performance, attention span and memory.
- Increases alertness, concentration, visual and motor coordination.
- Reduces fatigue and increases resistance to physical and mental stress.
- Results in better performance, reduced errors, increased stamina.

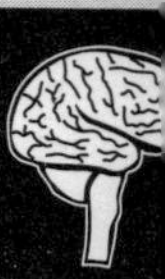

Gotu Kola***—Centella asiatica

- Increases mental performance, memory, retention, mood and sleep.
- Improves circulation to the brain; useful in developmental delay.
- Relaxes and energizes the senses. A traditional longevity herb.

Hawthorn**—Crataegus oxycantha

- Key in removing arteriosclerotic plaques from small arteries to brain.
- Strengthens capillaries, provides antioxidant protection to tissues.
- Improves heart output and strength, increases brain's oxygen supply.

Huperzine A***—Hyperzia serrata

- Extract from the club moss, used in Chinese medicine for centuries.
- Increases acetylcholine in the brain. Effective for dementia, Alzheimer's and age-related memory loss; improves learning, mental functioning.
- Acts 10 times longer than drugs used for Alzheimer's, without side effects and at a much lower cost. Suitable for long-term treatment.

Oats**—Avena sativa

- Treats nervous and mental exhaustion after illness, overwork or study, worry, anxiety, drug use, alcoholism, narcotics, effects of sexual excess.
- Promotes mental clarity, focus, memory, concentration, attention span.
- Helps correct insomnia, relieves nervous tremors, palpitations.

Periwinkle**—Vinca minor

- Powerful memory enhancer, increases mental alertness and cognition.
- Improves blood flow to brain; increases neurotransmitters, including dopamine, noradrenaline. Useful for senility, cerebral arteriosclerosis.
- Prevents arterial hardening, reduces blood clot risk. Helps insomnia.
- Increases cellular energy production, oxygen and sugar supply to brain.

Rosemary***—Rosmarinus officinalis

- Traditional memory-enhancing herb, shown to improve brain function.
- Potent free radical fighter, prevents breakdown of the neurotransmitter, acetylcholine. Promotes circulation, strengthens adrenals.

Schisandra***—Schisandra chinensis

- Nervous system toner/stimulant, increases mental clarity, reflex time.
- Helps memory, concentration, coordination, depression, irritability.
- Adaptogen herb; improves stress response, tones the liver and kidney.

Other promising herbs of the mint family that inhibit the enzymes that destroy the neurotransmitter acetylcholine include sage (*Salvia officinalis*), lemon balm (*Melissa officinalis*) and horsemint (*Monarda*). Common lime (*Citrus aurantifolia*) has also been shown to have a similar effects. Research on lemon grass has validated its memory-enhancing effects.

Menopause

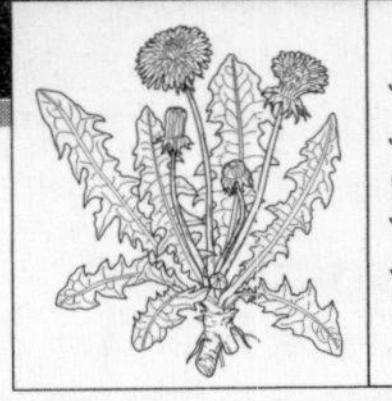

Select the herbs that are most suitable for your condition.

The Herbal Approach

As a normal part of the aging process, menopause affects all women eventually—50 million are postmenopausal in the year 2000. This presents a series of unique health challenges for females. In premenopause (perimenopause), irregular periods and PMS-like symptoms predominate. During menopause, 75% of women experience hot flashes and sweats. For postmenopausal women, the risks include increased bone loss and heart disease, as well as vaginal dryness, thinning skin and hair, depression and memory problems—all indicating accelerated aging. The entire process is due to a decrease in the ovaries' and adrenal gland's ability to produce adequate estrogen and progesterone. Yet hormone replacement (HRT) is questionable, causing a six-fold risk in uterine cancer, 50% increased risk of breast cancer and triple the rate of heart disease.

Specific herbs are used for relief of hot flashes, palpitations, excess bleeding, vaginitis, depression, etc. Many of these plants contain isoflavones or plant estrogens that are hormone precursors and regulators of natural estrogen and progesterone. These improve the function of the adrenals and ovaries. Women of third world countries (and Japan) with phytoestrogen-rich diets have almost no menopausal symptoms. Other herbs help the body utilize and metabolize hormones more effectively. Attention should also be paid to the liver, nervous and immune systems. Herbs should be taken for at least eight weeks to see results. See also ■ Amenorrhea ■ Anti-aging ■ Anxiety ■ Depression ■ High Blood Pressure ■ Immune Weakness ■ Insomnia ■ Liver Disorders ■ PMS.

Black Cohosh***—Cimicifuga racemosa

- Most popular natural alternative to estrogen therapy in Europe, shown to be as effective as HRT. Helps the body retains its own estrogen.
- Relieves hot flushes, depression, irritability, palpitations, ringing in the ears, headache, dizziness, vaginal atrophy and water retention.
- Controls excess bleeding, strengthens the heart, improves incontinence.
- Reduces LH (leutenizing hormone) levels, thereby increasing estrogen.

Chaste Tree***—Vitex agnus castus

- Improves progesterone to estrogen ratio; increases adrenal secretions (estradiol). Reduces excess prolactin secretion from the pituitary.
- Promotes normal menstrual cycle, lessens bleeding between periods.
- Counters hot flashes, night sweats, anxiety, too frequent periods.
- Must be used for several months (3 to 6 months) for optimal effects.

Dandelion**—Taraxacum officinalis
- Detoxifying liver tonic, clears out excess estrogen and other hormones.
- Reduces hot flashes. Strengthens the liver, promotes digestion.
- A gentle laxative, diuretic, for water retention without potassium loss.

Dong Quai**—Angelica sinensis
- Reduces flushing, sweats, bloating, water retention, vaginal dryness, insomnia, bladder weakness. Combats fatigue, with calming effects.
- Contains phytoestrogens that help correct menstrual irregularities, including absence of period, excess bleeding or painful menstruation.

False Unicorn**—Chamaelirium luteum
- Normalizing effect on hormonal system; stimulates ovarian function.
- Helpful in early menopause after hysterectomy or after using the pill.
- Produces estrogen/hormonal effects through its diosgenin content.

Fo-Ti**—Polygonum multiflorum
- For menopause or perimenopausal symptoms, restores balance to the hormonal system; stimulates ovary, increasing libido and stamina.
- A rejuvenation and longevity tonic, nourishing to the sexual organs.

Licorice*—Glycyrrhiza glabra
- Source of plant steroids (phytoestrogens), with hormone-like activity.
- Helps balance estrogen/progesterone ratio, induces ovulation.

Maca**—Lepidium meyenii
- In menopause, alleviates symptoms of low hormones, including flashes, vaginal lubrication, sexual function and libido, fatigue, night sweats.
- Works on hypothalamus and pituitary to reestablish hormone levels.

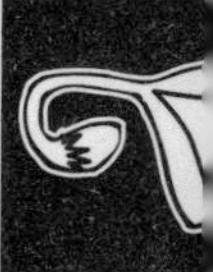

Motherwort**—Leonarus cardiaca
- Calms the nerves, relieves perimenopausal symptoms, stops cramping.
- Restores elasticity and lubrication to vaginal walls.
- Maintains hormonal balance, strengthens the heart and uterus.

Oats**—Avena sativa
- Eases tension, lowers cholesterol, improves circulation. Helps strengthen bones, relieves headache and depression. A longevity herb.

Red Clover***—Trifolium pratense
- Contains highest isoflavones, plant estrogens that balance hormones.
- Improves hot flashes, night sweats, vaginal dryness, loss of sexual desire, mood changes and depression. Also reduces menstrual cramps.
- May also protect against osteoporosis, heart disease and many cancers.

Wild Yam**—Dioscorea villosa
- Contains isoflavones; helps reduce menopause symptoms, decreases bone loss and inhibits excess clotting; improves elasticity of arteries.

Miscarriage

True Unicorn Root

Select the herbs that are most suitable for your condition.

The Herbal Approach

Miscarriage, medically termed spontaneous abortion, occurs in a remarkable 15% of woman, while about 25% have bleeding or cramping during the first four months of pregnancy. About 60% of miscarriages are part of a natural elimination process, where the fetus is seriously abnormal or absent. Thus ultrasound and other investigations are essential. Most miscarriages due to hormonal imbalance occur in the first trimester. Those that happen later, or in the second trimester, are often due to problems with the mother (e.g. diabetes, herpes, other viruses, or hypothyroidism). Bleeding and miscarriage can also occur if the placenta is in the wrong place (placenta previa) or separates prematurely from the uterus. The role of uterine fibroids is not clear, but they often do *not* interfere with pregnancy. Various toxic factors, especially heavy metal poisoning (i.e. mercury) can be underlying, undiagnosed causes.

Ideally, treatment should be under the guidance of a skilled doctor but self care is completely safe and without risk, and can be administered while seeking medical assistance. Herbs are appropriate as a preventive in habitual miscarriage, as well as for stopping threatened abortion. For acute miscarriage the remedies under Bleeding should also be consulted. If there is significant spasm the remedies under Dysmenorrhea or Colic/Cramps may be needed. Mother's Cordial is a traditional combination made of equal parts of *false unicorn*, *true unicorn*, *blue cohosh* and *black haw*, preferably in a non-alcoholic extract or capsule. This is excellent during the first trimester to prevent miscarriage, taking 10 drops daily. For habitual miscarriage, constitutional homeopathy also can also give brilliant results. *Caulophyllum* is excellent for the after-effects of miscarriage, including insomnia, exhaustion and depression. See also ■ Amenorrhea ■ Bleeding ■ Colic/Cramps ■ Dysmenorrhea ■ Infertility ■ PMS.

Black Cohosh***—Cimicifuga racemosa

- Effective for threatened miscarriage, both at third month or before term.
- Reduces spasm, pain, bearing down, back ache; helps stop bleeding.
- Normalizes cycle for irregular or absent menses after miscarriage.

Black Haw***—Viburnum prunifolia

- Strong antispasmodic; relaxes the uterus, prevents false labor pains.
- Stops threatened miscarriage or can be used for habitual tendency.
- Use acutely or as part of a Mother's Cordial. Lowers blood pressure.

Blue Cohosh***—Caulophyllum thalictroides
- For weak uterus, habitual or threatened miscarriage, bleeding.
- Relieves uterus spasms, with weakness and pain flying in all directions.
- Relieves symptoms after miscarriage: exhaustion, appetite loss, weak memory, insomnia, nervous tension and excitability. Helps arthritis.
- Regulates heavy menses, helps prevent and treat vaginal discharges.

Chamomile***—Matricaria recutita
- For threatened miscarriage, especially after anger or emotional upset.
- Strong antispasmodic; reduces bleeding; powerful anti-inflammatory.
- Helps with cramps, associated diarrhea, dizziness; prevents seizures.

Cramp Bark***—Viburnum opulus
- Antispasmodic for threatened miscarriage and bleeding tendency.
- Helps dysmenorrhea and cramping during pregnancy or after childbirth.
- Prevents miscarriage in the first trimester. Helps anxiety, irritability.

False Unicorn**—Helonias dioica
- For weak uterus; habitual miscarriage, prolapse, malposition, atony.
- Relieves feeling of heaviness, weight or soreness of womb, back pain.
- Suitable to problems from sedentary lifestyle or being overworked, exhausted. Helps relieve depression, irritability, improves sex drive.

Partridge Berry**—Mitchella repens
- Relaxant that promotes easy labor, yet prevents miscarriage, especially as part of Mother's Cordial. A urinary system tonic, useful in cystitis.
- Used during first or last trimester, good for labor or miscarriage.

Savine Juniper**—Juniperus communis
- Traditional medicine for threatened miscarriage, especially in the third month, or hemorrhage after miscarriage. Relieves cramps, bleeding.
- Use one or two drops of the green plant tincture, diluted in water.

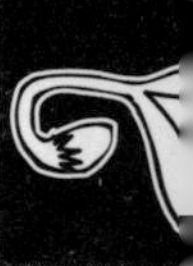

Trillium***—Birthroot/Trillium erectum or pratense
- Relieves uterus hemorrhage, bleeding between periods, uterine prolapse. Specific benefit for excess blood loss during menopause.
- Uterine tonic for pain in the back, hip and pelvis, as if broken apart.

True Unicorn Root**—Aletris farinosa/Star Grass
- Used as a uterine tonic to treat recurrent miscarriage, prolapse, sterility or frequent infections. Sense of uterine weight or heaviness.
- A tonic for fatigue, weakness, anemia, weight loss, loss of appetite, poor concentration, faintness associated with uterine or hormonal problems.

Wild Yam**—Dioscorea villosa
- Antispasmodic that reduces cramps or uterine colic in miscarriages.
- Pains are sharp and shooting, worse from bending forward or lying, and relieved by stretching. Best effect where progesterone levels are low.

MOUTH & GUMS

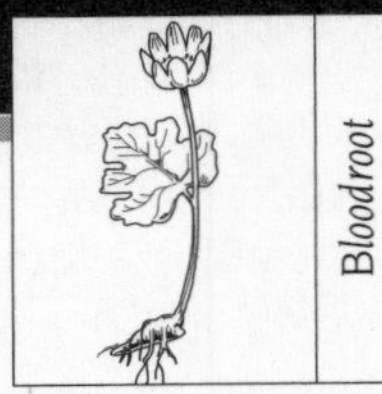

Select the herbs that are most suitable for your condition.

The Herbal Approach

The oral cavity is normally home to dozens of potentially nasty bacteria, including strep, various kinds of amoeba and even spirochetes (related to syphilis). These are normally kept at bay, aided by the immune system and good oral hygiene. But the mouth is also a reflection of overall metabolic health. The resistance of the mouth lining can be weakened by digestive disturbances, food allergies, intestinal dysbiosis, excess acidity or alkalinity and toxic factors (alcohol, tobacco, etc.), as well as deficiencies of everything from folic acid to amino acids. Once this happens, the mucus membranes become prey to resident bacteria, resulting in inflammation and infection. Note too that mercury has, as one of its main toxic effects, the creation of ulcers and inflamed, spongy gums.

Helpful herbs for mouth problems have anti-inflammatory and antimicrobial properties, as well as being soothing (demulcent) and pain relieving. Immune-supportive herbs and intestinal detoxifiers are important for follow-up and to prevent recurrences. Yet increasing health with vitamins and herbs will not be fully successful if exposure to heavy toxins continues. It is thus advisable to have metal fillings replaced with white filings by dentists who specialize in "biologically compatible" dentistry. See also ■ Infection ■ Inflammation ■ Stomach Conditions.

Bloodroot***—Sanguinaria officinalis
- Powerful astringent; a gargle or rinse for mouth ulcers, bleeding gums.
- Prevents tooth decay due to its ability to remove plaque from teeth.
- Chief ingredient in several over-the-counter anti-plaque mouthwashes.

Calendula***—Marigold/Calendula officinalis
- Promotes rapid tissue healing, anti-inflammatory, arrests bleeding.
- Healing and very soothing, as it decreases inflammation and swelling.
- Used in bacterial or viral infections to help canker sores, gum disease or inflamed tissues; excellent after dental or surgical work, mouth burns.

Chamomile***—Matricaria recutita
- Soothing anti-inflammatory for irritated and swollen membranes.
- Safe for children, excellent for teething. Prevents infection by staph.
- Promotes healing, tightens up gums in canker sores or gingivitis.

Echinacea**—Purple Cone Flower/Echinacea angustifolia
- General immune-boosting effects, taken internally as well as local rinse.
- Antibacterial, antifungal and anti-inflammatory, clears lymphatics.

Goldenseal***—Hydrastis canadensis
- Heals ulcers of the mouth and gums, destroys causative bacteria.
- Antibacterial and antiviral, used as a diluted mouth rinse.
- Astringent and cooling; tightens up swollen or boggy tissues.

Goldthread***—Coptis trifolia or chinensis
- Known as "canker root" because of its powerful effect on mouth ulcers.
- Antibacterial and antiviral, reduces inflammation, relieves pain.
- Heals inflamed membranes of mouth, eyes, similar to goldenseal.

Grapefruit Seed Extract***—Citrus aurantia
- Safe and non-toxic for gum infections, ulcers, gum boils or abscess.
- Internal and external treatment for a range of bacteria, yeast, parasites.

Licorice**—Glycyrrhiza glabra
- Licorice has been used since antiquity for canker sores.
- Coats and soothes mouth ulcers, promotes healing, in the form of DGL.
- Anti-inflammatory and antiviral for mucus membrane inflammation.

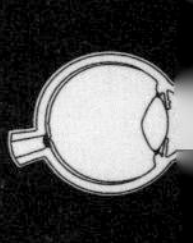

Myrrh***—Commiphora myrrha
- Powerful antimicrobial, astringent for gum disorders; tightens tissue.
- For gum abscesses or ulcerations, or after dental work; prevents infection and maintains gum integrity, soothes irritation of membranes.

Neem**—Azadirachta indica
- Ayurvedic herb that destroys bacteria involved with gingivitis. Use the leaf extract, taken as a mouthwash (2 to 12 drops) or in toothpaste.

Osha**—Ligusticum porteri
- Antiviral and antibacterial effect for mouth ulcers, cankers.
- Effective for stubborn, recurring cases. Provides immune support internally; a tea or diluted tincture is used as a local gargle or mouthwash.

Peppermint*—Mentha piperta
- As a gargle or mouth rinse has antimicrobial and antiviral properties.
- Due to its anti-inflammatory and cooling nature, peppermint relieves pain when applied topically to toothaches or inflamed gums.

Sage***—Red Sage/Salvia officinalis
- Soothes inflammation of the gingiva, mouth, tongue and throat.
- A healing gargle that is antibacterial, antiviral and antifungal.
- Tonifies and tightens gum tissue, soothes irritated, inflamed linings.

Tea Tree Oil***—Melaleuca alternifolia
- Destroys bacteria, fungi, etc., responsible for mouth ulcers, gingivitis, canker sores and thrush. Effective against drug-resistant bacteria.
- Use a few drops in water for an antiseptic gargle for above conditions.

Nausea

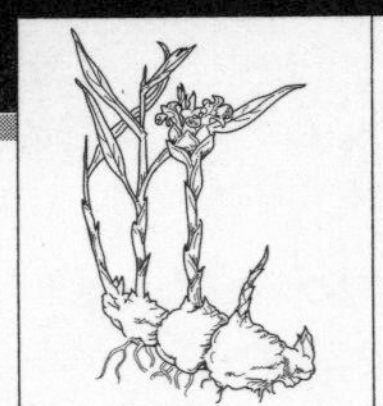

Select the herbs that are most suitable for your condition.

The Herbal Approach

Nausea can occur as a natural reaction from any stomach inflammation or irritation from bad food, a variety of drugs, alcohol, food additives, excess gas, food allergies, parasites or simple hunger. Conditions like pain, flu, headache, anxiety, stress or problems in the digestive tract or gall bladder produce similar results, and we all know through experience that odors and visual stimuli can do the same. Nausea of pregnancy occurs due to swelling of the stomach linings. Of an entirely different nature are disturbances in the inner ear, due to inflammation or motion (motion sickness). Vomiting can result in excess fluid loss and dehydration, and there is the risk of choking on acrid material.

Of the many herbs useful for nausea, *ginger* is the most researched and clinically effective. Unlike analogous drugs, anti-nausea herbs have the advantage of also improving digestion, calming irritation and inflammation, while relieving gas, cramping and other associated symptoms. However, underlying causes should still be addressed, using herbs that counter chronic infection, emotional stress or various toxins. See also ■ Alcohol Detox ■ Colic/Cramps ■ Ear Infections ■ Gas/Bloating ■ Indigestion ■ Infection ■ Liver Conditions ■ Stomach Conditions.

Cayenne***—Capsicum frutescens

- Anti-inflammatory; relieves nausea, vomiting, gas, indigestion.
- Promotes digestion, warms the stomach and stimulates appetite.
- Do not use in acute stages of inflammatory gastritis or stomach ulcer.

Chamomile***—Matricaria recutita

- Tranquilizing effects with action similar to drugs like Halcion, Valium.
- Reduces effects of stress-induced chemicals in the brain, while promoting healthy adrenal hormones (e.g. cortisol). Relieves pain, spasms.
- Also aids digestion, cramping, back pain. Promotes restful sleep.

Cinnamon*—Cinnamomum zeylandicum

- Relieves nausea, vomiting. Treats gastroenteritis, stomach flu, diarrhea.
- Antibacterial, antiviral and antifungal; expels gas, reduces spasms.
- Warming, astringent and stimulating to the digestion, reduces mucus.

Cloves*—Eugenia caryophyllata

- Relieves nausea, prevents vomiting. Reduces gastrointestinal spasms.
- Expels gas, bloating; antibacterial and antiviral, eliminates parasites.
- A few drops of the oil or infusion may be taken for quick nausea relief.

- Anesthetic and antiseptic properties; also stimulates the memory.

Curcumin***—Curcumin longa
- Alleviates nausea, gastritis; reduces acidity, increases mucus production and protects stomach. Anti-inflammatory action equal to cortisone.
- Improves liver and digestive function. Effective for motion sickness.

Fennel*—Foeniculum vulgare
- A digestive stimulant, relieves nausea, improves appetite.
- Relieves gas, flatulence and distention and subsequent pain.
- Relaxes the smooth intestinal muscles and quiets cramps and colic.

Galangal***—Alpinia officinarum
- Ginger-like, a remedy for nausea, vomiting, sea or motion sickness.
- Warms the digestive system, expels gas, helps pain, spasms, hiccups.

Ginger***—Zingiber officinale
- Best anti-nausea herb known; relieves nausea, vomiting after surgery, from chemotherapy, from coughs, etc. Relaxes stomach, relieves pain.
- Stimulates digestion and absorption, reduces diarrhea.
- For relief in the nausea of pregnancy (use only for short period of time).
- Motion sickness: very effective taken half hour (or days) before travel.

Marshmallow*—Althea officinalis
- Soothing demulcent that allays nausea and indigestion, heals stomach.
- Useful for acute or chronic inflammation of digestive linings.

Meadowsweet**—Filipendula ulmaria
- Anti-inflammatory; contains aspirin-like substances but without irritating stomach, due to tannins. Reduces acid indigestion, heals stomach.
- Astringent that combats diarrhea; irritable bowel; safe for children.

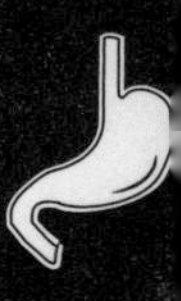

Patchouli**—Pogostemon cablin
- Fragrant Indian herb is an effective anti-nausea and anti-vomiting plant.
- Lessens stomach spasm, treats indigestion, poor appetite, diarrhea.

Peppermint**—Mentha piperta
- Promotes proper digestion. Reduces gas, flatulence and bloating.
- Peppermint oils are antibacterial, antiseptic and antifungal.
- Antispasmodic, helps intestinal cramping; calms inflamed gall bladder.

Raspberry Leaf*—Rubus idaeus
- A digestive astringent, valuable for nausea, vomiting and diarrhea.
- For morning sickness and nausea and to facilitate childbirth.
- Safe and non-toxic. Balances hormones, tones the uterus and ovaries.

OVERWEIGHT

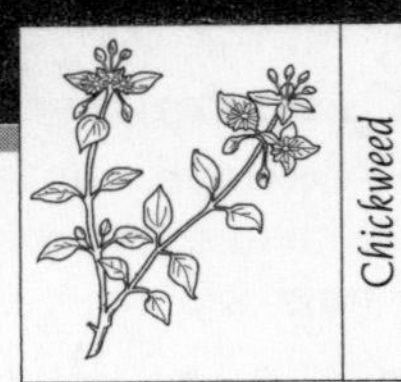

Select the herbs that are most suitable for your condition.

The Herbal Approach

Obesity affects 100 million adults, and as many as 20% of children ages 6–17. This dramatically increases the risk of heart disease, hypertension, gall bladder disease, diabetes, breast and colon cancer and a shortened life span. Being overweight is the result of a complex interplay of hormones, digestive function, liver health, toxicity and overall metabolism. Marginal thyroid problems are undiagnosed in 50% of people, blood sugar disorders such as hypoglycemia and syndrome X are frequent. A full-scale approach to weight loss often integrates a minimal carbohydrate, high-protein diet, nutritional supplements (chromium, carnitine, omega-3 fatty acids) and effective herbs.

The most important plants for obesity are *thermogenic*, raising the metabolic rate and burning off calories and adipose tissue (*ephedra, yohimbe, cayenne, bitter orange*). They can mobilize stored fats and transform them into more easily metabolized forms. Hormone-balancing herbs are also needed to influence the thyroid, pancreas and adrenals. Other weight fighters are adaptogenic, with broad effects on overall metabolism and stress-response mechanisms. See also ▪ Diabetes ▪ Detoxification ▪ Liver Conditions ▪ Menopause ▪ PMS ▪ Stress ▪ Thyroid Disorders.

Bitter Orange***—Zhi Shi/Citrus aurantia
- Induces thermogenesis; increases breakdown of fats and metabolic rate of cells, without any of the cardiovascular side effects typical of ephedra.
- Improves lean muscle mass, increases physical performance.
- Increases burning of calories after meals and overall metabolic rate.

Cayenne**—Capsicum frutescens
- Increases body heat or thermogenesis, burns fat-based calories.
- Increases metabolic rate, improves circulation, stimulates digestion.

Chickweed*—Stellaria media
- Traditional obesity remedy; internal cleanser that encourages weight loss through its diuretic action, eliminating waste through the kidneys.

Coleus***—Coleus forskohlii
- Promotes the breakdown of stored fats, inhibits formation of fat cells.
- Stimulates the thyroid gland. Counteracts obesity related to aging.
- Improves digestion and nutrient absorption; an immune stimulant.

Dandelion**—Taraxacum officinalis
- A powerful diuretic for water retention, yet prevents potassium loss.

- Liver detoxification; mobilizes fats from the liver. Balances hormones.

Ephedra*—Ma Huang/Ephedra sinica
- Increases thermogenesis, metabolism and reduces appetite.
- Reduces body weight. Effect is greatly enhanced by combining with caffeine and theophylline (i.e. coffee and tea). Adrenaline-like action.

Garcinia**—Malabar tamarind/Garcinia gambogia
- Slows production of fat, helps the body metabolize it more efficiently.
- Increases how much energy the body burns (i.e. basal metabolic rate).
- Reduces carbohydrate craving and appetite overall. Increases weight loss during dieting. Marketed as HCA (hydrocytric acid) or Citrin.

Gotu Kola*—Centella asiatica
- Reduces body mass, enhances adrenals and improves carbohydrate metabolism. An energizing metabolic enhancer. General detoxifier.

Guar Gum**—Cyanopsis tetragonoloba
- Water-soluble fiber, helps balance blood sugar and effects of insulin.
- Reduces number of calories absorbed, increases bowel function.
- Helps lose weight gradually, at about one pound weekly.

Guggul***—Commiphora mukul
- Increases body's metabolic rate, improves thyroid function, increases fat-burning activity of body, increases thermogenesis (heat production).
- Decreases blood cholesterol and triglyceride levels.

Kelp**—Bladderwrack/Fucus vesiculosis
- Iodine content improves thyroid function. Best for sluggish people with cold, clammy skin. Causes weight loss from areas with most fat.
- Gives lighter, more active feeling; indicated for goiter in obese people.

Maitake**—Grifola frondosa
- Promotes weight loss, improving the health of the liver and lungs.
- Neutralizes internally produced toxins and externally acquired poisons.
- Enhances immune function and lowers risks of cancer and diabetes.

Stevia**—Stevia rebaudiana
- An herbal sugar substitute, used all over the world, that is 300 times sweeter than sugar, no known toxicity. Blood sugar–lowering effects.

Yerba Mate***—Ilex paraguariensis
- Used extensively in Europe for obesity; reduces abnormal appetite, and thirst. Anti-diabetic effects; helps weight loss in diabetic patients.
- Improves sleep, digestion, mental clarity, depression, allergy.

Yohimbe**—Pausinystalia yohimbe
- A cerebral stimulant, increasing adrenal function, similar to ephedra.
- Thermogenic effects, breaks down fats, increases metabolism and heat.

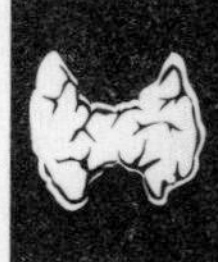

PAIN / NEURALGIA

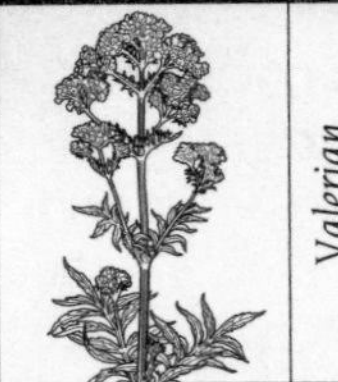

Select the herbs that are most suitable for your condition.

The Herbal Approach

Pain is a protective mechanism of the body, yet the most debilitating and challenging conditions. Pain fibers exist widely in skin. They are actually absent in many internal organs (brain, liver), while the capsule surrounding them is exquisitely sensitive to compression or expansion. Pain can occur as part of any condition, but especially due to the swelling and chemical messengers. Neuralgia is nerve pain, while nerve inflammation is termed neuritis. Special, and excruciating, types of neuralgia exist, such as facial neuralgia (tic doloreux), sciatica and arm pain (brachial neuralgia). These can occur due to nerve compression from the spine, scar tissue, toxic factors, alcohol, viruses (such as herpes), vitamin deficiencies, alcoholism or unknown, idiopathic causes.

The greatest pain-killer drugs in the world are herbal. Codeine and morphine are opium derivatives that are so powerful that they are both prescription drugs and highly addictive. H*enbane*, *mandrake* and many other well-known herbs have been used as anesthetics since antiquity. Yet less exalted herbs like *jamaican dogwoo*d and *lobelia*, are also extremely effective in common painful conditions arising anywhere in the body. Herbal pain-relievers are often also anti-spasmodic and anti-inflammatory, so that they go beyond symptomatic treatment alone. See also ■ Back Pain ■ Colic/Cramps ■ Headache ■ Herpes ■ Injury/Wounds.

Black Cohosh—Cimicifuga racemosa
- For radiating or electric-shock pains, intense aching. For neuralgia of heart, uterus, face, eyes, ribs, sciatic nerve, etc. Relieves depression.
- Reduces spasm, heaviness and stiffness of large muscles.

Cayenne***—Capsicum frutescens
- Internal and external use to reduce pain signals, increase endorphins.
- Use in injuries, after surgery, arthritis (reduces pain 30–50%), diabetic foot pain, headache, shingles, inflamed muscles, headache, neuralgia.

Chamomile***—Chamomilla recutita
- Contains anti-inflammatory compounds that ease pain and inflammation, especially in digestive pain, neuralgias, headache, arthritis.

Ginger***—Zingiber officinale
- Relieves the pain of arthritis, migraine headaches, burns, tooth pain.
- Decreases muscle spasms and stomach pain, promotes digestion.
- Broad anti-inflammatory action, relieves pain better than NSAIDs.

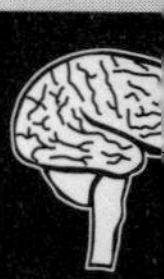

Jamaican Dogwood***—Piscidia erythrina
- Controls pain and relieves spasms, decreases tension, promotes sleep.
- Sedative action, effective for migraine, neuralgia, sciatica, facial neuralgia, abdominal pain or spasms, dysmenorrhea, spastic coughs, injury.
- Local use for hemorrhoid pain or toothache. Relaxant, calms nerves.

Kava Kava**—Piper methysticum
- Relaxes muscles, reduces internal and external spasms and cramps
- Pain reliever, plus enhances pain-reducing effects of aspirin and drugs.
- No hangover, tolerance, build-up, or addiction typical of medical drugs.

Lavender**—Lavandula officinalis
- Effective external use for pain, neuralgia; headaches, muscle tension.
- Eases the pain of burns, of arthritis aching and swelling and soreness.
- Tonifies the nerves, helps depression, calms anxiety, promotes sleep.

Lobelia***—Lobelia inflata
- Powerful muscle relaxant for muscles, bronchi, heart, uterus, cramps and spasms. Relaxant for asthma, coughs, spastic constipation.
- External use for arthritic pain, bites, stings, pain of bruises, or sprains.

Meadowsweet***—Filipendula ulmaria
- Contains salicylic acid, thus a source of aspirin and natural anti-inflammatory. Provides pain relief, without the side effects (gastric bleeding).
- Safe for children, soothes the digestion tract, lowers stomach acidity.

Prickly Ash***—Xanthoxylum americanum
- An antispasmodic herb, pain reliever for neuralgia, neuritis, specific to electric-like shooting pains, tingling and muscle cramps.
- Effective for swollen glands, fevers, intestinal infection, diarrheas.

Skullcap**—Scutellaria baicalensis or laterifolia
- For pain from over-stimulated states, chronic pain states, breast pain.
- Reduces spasms, nourishes nerves and encourages sleep. Useful in epilepsy, premenstrual tension, hysteria, schizophrenia and depression.

St. John's Wort**—Hypericum perforatum
- Internal and external use for neuralgic pain, trauma to fingers, toes, coccyx, pains of eyes, varicose veins, sunburns, herpes or shingles.
- Sedative effects; anti-inflammatory for sciatica, rheumatism, neuritis.

Valerian**—Valeriana officinalis
- Antispasmodic, eases intestinal cramps, muscle tension, anxiety.
- Promotes relaxing sleep; helps with insomnia, frequent awakenings.

Willow**—Salix nigra
- Contains natural aspirin as well as other synergistic anti-inflammatory and pain-relieving compounds for headache, arthritis and rheumatism.
- Slower, but more sustained effect. Gentler than aspirin.

Parasites

Olive Leaf

Select the herbs that are most suitable for your condition.

The Herbal Approach

Parasitic infections with single-celled protozoa, such as amoeba or giardia, or actual worms (roundworms, tapeworms) are a major cause of disease. They can be acquired from other people, food or pets, and many tropical species are now residents of northern regions. In spite of their widespread nature, their presence is often undiagnosed. And while the idea of a virus or bacteria is acceptable, we have a strong mental block to admitting to a parasitic infection. Once present, they not only cause many digestive symptoms, but slowly erode immune health and overall vitality. Others can migrate to the liver and deeper organs.

Herbal treatment requires herbs to destroy parasites, to expel them, and to heal the intestines and liver. Because of their life cycles, most parasites, whether protozoa or worms, need to be treated for 6 to 12 weeks. A changing, rotating series of herbs may also be needed. Note that a number of traditional anti-parasitic herbs are too toxic and not listed here. These include *pink root*, *wormseed*, and *kousso*. Gentle anti-parasitic foods include onions, figs, cinnamon, cloves and rhubarb. See also ■ Candida/Yeast ■ Colitis ■ Diarrhea ■ Immune Weakness ■ Infection.

Black Walnut**—Juglans nigra
- Treats intestinal worms. An intestinal tonic and important laxative.
- Improves indigestion, liver function. Tones the kidneys, benefits skin.

Elecampane**—Inula helenium
- Has effects against many parasites, along with bacteria and fungi.
- Marked effect against giardia, as well as amoeba and roundworms.
- Immune stimulant and respiratory tonic, expectorant for lung infection.

Garlic***—Allium sativa
- Effective against protozoa like amoebic dysentery, giardia, as well as viral and bacterial infections from staph, strep, proteus, salmonella.
- Destroys intestinal yeast and candida and an active anti-inflammatory.
- Garlic oil capsules can be inserted rectally for control of pinworms.

Goldenseal**—Hydrastis canadensis
- Antibiotic herb for many intestinal bacteria, fungi, protozoa and parasites/worms. Eliminates candida, trichomonas, strep, staph, E. coli.
- Treats shigella, salmonella, giardia and amoeba (histolytica).
- Similar effects with the related herbs: oregon grape and bayberry.

Grapefruit Seed Extract***—Citrus aurantia
- Effective against over 800 strains of viruses and fungi, 100 strains of

bacteria. Destroys various protozoa, Inhibits candida, E. coli overgrowth.
- Does not damage or destroy bifidobacteria (healthy intestinal flora).
- Improves symptoms of gas, constipation, abdominal pain, insomnia.

Male Fern Root*—Dryopteris filix mas
- Able to kill worms and expel tapeworm, used only under supervision.
- Taken in the morning, followed by a laxative in the p.m. or next a.m.

Olive Leaf***—Olea europaea
- Combats amoebic dysentery, giardia, pinworms and most parasites.
- Broad-spectrum antifungal, anti-candida, antiviral, antibacterial activity, used against malaria, dengue fever. Provides immune support.

Papaya Seed**—Carica papaya
- Protein-digesting enzyme acts on tapeworm, pinworm, roundworm, etc.
- Concentrated papain capsules (or bromelain extracted from pineapple plants) are taken while fasting. Has additional laxative effect.

Pomegranate**—Punica granatum
- Traditional use to expel tapeworm, roundworm. Has astringent properties to heal the intestines and gently moves the bowels.
- Can cause nausea and vomiting; follow with an enema or cathartic.

Pumpkin Seeds**—Curcubita pepo
- Specific treatment for tapeworms (beef, pork or fish) and pinworms.
- Twelve ounces of pumpkin seed are taken after a twelve-hour fast, followed in one hour by warm drinks and a cathartic.

Quassia**—Picrasma/Quassia excelsa
- Expels pinworms, threadworms; also effective against amoeba.
- A bitter herb that stimulates appetite and digestive secretions and has a laxative effect; used as an internal medicine and as an enema.

Tansy*—Tanacetum vulgare
- Antifungal, antibacterial and anti-parasitic effects against threadworm, roundworm. Potential toxicity in large doses or with prolonged use.
- A bitter digestive tonic and stimulant, helps expel gas.

Wood Sage*—Cat Thyme/Teucrium scorodonia
- Eliminates, thread or round worms. Calms nervousness, irritability, sleeplessness. Promotes digestion and relieves gas and heartburn.

Wormwood***—Artemesia annua
- Has lethal effects on many parasites, especially amoeba, giardia.
- For disturbed intestinal flora or toxic mix of organisms (dysbiosis).
- Very gentle action, even for sensitive people.
- Decreases bloating, normalizes stool, improves overall well-being.

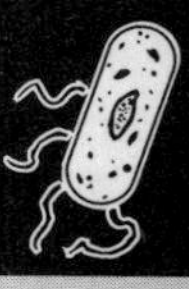

PMS

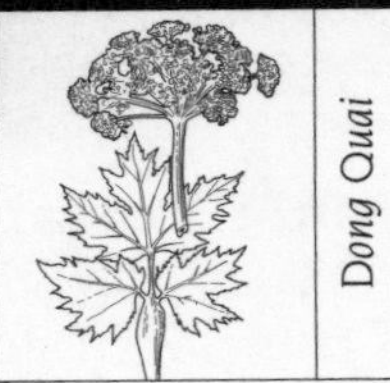

Select the herbs that are most suitable for your condition.

The Herbal Approach

Premenstrual syndrome is the most common gynecological complaint affecting up to 60% of women. Well-known symptoms of depression, anxiety, sweet craving, bloating, etc., are due to imbalances in hormones and brain neurotransmitters, including serotonin and dopamine. PMS can be divided into four categories, but in most cases there is a dominance of estrogen in relation to progesterone, causing typical mood swings and water retention. This may be due to excess estrogen production or the liver's inability to clear it from the system. Estrogen-like environmental toxins (PCBs, pesticides, DDT) also play a major role, as do deficiencies of magnesium, chromium, essential fatty acids, B6 and other key nutrients. Low blood sugar and faulty liver function must be corrected, and a high-protein, high-fiber, low-sugar, non-dairy diet is essential. A diet rich in plant-based phytoestrogens is excellent, but soy should be avoided, as it has been shown to increase estrogen excessively.

The herbal approach uses botanic medicines that favorably influence the estrogen-progesterone ratio through a variety of mechanisms. The final result is the reestablishment of the body's ability to produce a balanced and timely supply of hormones throughout the menstrual cycle. Liver strengthening herbs are also essential, and general tonics are extremely helpful for long-term cure (e.g. *ashwaganda, schisandra*). See also ■ Anxiety ■ Breast Inflammation ■ Depression ■ Dysmenorrhea ■ Fatigue ■ Gas/Bloating ■ Headache ■ Insomnia ■ Liver Conditions.

Black Cohosh*—Cimicifuga racemosa
- Relieves premenstrual tension, menstrual cramps and water weight.
- Normalizes the cycle, relieves cramping before and during menses.
- Sedative qualities help irritability, nervousness and depressive states.

Bupleurum**—Bupleurum chinense
- A well-known Chinese herb for PMS symptoms associated with a congested liver or a history of caffeine, alcohol or drug overuse.
- Helps with abdominal bloating, nausea, breast swelling, constipation, diarrhea, indigestion, irritability, depression and overstimulated nerves.

Chamomile*—Matricaria recutita
- Sedative that relieves uterus spasms, back pain. Calms irritability, anxiety, tension, muscle spasm; tranquilizes and promotes restful sleep.
- Help with indigestion, gas, bloating or diarrhea during PMS.

Chaste Tree***—Vitex agnus castus
- Regulates hormonal cycle, reduces pituitary gland prolactin, increases progesterone levels. Reduces FSH and estrogen if used for 3–6 months.
- Reduces anxiety, irritability, insomnia, headache, mood changes, tension, breast tenderness, water retention, bloating and sweet cravings.
- Large scale studies show good to very good results in 90% of women.

Dandelion Root***—Taraxacum officinale
- Powerful diuretic that clears excess water weight and bloating.
- Does not deplete potassium like other diuretics; safe in heart disease.
- Assist the liver in clearing estrogen dominance, thereby reducing PMS.

Dong Quai***—Angelica sinensis
- Relieves pain, cramps, headache, mood swings, insomnia, constipation.
- Phytoestrogens in dong quai balance the menstrual cycle and hormone levels—will lower them if too high or increase them if too low.
- Regulates blood sugar, helps anemia and is a tonic for low energy.
- Combats toxic and carcinogenic environmental estrogens (pesticides).

Licorice**—Glycyrrhiza glabra
- Contains phytoestrogens that regulate estrogen and progesterone ratios to relieve symptoms of anxiety, headaches and exhaustion.
- Decreases breast tenderness, abdominal discomfort and ankle swelling.

Maca***—Lepidium meyenii
- Increases or decreases ratios of hormones according to what the body needs. Promotes proper hormonal metabolism and production.
- Decreases acne, increases fertility, normalizes libido and is nutritive to the body; high vitamin, mineral and amino acid content.

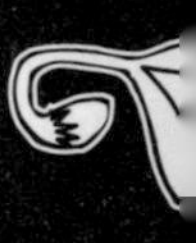

Skullcap**—Scutellaria laterifolia
- A wonderful PMS nervine to calm symptoms of irritability, depression sensitivity, mood alterations, sleep disturbances and anxiety.
- Relieves muscle spasms and tension; works best taken for some time.

Vervain**—Verbena officinalis
- For PMS symptoms associated with hormonal fluctuations and abnormal bleeding patterns. Sedates an overactive mind and disturbed sleep.
- Relieves tension headache, nervousness, irritability and sadness.

Wild Yam***—Dioscorea villosa
- Useful to take during the progesterone-dominant phase of the menstrual cycle, from ovulation to menstruation. A muscle and nerve relaxant.
- Helps correct low progesterone and high estrogen ratio.
- Contains steroid precursors, used by the body to make both sex hormones and adrenal cortisol; source of commercial estrogen products.

PROSTATE CONDITIONS

Select the herbs that are most suitable for your condition.

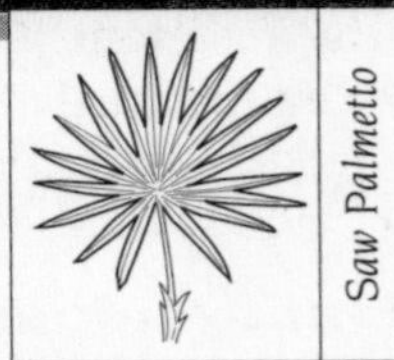

The Herbal Approach

Benign prostate hypertrophy (BPH) or enlargement occurs when testosterone is converted to dihydrotestosterone (DHT) and accumulates in that gland. The causes of conversion of testosterone to DHT are both nutritional (deficiencies of zinc, B6 and essential fatty acids) and toxic (cadmium and hormone-mimicking pesticides). Chronic bacterial or parasitic infections also play an important role. With half of all men experiencing prostate problems by the age of fifty (and 2 million cases of prostatitis at any one time), prostate surgery accounts for 400,000 operations a year. Side effects, especially impotence, are common. Yet in Germany, 90% of BPH is treated with plant medicines. Zinc, essential fatty acids, bee pollen and herbs like *saw palmetto berries* have been shown to shrink the prostate in 90% of men, if used for a full year, while medical drugs (such as Proscar) work in only 37%. Thus surgery is a last resort strategy when symptoms of urinary blockage become dangerous.

The herbs listed here are effective for prostate problems arising through age, as well as chronic infection or inflammation. *Saw palmetto* is the most well researched and broadly used for BPH, while *pygeum* is a close second and is excellent for prostatitis. The other plants can be combined for maximum effects. For optimal results, these herbs need to be taken for 3 to 12 months. Improvements can be expected in symptoms like dribbling, painful urination and sexual weakness or impotence. See also ■ Bladder Infection ■ Impotence/Male Infertility.

Goldenseal**—Hydrastis canadensis
- Powerful antibiotic effect for prostatitis; acts on wide range of bacteria.
- Soothes and heals the urinary tract. Helps shrink swollen prostate.
- Tonifies the prostate linings, strengthens against invading organisms.

Lycopene**—Tomato/Lycopersicum esculentum
- Bioflavonoid extract of tomato that reduces dribbling or frequency.
- A powerful antioxidant, specifically protects against prostate cancer.
- Concentrated in the adrenals, increases stress resistance, endurance.

Nettles**—Urtica dioica
- Root contains plant sterols that help reduce prostate enlargement.
- Anti-inflammatory, detoxifying and high in bioflavonoids and iron.
- Strong diuretic, yet is high in potassium. Relieves urgency and pain and other symptoms associated with prostate enlargement.

Pipsissewa**—Chimaphila umbellata
- North American herb used as a urinary disinfectant for cystitis and urethritis, it also has diuretic effects. Prevents atrophy of the testicles.
- For prostate enlargement with a sense of sitting on a ball or lump.

Pollen**—Bee Pollen
- Shown to shrink enlarged prostate, especially if taken in early stages.
- Effective for prostatitis, curing 40% and improving 80% within 6 months.
- Eliminates associated mild to moderate urinary problems, nocturia.

Pumpkin Seed**—Cucurbita pepo
- Long used as a traditional treatment for the prostate, partly because of zinc content, partly because of its concentrated essential fatty acids.
- Promotes anti-inflammatory prostaglandins, reduces swelling.
- A tonifying diuretic; often used in products as pumpkin oil extract.

Pygeum***—Pygeum africanum
- Reduces size of prostate in both acute swelling and chronic prostatitis.
- Anti-inflammatory and decongestant; also removes cholesterol deposits from prostate and has diuretic effects, improves urinary flow.
- Like saw palmetto, reduces effects of testosterone on the prostate.

Red Clover**—Trifolium pratense
- Traditional blood cleanser and free radical fighter, benefits prostate disorders and men's health; contains ten times the isoflavones as soy.
- Inhibits the formation of DHT, eliminates pesticides, fights cancer.

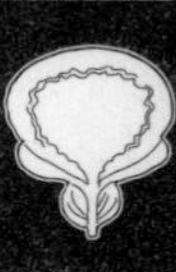

Saw Palmetto***—Sabal Serrulata
- Best long-term treatment for prostatic hypertrophy (BPH), extensively used as a prescription drug in Europe to avoid the need for surgery.
- Reduces the size of enlarged prostate, also reducing inflammation.
- Improves flow, reduces pain, nocturnal urination, retention, hesitancy, difficulty starting urination and dribbling. May reduce risk of cancer.
- Helps with impotence, reduced sex drive, atrophy of the testes.
- Effective in 90% of men in 4–6 weeks, but should use for 6 to 12 months.

Tribulus**—Ikshugandha/Tribulus terrestris
- Treats prostatitis, prostate enlargement and seminal emissions.
- Helps low sex drive, impotence, infertility; improves heart, liver, kidney.
- Markedly stimulates male libido, increases testosterone levels.

SINUSITIS

Select the herbs that are most suitable for your condition.

Eucalyptus

The Herbal Approach

Sinusitis is one of the most common chronic disorders in the United States, affecting 40 million Americans. The hollow sinus cavities can become inflamed or infected from a variety of sources. The most common culprits are respiratory and food allergies, along with viruses and bacteria. These guardians of the respiratory pathways are also being constantly challenged, as the first line of defense against a barrage of inhaled environmental toxins and pollutants. Apart from the pain and discharge of sinusitis, a chronic post nasal drip can leak toxic secretions into the throat or lungs, causing recurrent problems in those areas.

The herbal approach is to use antimicrobial remedies, (*goldenseal, echinacea*), along with decongestants and astringents (*euphrasia, elderflower*) that both drain and dry up secretions from the sinus cavities. While many of these herbs are taken internally, others, like *myrrh*, can be used as a nasal wash or as a steam inhalation (*tea tree oil*). See also ■ Colds & Flu ■ Hayfever/Allergy ■ Immune Weakness ■ Infection.

Cayenne*—Capsicum frutescens
- Can markedly reduce symptoms of nasal obstruction and discharge.
- Decongests sinus tissues, decreases swollen sinuses through its anti-inflammatory action, reduces irritation from environmental pollution.

Echinacea***—Echinacea angustifolia
- Antibacterial and antiviral effects for both prevention and treatment.
- Stimulates immune cells, enhances removal of bacteria and debris.
- Accelerates healing time if taken during an acute or chronic infection.

Elder**—Sambucus nigra
- Use for clearing mucus congestion, chronic sinusitis and ear infections.
- Ideal for children; antiviral properties reduce flu and cold symptoms.
- Clears mucus build-up. Increases resistance to hay fever and colds.

Ephedra**—Ephedra sinensis
- Relieves sinus swelling and nasal congestion, especially from allergy.
- Opens up bronchial tubes, relieves wheezing in asthma and bronchitis.
- Anti-inflammatory, anti-allergic and heat-producing effects.

Eucalyptus**—Eucalyptus globulus
- A vapor bath of leaves or oil opens clogged sinuses, drains mucus.
- A hot compress can be placed directly on sinuses as a decongestant.

- Antiseptic for cold flus and fever, encourages sweating, lowers fevers.

Eyebright***—Euphrasia officinalis

- Powerful astringent for drying up mucus secretions of the nose, sinus.
- Anti-inflammatory, for mucus congestion or sinusitis after colds, flu.

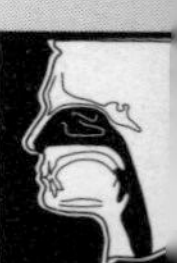

Garlic***—Allium sativum

- Destroys numerous bacteria, fungi, viruses; antioxidant, anti-inflammatory, antihistamine and immune-stimulating for sinusitis, colds, flu.

Ginger***—Zingiber officinale

- A pungent decongestant, opens nasal passages, clears mucus conditions in colds and flus, relieving body aches, pains and headaches.
- Fresh ginger is more effective than dried for sinusitis, acute conditions.

Goldenseal***—Hydrastis canadensis

- Antibacterial effects against a wide variety of organisms, strep, staph.
- Helps expel thick or hardened mucus, eventually drying up these secretions. Healing effect on damaged linings of the nose, throat, bronchi.

Horseradish***—Armoracia rusticana

- Stimulating herb, like cayenne, that encourages flow of mucus.
- Apply externally as a poultice to the sinuses to clear congestion.
- Eases watery, irritated membranes of the nose, sinuses, mouth, eyes.

Myrrh**—Commiphora myrrha

- Used locally, has strong antibacterial properties; myrrh's tannins have astringent properties with a drawing effect on swollen or boggy tissues.
- Benefits nasal congestion with excess mucus and runny nose.

Osha**—Ligusticum porteri

- Antiviral, antibacterial expectorant, best taken at start of infections.
- Helps acute and chronic mucus build-up and relieves associated sore throats or coughing. Clears lingering sinus mucus after cold, flu.

Peppermint Oil/Thyme Oil***—Mentha piperta

- Use the diluted oil as a sinus or chest rub for congestion.
- Reduces fever through inducing perspiration and breaking up mucus.
- The oil is a powerful antibacterial, antifungal and pain reliever.

Tea Tree Oil**—Melaleuca alternifolia

- Effective antibacterial, antifungal, antiviral and immune stimulant.
- Use as a steam inhalation or vaporizer, with several drops in hot water.

Usnea**—Lichen/Usnea species

- A broad-spectrum antifungal and antibacterial for sinusitis, coughs.
- Used also with acute infections such as colds or flus, relieving symptoms and enhancing immunity. Combines well with echinacea, etc.

SKIN CONDITIONS

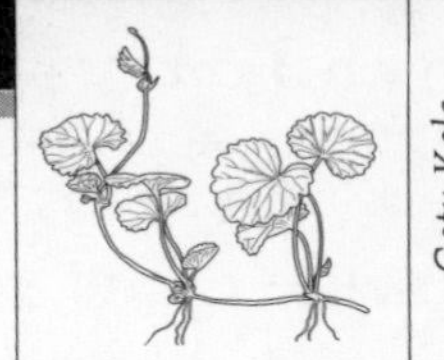

Select the herbs that are most suitable for your condition.

The Herbal Approach

A remarkable protective barrier between the outside world and our inner physiology, the skin is the largest organ in the body. As a main detoxification organ, when other cleansing organs like the liver and colon are compromised, it will respond with eruptions, discharges and other abnormalities. Of the many possible skin conditions, eczema or atopic dermatitis is the most common. Often related to respiratory allergies, eczema takes a variety of forms, with a mix of itchiness, blistery eruptions and dryness and cracking. Dermatitis is also a common side effect of drugs, as well as chemical sensitivities. Psoriasis, on the other hand, is an immune abnormality that affects about 4% of the population with a build-up of silvery scales and red patches of inflammation. About 7% of sufferers develop mild to severe forms of arthritis.

Because of the strong cross-over of herbal treatments for skin problems, all of the above conditions are dealt with here. These conditions are treatable—and curable—by herbal and nutritional therapy. Treatment must also be directed to underlying liver and immune imbalances, and bowel toxicity. In psoriasis, avoid alternatives, like *burdock*, *elecampane* and *echinacea*. See also ▪ Acne/Abscess ▪ Detoxification ▪ Herpes ▪ Infection ▪ Inflammation ▪ Injury/Wounds ▪ Liver Conditions.

Aloe***—Aloe vera/barbadensis
- Topical gels or creams protect and soothe while encouraging healing.
- Help in rashes, burns, ulcers, wounds. Reduces pain, itching, burning, irritation. Shown to heal chronic psoriasis in 83% of patients.

Bitter Melon**—Momordica charantia
- Inhibits guanylate cyclase enzyme, thus improves the cellular turnover rate, decreasing psoriasis eruptions. Also a liver and colitis remedy.
- Used as an external paste to soothe irritation and soreness.

Burdock***—Arctium lappa
- A traditional detoxifier and blood cleanser for many skin conditions.
- Treats acne, boils, eczema. Also acts as a liver tonic and stimulant.
- Tones the stomach, promotes perspiration; a detoxifying diuretic.

Calendula***—Calendula officinalis
- Soothing external cream and internal treatment; promotes healing, calms itching. Non-suppressive relief for eczema, psoriasis, rashes.
- Antiseptic properties for ringworm, diaper rash, cradle cap, etc.
- Treats wounds, burns, bruises; moisturizes skin, prevents scarring.

Cardiospermum**—Cardiospermum halicacabum
- The ointment (Florasone) is proven effective in research and practice.
- Highly beneficial in a variety of eczemas and atopic dermatitis. Equal effects to some pharmaceutical drugs, with fewer adverse effects.
- Improves or cures redness, itching, swelling, skin fissures and scaling.

Cayenne**—Capsicum frutescens
- Antioxidant that increases circulation and warmth to the skin.
- Decreases pain and reduces inflammation associated with psoriasis.
- The cream results in less scarring and redness in psoriasis, with reduced scaling, thickness, itchiness and puffiness. Do not use on open wounds.

Chamomile**—Matricaria recutita
- Topical cream or ointment can reduce or eliminate dermatitis, eczema.
- In Europe, used as an internal and external anti-inflammatory and pain reliever for psoriasis. Treats colic, gastroenteritis, nervous irritability.

Chickweed**—Stellaria media
- A soothing skin ointment or compress for dry, irritated, itchy skin.
- A treatment for eczema, psoriasis, boils, abscesses, ulcers. Decreases inflammation, repairs damaged skin and helps speed healing.

Coleus***—Coleus forskohlii
- Coleus assists the body in recalibrating cellular and enzyme messages, thus regulating the pattern of skin imbalances, especially psoriasis.
- Balances, regulates skin chemistry; decreases inflammation, allergy.

Elder**—Sambucus nigra
- A soothing cream for chronic skin conditions such as eczema, poison ivy rashes, skin inflammation, wounds, burns and old ulcers.
- Dries up swollen tissues and vesicles; assists in sloughing dead skin.

Evening Primrose**—Oenothera biennis
- Improves skin health and appearance when applied externally or taken internally, provides essential fatty acids and GLA for cell integrity.
- Proven effective for weeping eczema, atopic dermatitis and allergic skin conditions, symptoms of dryness, itching redness and swelling.

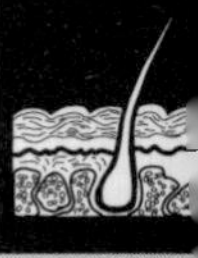

Gotu Kola***—Centella asiatica
- Treats a wide range of skin diseases, especially thickened skin or scaly rashes; Useful in psoriasis and eczema, itching, lupus, acne, herpes.
- Improves connective tissue formation, reducing scar tissue, cellulite.

Licorice**—Glycyrrhiza glabra
- Topical use or internal DGL form is soothing to skin and mucus membranes, possesses antibacterial and antiviral properties.
- Use topically as a demulcent for external itching and inflamed tissues and for herpes simplex and zoster. Helps prevent infection to wounds.

Lycium**—Chinese Wolfberry/Lycium chinense
- Chinese medicinal fruit, rich in immune-stimulating polysaccharides.
- In one study, psoriasis improvements were seen in 75% of cases after two months of use, while 20% showed complete remission of lesions.

Neem***—Azadirachta indica
- High in fatty acids, an Ayurvedic herb for eczema, psoriasis and rashes.
- Can be used preventively in those susceptible to skin diseases.
- Use topical oil or cream (with 2% neem) and internally in capsule form.

Olive Leaf**—Olea europea
- Use externally for dry skin and scalp, abrasions and minor scrapes.
- Skin antiseptic, destroying fungal infections (ringworm), viral infections (herpes, shingles) and bacteria (abscess, pimples, infected wounds).

Oregon Grape***—Berberis aquifolia
- Treats psoriasis or eczema, pimply skin, scales, itching, acne and poor complexion, vitiligo, herpes or eruptions on the scalp, face or neck.
- Tonic and detoxifier for the liver, gall bladder and digestive system.

Red Clover**—Trifolium pratense
- Used as an effective remedy for chronic skin conditions, psoriasis and eczema in children. An immune enhancer and hormone balancer.
- Traditional blood purifier, alterative with known anti-cancer properties.

Sarsaparilla**—Smilax officinalis
- Benefits eczema and psoriasis; in one study cured 50% of cases in two months. Detoxifying herb, cleanses the liver, binds intestinal toxins.
- Anti-inflammatory effects for dry, itching or cracked skin.

Tea Tree Oil***—Melaleuca alternifolia
- Potent topical disinfectant; accelerates healing, prevents scarring.
- Helps with impetigo, psoriasis, acne, furuncles, eczema, nail infections, ringworm, carbuncles, corns, wounds, burns and herpes.

Wild Pansy**—Viola tricolor
- A cleansing herb for skin conditions, chronic eczema, children's rashes.
- A wash for itching, scaling skin, psoriasis, chapped dry skin and hives.
- Use when skin is difficult to heal, with scabbing, cracking, impetigo.

Witch Hazel**—Hamamelis virginiana
- Soothing and cooling lotion, decreases inflammation and bleeding.
- Astringent for all skin disorders with itching, redness and pain, including hives, atopic dermatitis. Drugstore products are not as effective.

Yellow Dock**—Rumex crispus
- External compress used to discharge pus and infection from the skin.
- Eliminates waste products, toxins from the skin and deeper tissues.
- Combine with burdock and dandelion for blood and liver detoxification.

SKIN HERBS

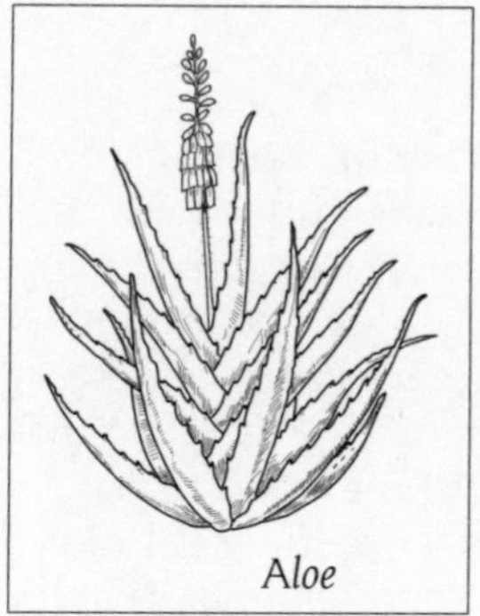
Aloe

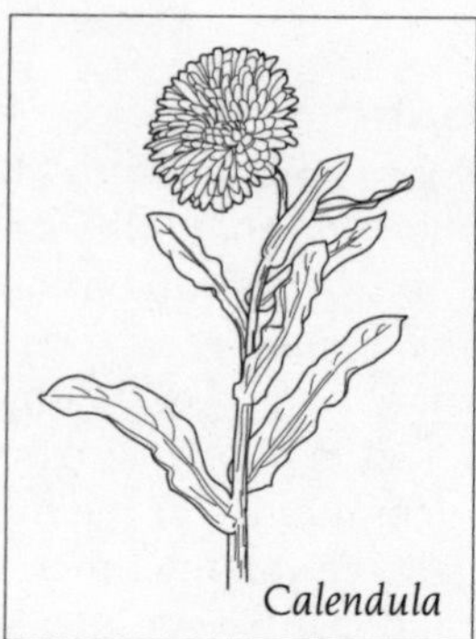
Calendula

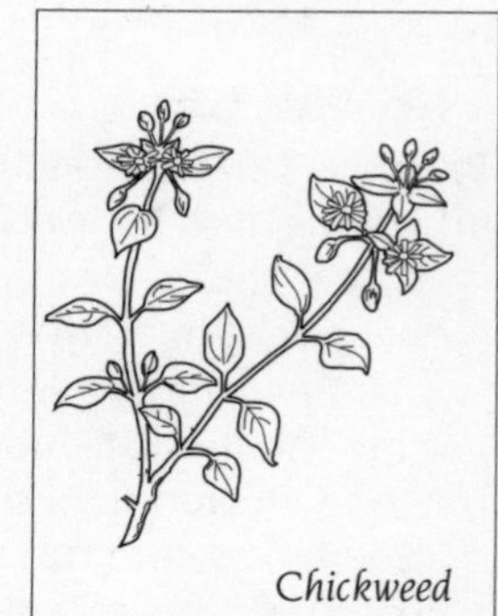
Chickweed

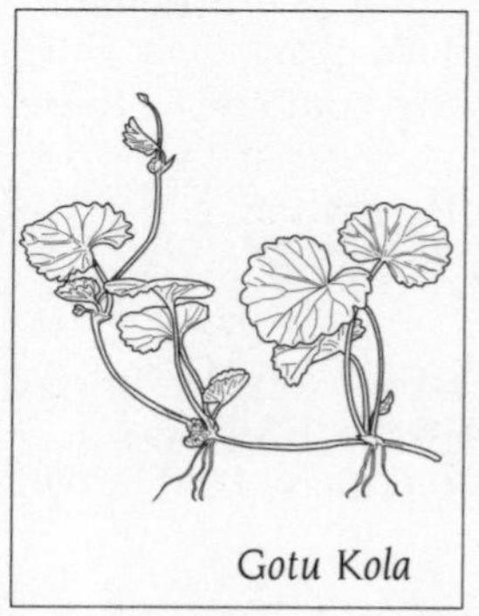
Gotu Kola

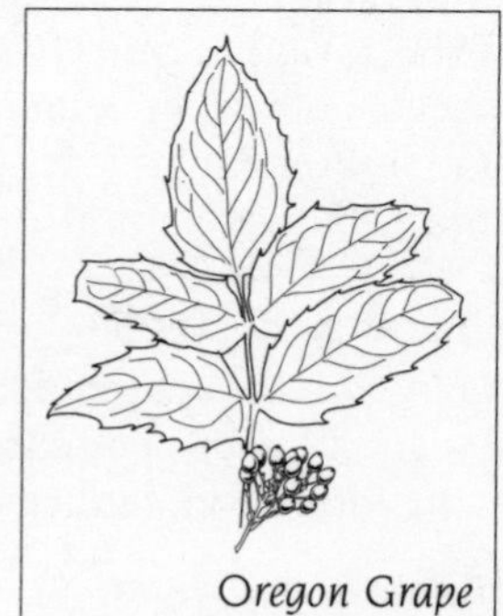
Oregon Grape

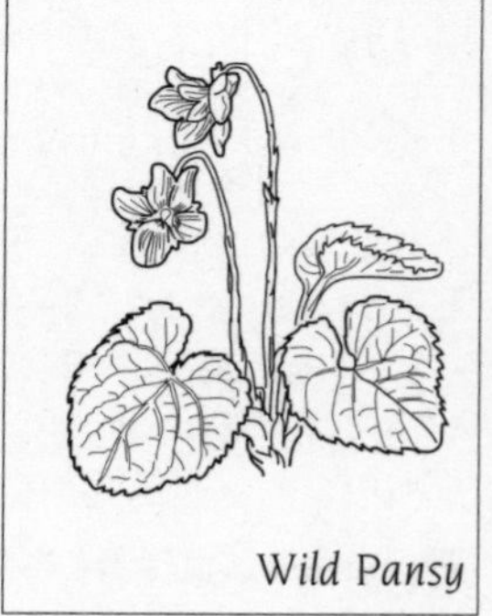
Wild Pansy

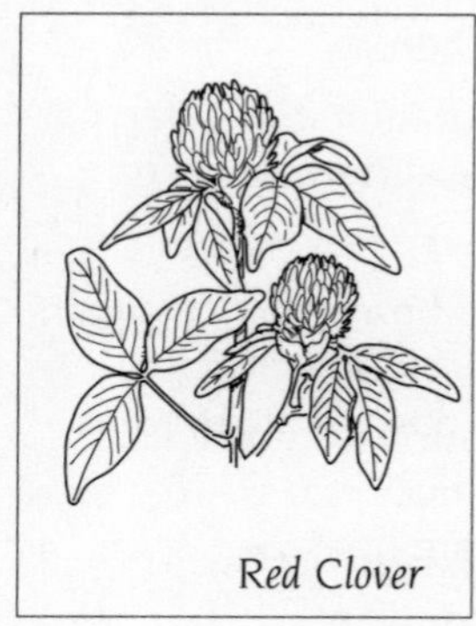
Red Clover

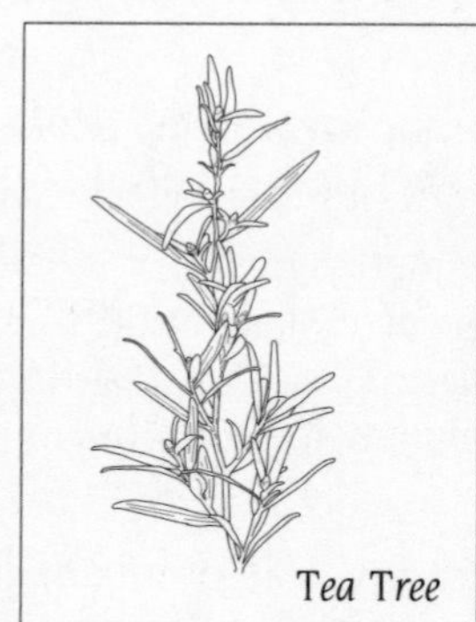
Tea Tree

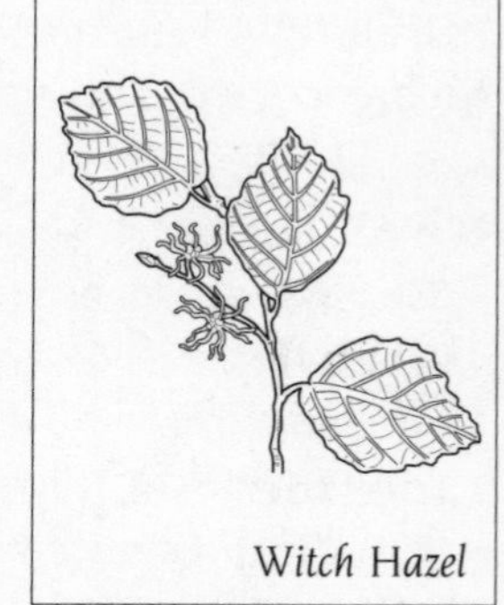
Witch Hazel

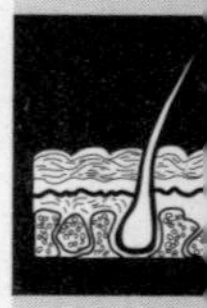

SORE THROAT

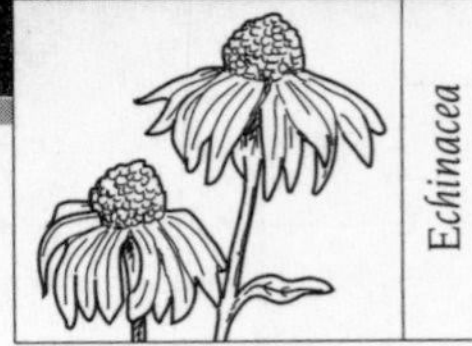

Select the herbs that are most suitable for your condition.

The Herbal Approach

Because we tend to associate sore throat with strep or other bacterial infections, it is important to note that 90% of these conditions are viral in nature. This means that antibiotics will be completely ineffective! Allergies and post nasal drip are common predisposing causes, and acid reflux can be the culprit in recurring cases. Another important factor is mercury filings. The hard scientific fact is that this toxic metal causes inflammation and ulceration of the membranes of the mouth, gums and throat.

Herbs for sore throats serve varying functions. Powerfully antibiotic plants like *myrrh*, *poke root* and *sage* have a justifiably strong reputation for quelling acute throat infections. Others, including *slippery elm* and *mullein*, are demulcent, soothing and protective to irritated linings. Anti-inflammatory effects of most of these plants quickly reduce symptoms while some, like *kava*, provide specific pain relief. Many herbs combine all these properties with antiviral and antioxidant effects in a synergistic way. See also ■ Colds & Flu ■ Ear Infections ■ Infection ■ Inflammation.

Echinacea***—Echinacea angustifolia
- Antiviral and antibacterial action for acute infection and prevention.
- Improves lymphatic drainage of infection areas, speeds healing.
- Immune booster, increasing interferon; reduces duration of sore throat.

Horseradish**—Armoracia rusticana
- Antibacterial effects for sore throat and upper respiratory infection.
- Promotes discharges, expels tough mucus, reduces fever, causes sweat.

Isatis**—Isatis tinctoria
- A broad spectrum antibiotic for treating acute inflammations: laryngitis, high fever, heat and dry throat. Cools, soothes and decongests.

Kava Kava**—Piper methysticum
- Used as a gargle, has topical analgesic effects, soothes the mucus membranes in sore throats, tonsillitis, canker sores and toothaches.
- Relaxant and pain relieving; helps with insomnia due to throat pain.

Licorice**—Glycyrrhiza glabra
- A soothing demulcent, for dry, sore or inflamed tissues associated with a sore throat. Antiviral properties and immune stimulant.

Lomatium**—Lomatium dissectum
- Used as a gargle for throat infection; treats various stages of illness.

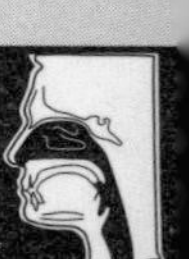

• Antibacterial, antifungal.and especially antiviral. Works best for stubborn respiratory infections. The isolate may work better for some.

Mullein**—Verbascum thapsus
• Coats the throat with a protective, mucus residue, soothes irritation.
• Expectorant, clears phlegm. Relieves tickling coughs, hoarseness.

Myrrh***—Commiphora myrrha
• Antiseptic and anti-inflammatory; effective for chronic sore throat, tonsillitis. Promotes healing of mouth and gum disease, swollen glands.
• Astringent, decongestant, expectorant that tightens lining membranes.

Oregano Oil***—Origanum vulgare
• Relieves tonsillitis, laryngitis; traditional use by European singers.
• Antifungal, antibacterial, specifically combats respiratory allergies.

Osha***—Ligusticum porteri
• Antiviral, antimicrobial and expectorant; best at first sign of infection.
• Sore throats with coughing in colds and flus; phlegm conditions of an acute or chronic nature. Helps recuperate from vomiting, indigestion.

Poke Root**—Phytolacca decandra
• Relieves throat inflammation and infection; reduces swollen glands, tonsils and adenoids. Relieves soreness, exhaustion of viral infection.
• Clears mucus, post-nasal drip and hawking. For arthritis *after* tonsillitis.

Poplar**—Balm of Gilead/Populus candicans
• Antibacterial, antifungal expectorant and anti-inflammatory herb.
• Soothing effects for sore throats, tonsillitis, bronchitis and dry coughs.
• Contains salicin, a natural form of aspirin; reduces fever, swelling.

Queen's Delight**—Stillingia sylvatica
• Useful in both acute and chronic sore throats, laryngitis, bronchitis.
• A lymph cleanser that detoxifies swollen lymph glands, stimulates white blood cells to respond to infection. Counteracts mercury, treats ulcers.

Sage***—Salvia officinalis
• Strong antiviral, antifungal, antibacterial due to menthol content.
• Used as a gargle for sore throats, helps with stuffed nose and coughs, mouth sores and gingivitis. Astringent; tonifies throat membranes.

Slippery Elm**—Ulmus fulva
• A soothing demulcent for sore throats, coughs and respiratory tract irritation. Moistens and relieves pain and inflammation of mucus linings.

Wild Indigo**—Baptisia tinctoria
• A deep-acting antiviral and antibiotic for focused infections, chronic sore throats or tonsillitis, enlarged lymph nodes; an immune stimulant.
• Lymphatic and tissue cleanser for deep toxicity, debility, poor healing.

SPORTS FITNESS

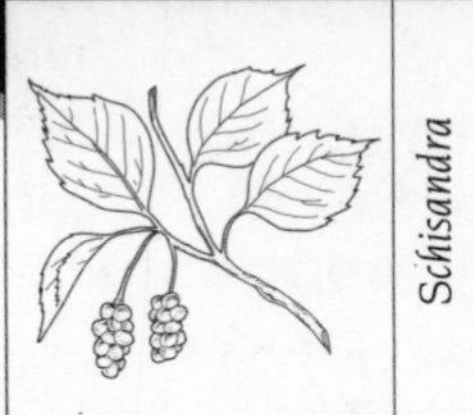

Select the herbs that are most suitable for your condition.

The Herbal Approach

From the ancient games of the Greece, Asia and the Mayan civilizations, to modern day Olympics, the form and style of sports have varied tremendously. What has remained consistent is the desire to compete and to excel, pushing the limits of human skills and physical prowess. Today, sports medicine is a growth industry with over 40,000 team doctors assigned to schools, colleges, and professional teams, and hundreds of sports clinics and centers all over the country. Physical training methods for both professionals, amateurs and weekend warriors has reached new heights.

Yet herbal medicines have something quite different and unique to offer. While steroids and stimulating drugs have long-term damaging effects, the herbs listed below have extraordinary benefits, without these risks. Many tonic and adaptogen herbs have been shown to improve overall physical performance and endurance, as well as specific factors such as recovery time, pulse rate, vital lung capacity, back strength and muscle power. In research done on runners, gymnasts, wrestlers and trainers, herbal energizers show improvement in athletic performance across the board. See also ■ Anti-aging ■ Fatigue ■ Injury/Wounds ■ Stress.

Amalaki**—Emblica myrobalan
- Ayurvedic tonic herb that increases lean body tissue mass while reducing body fat. Increases energy, clarity and combats weakness, fatigue.
- Improves circulation, digestion and promotes elimination of wastes.

Ashwaganda**—Withania somnifera
- Adaptogen herb that works on muscles and nerves to increases performance in athletes; enhances psychomotor coordination, reaction time.
- Protects and overcomes the effects of overwork, fatigue, anxiety, sexual debility. Tones the liver, kidney, immune system; balances hormones.

Cordyceps**—Cordyceps sinensis
- Enhances athletic performance, increases oxygen intake to the lungs.
- Tones the immune system and male organs, improves sexual vitality.
- Increases sperm activity; used in states of exhaustion and low vitality.

Codonopsis**—Codonopsis pilosula
- Tonifies chi, increases energy, stamina, vitality and overall metabolism.
- Strengthens the limbs, blood, lungs and spleen's digestive functions.
- Similar but gentler than ginseng, which can be overly stimulating.

Ginseng**—Panax ginseng
- Increases stamina, endurance, as well as stress resistance. Elevates testosterone and increases adrenal function, including cortisol levels.
- Immune booster; do not use while taking any steroid (e.g. prednisone).

Jianogulan**—Gynostemma pentaphyllum
- Enhances physical strength, stamina and endurance; improves fat metabolism and cholesterol levels. Enhances the immune system.
- Regulates blood pressure, hormone balance and reduces inflammation.

Maca***—Lepidium meyenii
- Boosts energy, stamina, endurance and increases athletic performance.
- Adaptogenic, benefitting the entire system in times of stress or when extra energy is needed. Balances female and male hormone levels.

Rhodiola**—Golden Root/Rhodiola rosea
- Increases levels of protein and RNA in skeletal muscle. Increases activity of protein-digesting enzymes, thus increasing muscle mass.

Sarsaparilla**—Smilax officinalis
- Possesses a testosterone-inducing effect on the body, increasing lean muscle mass and improving strength and athletic performance.
- Aphrodisiac effects due to hormonal rebalancing and tonification.

Schisandra***—Schisandra chinensis
- In tests, 74% of runners obtained their best results when using this herb.
- A supreme adaptogen, balancing all systems; powerful liver healer.
- Improves reflexes, strength and endurance, decreases recovery time, while preventing muscular damage from extreme exercise.

Siberian Ginseng***—Eleuthrococcus senticosus
- In tests on athletes, improves efficiency, endurance; decreases fatigue.
- Produces striking improvements in performance, reduces occurrence of illness and lowers risk of injury-related infection during stress.

Suma***—Pfaffia paniculata
- Increases protein production dramatically; superior to anabolic steroids without their risks; increases physical endurance and muscle mass.
- Reduces muscle fatigue and inflammation, lessens need for insulin.

Tribulus***—Tribulus terrestris
- Increases energy, stamina, speeds muscle recovery after exercise.
- Increases body's testosterone levels naturally. Reduces fluid and sodium retention while reducing blood pressure.

Yerba Mate**—Ilex paraguariensis
- Increases energy, decreases muscle fatigue and lactic acid build-up.
- Balances the nervous system; a rejuvenator during stress and fatigue.
- Controls the appetite, stimulates adrenal cortisol and liver function.

STOMACH CONDITIONS

Select the herbs that are most suitable for your condition.

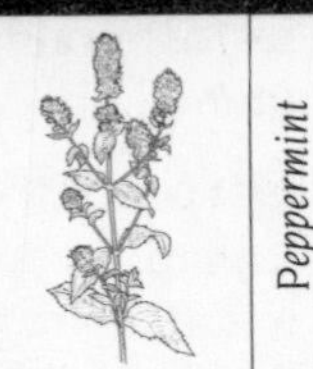

The Herbal Approach

Factors causing simple indigestion, gastritis or ulcers are numerous: bad food, bacteria, alcohol, tobacco and stress. Anti-inflammatory drugs, like aspirin, are also a primary cause of stomach irritation and bleeding. Yet 80–95% of all ulcers are related to infection with *helicobacter pylori*. Thus while antacid therapy drugs account for $4 billion in annual sales, they are not particularly effective and often contain toxic aluminum salts. Additionally, heartburn is often due to acid *deficiency*, with symptoms arising from stomach fermentation.

Herbal remedies for stomach problems, including ulcers, are a combination of soothing demulcents, healers (vulneraries) and anti-inflammatory medicines. Some are particularly effective for destroying harmful bacteria. Hiatus hernia, or spastic reflux in the esophagus, may require relaxing, antispasmodic herbs. The most effective traditional herbal combination for irritation and ulcers is Robert's Formula, consisting of *goldenseal, marshmallow, geranium* and *slippery elm* or *comfrey*. *Licorice*, in the form of DGL, is also a favored contemporary approach. In order to kill off helicobacter, supplements with the mineral *bismuth* are often essential. See also ▪ Colic/Cramps ▪ Colitis/IBS ▪ Diarrhea ▪ Nausea ▪ Parasites.

Anise**—Pimpinella anisum
- Improves appetite and helps digestive function when taken after a meal.
- Use in dyspepsia, heartburn, indigestion, with spitting up of mucus.
- Relieves nausea, gas, infant colic, cramps and rumbling in abdomen.

Artichoke**—Cynara scolymus
- In dyspepsia, indigestion or irritable stomach is effective in 85% of people within one month. Helps abdominal pain, heartburn, bloating.
- Relieves constipation, diarrhea, nausea, vomiting. Improves liver health.

Calamus***—Sweet Flag/Acorus calamus
- Important for stomach inflammation, ulcer tendency. Relieves gas and colic; demulcent and antispasmodic, calms the whole digestive system.
- Improves appetite, helps associated headache, distention, fatigue.

Cayenne**—Capsicum frutescens
- Increases appetite; a digestive tonic that relieves gas and indigestion.
- Useful where there are deficient secretions, in sluggish person with slow metabolism. Not for use in acute stages of gastritis or stomach ulcer.

Chamomile**—Matricaria recutita
- Neutralizes heartburn, gas and bloating; relieves abdominal cramps.
- Ideal for "nervous stomach," diarrhea with indigestion. Antispasmodic.
- Soothes inflamed and irritated stomach linings; calming and sedative.

Gentian**—Gentiana lutea
- A bitter tonic that stimulates the stomach and gall bladder secretions.
- Tones intestinal membranes, regulates and strengthens digestion.
- Heartburn from lack of stomach acid, weak digestion; not for gastritis.

Geranium***—Geranium maculatum
- One of the best herbs for ulcers; tightens and rapidly accelerates healing of tissues. Relieves pain, decreases acidity, checks hemorrhage.

Ginger***—Zingiber officinale
- Relieves gastritis, indigestion and gas, helps heal or prevent ulcers.
- Anti-inflammatory and antibacterial; most effective anti-nausea herb.
- Stimulates digestive enzymes and digestion of fats. Natural antibiotic.

Goldenseal***—Hydrastis canadensis
- Destroys bacteria that cause gastritis, stomach irritation and ulcers.
- Stimulates digestion, initiates normal liver function.
- Promotes rapid healing of ulcerated, inflamed stomach linings.

Licorice***—Glycyrrhiza glabra
- Soothes inflamed stomach linings, promotes protective mucus.
- Inhibits H*elicobacter pylori*, the bacteria that causes stomach ulcers.
- DGL form is safe for long-term use and is as effective as Tagamet.

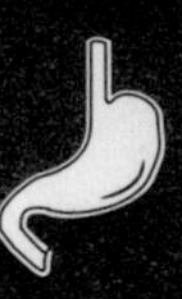

Marshmallow**—Althea officinalis
- A soothing demulcent for irritated and inflamed digestive linings.
- Effective for indigestion, gastritis, ulcers and relieving nausea.

Meadowsweet**—Filipendula ulmaria
- Has anti-inflammatory salicylates, but without irritating the stomach.
- Reduces stomach acidity, heartburn, nausea; heals stomach, aids ulcers.
- Safely controls gastritis, heartburn; combats diarrhea, irritable bowel.

Papaya*—Carica papaya
- Slightly unripe papaya or papain tablets are rich in digestive enzymes.
- Helpful in acid reflux, hiatus hernia, belching and protein maldigestion.

Peppermint***—Mentha piperta
- Contains volatile oils like menthol, relieves indigestion, gastritis, stomach ulcer. Antibacterial, neutralizes excess acidity, relaxes spasms.

Slippery Elm*—Ulmus fulva
- Soothing and healing mucilaginous demulcent for inflamed conditions.
- Nutritional gruel for poor digestion, malabsorption, recovery from toxins.

STRESS

Select the herbs that are most suitable for your condition.

Wild Yam

The Herbal Approach

"Stress is the spice of life," said Hans Selye, the famous researcher who first investigated the physical effects of stress. Everything that disturbs our equilibrium and requires an adaptive response is a stressor. These add the variety to life's journey, but the accumulation of psychological and physical impacts often becomes overwhelming. The organism has complex nervous, immune and hormonal mechanisms to deal with small and large stresses. In spite of these efforts, a whole pantheon of stress-induced illnesses exist, and most chronic illnesses—migraines, colitis, anxiety, depression, immune suppression, fatigue, arthritis, fibromyalgia and asthma—contain a stress element.

Herbs that help with the stress response are *tonic* and *adaptogenic*, helping various systems and organs increase or decrease their activity, as required. This class of herbs is well represented here, each with their own way of fortifying the adrenal glands, brain and metabolism to overcome the accumulation of biological stress. N*ervines* also aid in this work of healing the damage done and establishing a strong basis for fending off further assaults. Most stress-reducing herbs need to be taken for several months for optimal resistance-building effects. Tonic herbs are best taken as the whole herb, rather than as an isolated, standardized extract.

Ashwaganda***—Withania somnifera
- Mediates the effects of stress; improves mental, physical performance.
- An adaptogen that overcomes effects of overwork, fatigue, anxiety, sexual debility. Corrects depressed immunity and hormonal imbalance.

Cordyceps***—Cordyceps sinensis
- Contains building blocks for DNA, RNA repair; overcomes fatigue.
- Strengthens and restores body after exhaustion, rebuilds vitality.
- Promotes immunity, sex drive, improves endurance, clears the lungs.

Ginseng***—Panax ginseng
- Adaptogen that accents ability to cope with mental and physical stress.
- Reduces fatigue and debility from long stress, unbalanced sleep.
- Improves alertness, concentration; tones the immune system, adrenals.

Gotu Kola**—Centella asiatica
- An Ayurvedic adaptogen that helps ability to cope with stress, fatigue.
- Nervous system rejuvenator and longevity herb; reduces anxiety states.
- Improves concentration, memory; augments adrenals and immunity.

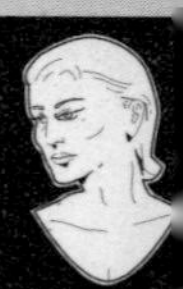

Holy Basil***—Ocimum sanctum
- Adaptogen that lowers stress levels and helps the body respond appropriately; an overall tonifying and invigorating herb, increasing vitality.
- Protects the heart, lowers blood pressure, decreases high blood sugar.

Licorice**—Glycyrrhiza glabra
- An adrenal tonic, increasing cortisone. Protects against the damaging effects of stress, enhances immunity; anti-inflammatory, antihistamine.
- Improves hormonal balance, increases energy, normalizes blood sugar.

Maitake***—Grifola frondosa
- Adaptogen mushroom, capable of improving the body's stress response.
- A powerful immune stimulant, protecting against a variety of toxins.
- Anti-tumor, antiviral, anti-aging; lowers blood pressure, cholesterol.

Oats**—Avena Sativa
- A nutritive brain tonic for effects of stress, exhaustion, sexual weakness, worry, over study, recuperation after illness, overuse of stimulants.
- Improves memory, mental acuity, insomnia. Weans off drugs, alcohol.

Reishi***—Ganoderma lucidum
- A longevity tonic that augments the nervous and immune systems.
- An adaptogen that enhances immunity; anti-inflammatory, antioxidant.
- Relieves fatigue, anxiety, insomnia. Tones the heart, liver, digestion.

Schisandra***—Schisandra chinensis
- A tonic and adaptogen that counters the effects of stress, fatigue.
- A nervine that improves endurance, enhances ability to do mental and physical work, increases efficiency. Liver tonic, protects from toxins.

Siberian Ginseng***—Eleuthrococcus senticosus
- Tones the adrenals, increases resistance to stress-induced illness.
- Immune stimulant, improves both physical and mental performance, alertness, stamina. Speeds convalescence and tones a weak organism.

Suma***—Pfaffia paniculata
- Increases resistance to stress, endurance. Anti-inflammatory and pain relieving, speeds healing, reduces fatigue, regulates hormones.

Wild Yam**—Dioscorea villosa
- A hormonal tonic, muscle and nerve relaxant and antispasmodic.
- Provides precursors for production of adrenal and sex hormones.
- Helps correct low progesterone and high estrogen ratio in PMS.

Yerba Mate***—Ilex paraguariensis
- Increases mental clarity; caffeine-like, but without overstimulation.
- Balances the nervous system. Improves sleep, digestion. Antioxidant.
- Improves depression, reduces allergy, increases oxygen to heart, brain.

THYROID DISORDERS

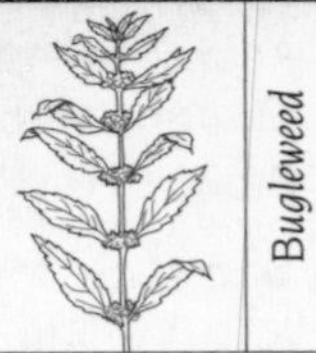

Select the herbs that are most suitable for your condition.

The Herbal Approach

Thyroid problems are not only on the increase, but go undiagnosed in the majority of cases. Both undue fatigue and lethargy on the one hand or hyperactivity and anxiety on the other require one to rule out thyroid problems. However, current blood tests often do not accurately reflect these conditions. While there is often a genetic predisposition toward thyroid disorders, toxic factors are what usually send it over the edge. This includes heavy metals (especially mercury), as well as chronic allergies and radioactive pollutants, which are still very much with us. Yet all thyroid disorders are related to an autoimmune response, with the body developing antibodies to its own thyroid tissue. This may produce overactivity, or there can be enough damage to create hypothyroidism.

There are a number of herbs, as well as specific nutrients, like tyrosine and selenium, that can substantially improve thyroid function. In borderline states of low thyroid, a course of therapy directed toward the gland, as well as underlying allergies and toxins, often produces excellent results. In overactive states, treatment is also directed toward reducing hyperactive immune function. Supplementation with synthetic or animal thyroid can be resorted to if natural methods of rebuilding thyroid function fail. Similarly, destroying the thyroid with radioactive materials or surgery should be a last resort in hyperthyroidism. See also ■ Detoxification ■ Fatigue ■ Immune Weakness ■ Overweight.

Bitter Herbs—Dandelion, Gentian/Taraxacum, Gentiana

- Stimulates a low thyroid, increases metabolism, balances lipid levels.
- Digestive stimulants assists the breakdown and absorption of nutrients.
- Tonify the liver and gall bladder, relieve heartburn and indigestion.

Bugleweed***—Lycopus virginiana

- Used for hyperthyroidism, enlarged thyroid, exopthalmos and associated heart or lung troubles. Calms palpitations, tight chest, heart pain.
- Sedative, anti-inflammatory and astringent, for urinary incontinence and internal bleeding irritating nervous coughs.

Coleus***—Coleus forskohlii

- Forsklin has been shown to increase the production of thyroid hormone and also stimulate its release. Enhances immune function.
- Stimulates fat breakdown and inhibits the synthesis of fat from fat cells.
- Helps depression, heart function and digestive activity.

Gotu Kola***—Centella asiatica

- Used in autoimmune and connective tissue disorders, including Hashimoto's thyroiditis. Good for nervous system disorders.
- Decreases cellular inflammation, improves circulation, venous tone, wound healing, mental functioning. Normalizes hair and nail growth.

Guggul***—Commiphora mukul

- Stimulates the thyroid, benefits endocrine abnormalities, irregular menstrual cycles and aids the nervous system. Prevents arteriosclerosis.
- Lowers cholesterol, normalizes blood lipids, prevents blood clots.

Hai Zao***—Sargassum fusiforme

- Used in Chinese medicine for goiter, caused by low iodine; helps to improve general thyroid function and prevents thyroid disease.
- Used in Hashimoto's thyroiditis. Treats edema and enlarged glands.

Irish Moss**—Chondrus crispus

- A sea herb, high in iodine and trace minerals and part of herbal, vitamin and mineral formulas that assist in debility and anemic states.
- Use in lung diseases, muscle wasting and impaired immunity.

Kelp***—Bladderwrack/Fucus versicolor

- Source of trace minerals, useful in low or enlarged thyroid; activates thyroid functioning, often boosts T4 levels if borderline. Treats goiter.
- Increases basal metabolic rate, lessens edema, balances blood lipids.

Meadowsweet—Filipendula ulmaria

- Has anti-thyroid effects, calming down a hyperactive thyroid gland.
- A sedative herb, relieves nervousness, restlessness, palpitations, mild depression and irritability as well as hyperactivity in children.

Motherwort**—Leonarus cardiaca

- Indicated for swollen or hyperactive thyroid; regulates menses, is a uterine stimulant, treats depression/anxiety. Helps thyroid at menopause.
- Eases palpitations, strengthens the heart, lessens rheumatic pain.

Myrrh***—Commiphora myrrha

- Similar to guggul, stimulates the thyroid gland by unknown action.
- Speeds up sluggish intestines. Possesses antimicrobial, antiseptic and astringent properties, for infections of skin, gums, throat and chest.

Siberian Ginseng**—Eleuthrococcus senticosus

- Enhances thyroid gland functioning and balances hormone levels.
- Improves response to stressful events, increases emotional well-being.
- For persons under high stress with fatigue and taxed immune system.

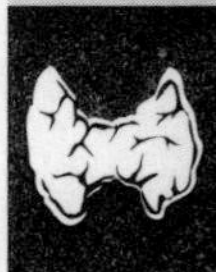

TOBACCO DETOX

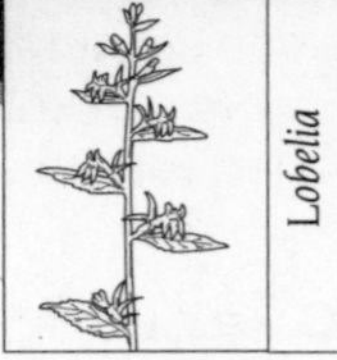

Select the herbs that are most suitable for your condition.

The Herbal Approach

The current "new" revelations regarding the hazards of smoking are curious, since tobacco's effects on the heart and lungs, and its carcinogenic and addictive properties, have been described by medical observers for at least 150 years! Smoking contributes to 20% of all deaths a year, cutting 25 years off the lifespan of users. It kills 3 million smokers worldwide per year, while second-hand smoke also causes 3,000 cases of lung cancer annually and kills another 40,000 bystanders from heart disease.

Herbs can be extraordinarily effective for quitting tobacco. They actually reduce cravings, especially in the case of *lobelia* and *plantain*. Naturally, there are herbs that also help associated coughs, mucus congestion and sore throats. Some are particularly useful in protecting and healing the linings of the nose, throat, bronchi and lungs after cessation of smoking. On deeper levels, they provide immune and adaptogenic support, strengthening the adrenals and nervous system. For craving and addiction, attention should be given to nervines, both those listed here and under Anxiety, especially *kava kava*. See also ▪ Anti-aging ▪ Anxiety ▪ Depression ▪ Detoxification ▪ Fatigue ▪ Heart Conditions ▪ Stress.

Cayenne***—Capsicum frutescens
- Desensitizes the respiratory linings to tobacco and chemical irritants.
- Antioxidant capabilities stabilize lung membranes, preventing damage.
- Warming, peppery taste; distracts attention from cigarette cravings.

Coltsfoot**—Tussilago farfara
- Demulcent and detoxifying; soothes the respiratory membranes.
- Expectorant that relieves congestion, even in elderly and weakened conditions. Regenerates cilia after exposure to chemicals or irritants.

Ephedra*—Ephedra sinensis
- Helps heavy smokers reduce number of cigarettes, helps lobelia and other herbs work better, relaxes bronchi, clears nasal obstruction.
- In allergic hypersensitivity opens the bronchi, helps ease breathing.

Ginger***—Zingiber officinale
- Prevents nausea and helps quitting. Use with lobelia to reduce possible stomach irritation from that herb. Reduces inflammation, anxiety.
- Antioxidant; prevents damage from the chemical residues of smoke.
- Anti-inflammatory, decreases bronchial constriction and irritation.

Licorice**—Glycyrrhiza glabra
- Demulcent, antiviral and antibacterial; supports the immune system, protects the lungs and mucus membranes while they rebuild.
- An adaptogen and adrenal toner; increases energy and stress response.

Lobelia***—Indian Tobacco/Lobelia inflata
- Relieves withdrawal, including irritability, hunger, poor concentration.
- Contains alkaloids similar to nicotine; occupies same brain receptor site and exerts nicotine-like effects. Decreases craving, creates aversion.
- Bronchial antispasmodic that relieves asthma, emphysema, nausea.

Mullein**—Verbascum thapsus
- Soothing demulcent, reducing congestion, encouraging expectoration.
- Benefits inflamed membranes; helps in rebuilding the lung linings.
- Eases sore throats, bronchitis, tracheitis, wheezing and asthma.

Oats***—Avena sativa
- Reduces or eliminates craving for tobacco and other narcotic alkaloids.
- Reduces number of cigarettes desired, even in those not trying to quit.
- Eases anxiety, provides mental and physical energy, improves clarity.

Plantain***—Plantago officinalis
- Creates aversion to tobacco and nicotine, especially chewing.
- Helps depression, irritability, restlessness and insomnia from tobacco.
- Both demulcent and astringent, soothing irritated membranes; useful in coughs, pharyngitis or loss of voice. Reduces noise sensitivity.

Skullcap**—Scutellaria laterifolia
- Sedative and anxiety-reducing; decreases cravings, relieves tension, improves mental clarity. Helps reduce spasms, relieves insomnia.
- Useful in depression and serious mental debility, nourishes and restores the nervous system at a deep level.

Spikenard*—Aralia racemosa
- A lung tonic and expectorant, nourishes and heals the respiratory tract.
- Encourages productive coughs to rid the body of excess mucus.
- An adaptogenic herb, assists the body with stress, easing withdrawal.

Valerian**—Valeriana officinalis
- Relieves the tension and anxiety associated with nicotine withdrawal.
- Promotes sleep, decreases time to fall asleep, quiets disturbed dreaming and lessens awakenings. Relaxes muscle spasticity, cramps.
- Preferable to tranquilizers or barbiturates due to effectiveness and safety.

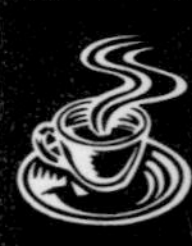

Yerba Santa**—Eriodictyon californicum
- Dilates the bronchi, expels mucus, relieves wheezing and tightness.
- Antibacterial for sore throat, laryngitis, chronic bronchitis, flu, colds.
- Tones the respiratory system, while improving digestion and appetite.

VAGINITIS

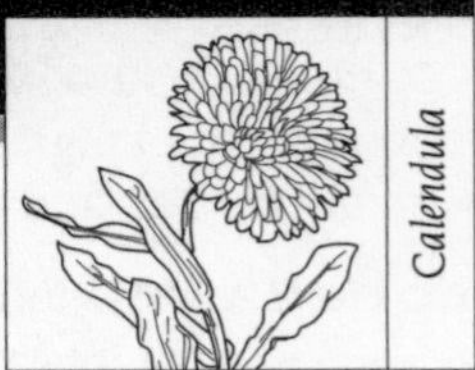

Select the herbs that are most suitable for your condition.

The Herbal Approach

Similar to the intestinal tract, the vaginal canal contains a wide variety of organisms and biochemical secretions in a subtle balance. Disturbance of this balance results in vaginal dysbiosis, an unhealthy mix of disease-producing bacteria, which often results in vaginal inflammation or infection (vaginitis). T*richomonas* is a small protozoa that causes one-third of cases, the rest being related to bacterial *gardnerella* or *candida* type of yeast. Other organisms, like strep, staph and E. coli can form mixed infections. Chlamydia and gonorrhea are more serious sexually transmitted infections. Antibiotics, which destroy healthy bacterial flora, predisposes toward yeast infections, as does anything that increases the sugar content of vaginal cells. This includes use of the pill, diabetes, pregnancy and as a normal part of the menstrual period. Postmenopausal women are also susceptible to changes in secretions and immune health.

Herbs for vaginitis are natural antibiotics, attacking parasitic, bacterial and fungal infections. The advantage is that microorganisms do not develop immunity to them, and they are far safer than medical alternatives. Additionally, demulcent and vulnerary herbs assist in soothing and healing the damaged vaginal linings, while promoting tissue repair. See ▪ Acne/Abscess ▪ Immune Weakness ▪ Infection ▪ Menopause ▪ Warts.

Calendula**—Calendula officinalis
- Antiseptic, antiviral and anti-inflammatory; useful in vaginitis from candida, bacterial, or in HPV (warts). A soothing ointment or suppository.
- Promotes tissue healing; good for connective tissue support with less risk of scarring. Beneficial for minor infections of the epithelial tissue.

Echinacea**—Echinacea angustifolia
- Shown to be effective against candida, trichomonas and many bacteria.
- An immune stimulant, increasing interferon, macrophages and T cells.
- Also has anti-inflammatory effects; best for short-term, intense use.

Garlic***—Allium sativa
- Potent antibacterial with antiseptic properties against a wide variety of organisms, including parasites, candida, and other typical pathogens.
- A component of vaginitis suppositories, capsules and internal rinses.
- Can also be used internally for immune-boosting and antibiotic effects.

Goldenseal***—Hydrastis canadensis
- Effective for thick yellow discharge due to staph, strep and other organisms. Helps heal the mucus membrane linings of the vagina.
- Promotes healing of ulcers, inflammation of cervix, HPV (warts).

Myrrh**—Commiphora myrrha
- Disinfectant to vaginal membranes; destroys bacterial or fungal growth.
- Strong astringent that tones tissue swollen by infection or irritation.
- For all disorders of mucus membranes: gums, throat, lungs and GI tract.

Oregano Oil**—Origanum vulgare
- Powerful antiseptic ability; destroys fungi and yeasts, protozoa, parasites and bacteria. Anti-inflammatory for irritated mucus membranes.
- Can be used as internal capsules and as an external wash or douche.

Oregon Grape***—Mahonia/Berberis aquifolia
- Used to treat amoebiasis, parasites, bacteria, yeasts. Berberine is a powerful antimicrobial and skin remedy. Antioxidant, anti-inflammatory.
- Helps clear cellular wastes, as well as improve the tissues.

Pau D'Arco**—LaPacho/Tabebuia avellanedae
- External and internal use for vaginitis due to candida, virus or bacteria.
- Fights infections, assists the immune system. Helps clear congested lymph tissue and glands, reduces tissue swelling.

Slippery Elm**—Ulmus fulva
- Used as a douche or suppository, acts as a healing demulcent.
- Coats inflamed membranes, relieving itching, irritation, inflammation.

Tea Tree Oil***—Melaleuca alternifolia
- Use ten drops in water as a douche or in vaginal suppositories.
- Effective against a wide range of vaginitis infections, including candida, yeast, trichomonas and even antibiotic resistant bacterial strains.

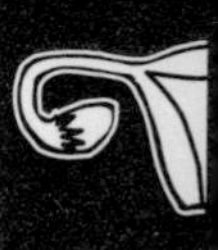

Usnea***—Lichen/Usnea species
- Antimicrobial action extends to bacteria, fungi, virus and parasites.
- Effective for trichomonas, gardnerella and chlamydia, staph and strep.
- Effective antifungal, treats candida locally and systemically.

Yarrow**—Achillea millefolium
- Astringent, quickens healing time, promotes growth of new tissue.
- Antiseptic, antifungal; both fights infection and relieves pain.
- Improves the tone of the mucus membranes of the vagina and uterus.

VEINS/CIRCULATION

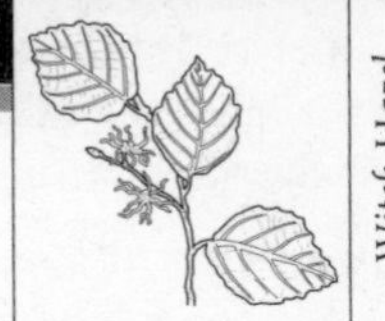

Select the herbs that are most suitable for your condition.

The Herbal Approach

Herbs for the circulatory system have a cross-over effect. They affect both the arterial system, leading from the heart to all the tissues and organs, and the venous system, draining the blood and returning it to the heart. Problems with the arteries affect 3/4 of a million Americans, either from arteriosclerotic narrowing of the arteries (Burger's disease), diabetes, or spasm of these vessels, as in Raynaud's disease. These can all be very painful, as the tissues become starved of oxygen. Vein problems affect almost 25% of women. This includes varicose veins, where the interior valves in the vessels become damaged and, eventually, enlarged, tortuous and hardened. Vein inflammation or *phlebitis* may occur, or clots may form in them (*thrombosis*). Prevention of damage to the elastic tissue in the arterioles and veins would be ideal, with antioxidants like grape seed bioflavonoids and vitamin C. Herbal medicines help stimulate circulation through small arteries, veins and capillaries. They also act to protect and heal the vessel linings and valves, with their antioxidant and anti-inflammatory effects. For varicose veins, it is essential to relieve the back pressure in the liver, kidneys or uterus that underlies the problem. See also ■ Bleeding ■ Inflammation ■ Injury/Wounds ■ Hemorrhoids.

Bilberry***—Vaccinium myrtillus
- Antioxidant and anti-inflammatory, improves circulation, strengthens blood vessels; protects vein and artery walls from free radical damage.
- Useful for phlebitis, varicose veins, hemorrhoids, Raynaud's, diabetic retinopathy, blood clots, post-surgical bleeding; helps arteriosclerosis.

Butcher's Broom***—Ruscus aculeatus
- Proven through traditional and modern practice to be effective in treating varicose veins, phlebitis, vascular insufficiency, hemorrhoids.
- Anti-inflammatory; constricts the veins and reduces their permeability.

Cayenne**—Capsicum frutescens
- When applied externally, causes increased blood flow to the skin.
- Beneficial for atherosclerosis and those prone to blood clotting.
- A warming stimulant for a sluggish circulatory system.

Coleus**—Coleus forskohlii
- Arterial vasodilator, lowering blood pressure, improves heart action.
- Increases blood flow in arteries, helps vascular insufficiency, thins the blood; useful in arteriosclerosis. Helps coronary heart disease, angina.

Daisy***—Bellis perennis

- Taken internally and externally for varicose veins; relieves pain, swelling.
- Helps varicosities during pregnancy. Relieves heavy, tired limbs.
- Particularly effective in areas of old injuries, sprains, trauma to veins.

Garlic**—Allium sativum

- Lowers blood pressure, reduces cholesterol and relieves pain of poor arterial supply (intermittent claudication). Helps prevent blood clots.
- Reduces blood lipids, thins the blood, causing better circulation.

Ginger**—Zingiber officinale

- Helps prevent blood clots. Promotes circulation to the hands and feet.
- Blood-thinning qualities similar to aspirin, with no side effects.
- Increases the circulation and brings blood to the surface of the skin.

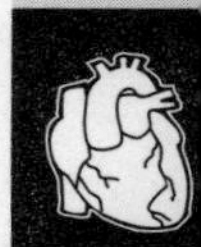

Ginkgo***—Ginkgo biloba

- Effective for intermittent claudication, leg cramps (at night or after exercise), Raynaud's disease and diabetes-related circulatory problems.
- Increases blood flow to brain and extremities without generating heat.
- Better results for circulation to the limbs than any herb or medical drug.

Gotu Kola***—Centella asiatica

- Dilates arteries, improves flow through veins; improves symptoms in 80%. Strengthens and repairs vein and artery walls, reduces hardening.
- Helps varicose veins, phlebitis, leg cramps, ulcers, swelling, heaviness.

Hawthorn***—Crataegus oxycantha

- Heart tonic that improves angina, hypertension, coronary artery disease, high or low blood pressure, congestive heart failure, arrhythmias.
- Improves blood flow to the limbs, improves walking performance.

Horse Chestnut***—Aesculus hippocastanum

- For chronic poor circulation, strengthens and tones the blood vessels.
- Effective internally and externally for varicose veins, phlebitis, varicose ulcers, blood clots, night cramps, varicosities of pregnancy.
- Reduces swelling, pain, itching, tenderness, fatigue and heaviness.

Khella*—Ammi visnaga

- Very effective in dilating arteries, including coronary; relieving symptoms of angina, improves exercise tolerance, normalizes EKG tests.

Stone Root*—Collinsonia canadensis

- Improves varicose veins of limbs, phlebitis, itching, heaviness in legs.
- For kidney stones, water retention, kidney congestion, vein pressure.

Witch Hazel***—Hamamelis virginiana

- Important remedy for varicose veins, ulcers or phlebitis; use externally.
- Tightens tissues, anti-inflammatory and stops all kinds of bleeding.
- Useful during pregnancy. Also effective for bruising, hemorrhoids.

WARTS

Select the herbs that are most suitable for your condition.

White Cedar

The Herbal Approach

Next to acne, warts are the most common skin complaint, occurring in 75% of people. Warts are caused by a variety of related, slow-acting viruses (HPV or human papilloma virus). They can spread to other parts of the body or to others through direct contact or via showers, damp floors, etc. Warts commonly occur on the hands and feet (plantar warts), face and trunk, but may also appear around the genitals or anus. In women, the same virus affects the cervix, often without the appearance of external warts, and is the main cause of cervical dysplasia, leading toward cancer. Warts that appear in those over age forty-five, or that suddenly change in color or size, should be checked to rule out skin cancer. Medically, warts are removed by lasers, liquid nitrogen, surgery or caustic chemicals. Most disappear on their own within two years, but also frequently recur. From a holistic viewpoint, warts are part of an underlying susceptibility that both herbs and homeopathics can eradicate.

There are dozens of effective traditional herbs for removing warts. Many destroy the wart or literally digest it (*pineapple, celandine*). Others have a direct antiviral effect as well. Generally, treatment should be done twice daily and can require several weeks for full effect. In the author's experience, fresh milkweed (*Ascelpias syriaca*) is the most effective of all, usually working after only one or two applications of the milky juice of the fresh plant. NOTE: For most external treatment, protect the surrounding skin with oil, vaseline or zinc ointment. If irritation occurs with any of the treatments, discontinue. Use a less concentrated dose, or use an alternative. See also ■ Immune Weakness ■ Skin Conditions.

Aloe***—Aloe vera/barbadensis
- Fresh aloe juice is applied directly to dissolve warts and tone the skin.
- Healing effects for irritated skin, ulcers or after laser or surgical removal.

Birch Bark*—Betula lenta
- Contains salicylate and antiviral compounds, similar to many over-the-counter wart compounds. Apply directly to wart as a tea or paste.

Bittersweet**—Solanum dulcamara
- A very effective herb for warts of the hands, face. Treats flat as well as large or smooth warts. External application of juice or tincture.

Bloodroot*—Sanguinaria canadensis
- The fresh red juice of the root, or paste made from the powdered root, is applied locally to dissolve hard tissues. Like birch, can be irritating.

Castor Oil**—Ricinus communis

- Cover wart in castor oil and a hot water bottle for warts, cysts. Detoxifies the tissues. Use externally on bruises and sprains; softens scars.

Celandine**—Chelidonium majus

- The fresh yellow juice, tincture or decoction of the root can be applied directly to the wart area. Use daily for best results.
- Surround the periphery with vaseline or oil to protect it from irritation.

Garlic/Ginger**—Allium sativum/Zingiber officinale

- Contain protein-digesting, antiviral and anti-inflammatory properties.
- Can be used individually, or together, applied in crushed form or paste. for several hours daily or overnight, unless the skin becomes irritated.

Houseleek**—Sempervivum tectorum

- Externally for warts, insect bites, infections, growths in the mouth.
- It is recommended for herpes zoster and has been used on cancers.

Juniper**—Juniperus communis

- External treatment for warts, especially with itching and burning.
- Particularly for warts around anus and genitals (use internally as well).

Lemon Peel*—Citrus limon

- Citric acid and antimicrobial properties of the plant can reduce warts.
- The inner surface of the fresh peel is applied overnight for some weeks.

Milkweed***—Ascelpias tuberosa

- A weed that is widespread across North America; the fresh milky sap of the leaf or stem is applied directly to warts once daily.
- Usually works dramatically; non-irritating; does not affect normal skin.
- Dandelion is used in the same way, though not with as effective effects.

Olive Leaf**—Olea europaea

- Fights chronic viral conditions, including HPV. Immune strengthening.
- Take tablets internally and apply a crushed one to the local area.

Proteolytic Enzymes***

- Papaya (papain), pineapple (bromelain), banana peel and figs contain enzymes that digest proteins and dissolve warts in a safe manner.
- The fresh plant, sap (figs) or concentrate (papain) can be applied; any of these can be wrapped or taped on to the wart area for several hours.

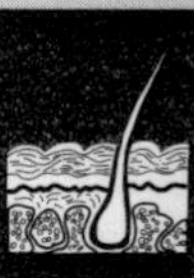

White Cedar***—Thuja occidentalis

- Important for the tendency toward warts, growths, benign tumors.
- Best for cauliflower, moist, large, broad or rapidly growing warts with stalks (fig warts), for easily bleeding or oozing warts, brown or red naevi.
- For warts of the face, lips, nose, feet, neck, genitals, anus. Small crops.
- Use thuja oil externally only. May take 1–2 drops of tincture internally.

Part 4

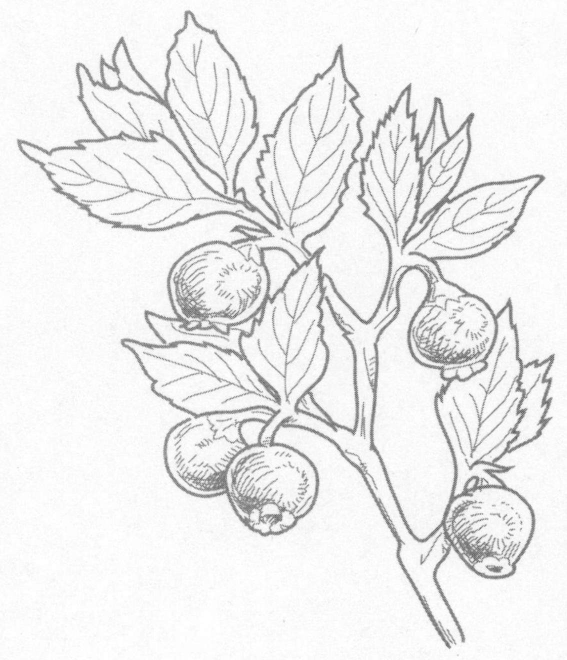

Herbal Sources, Dosage & Safety

NOTE: In the dosages given below, 1 ml is equivalent to one dropperful of liquid or tincture.

A

Alfalfa—Medicago sativa

Source: This member of the pea family is a gentle tonifier, restorative and nutritive herb. The leaves and flowers contain a variety of vitamins and minerals which build strength and vitality in weakened or anemic conditions.

Standardization: None.

Dosage: Capsules: 500–1000 mg, up to 9 capsules daily. Tincture: 1–3 ml, 4 times daily.

Safety: Possible exacerbation of lupus, but human studies have not confirmed this. Avoid alfalfa if using blood thinners. Avoid eating the seeds or sprouts as they contain canavanine and/or toxic saponins.

Aloe—Aloe vera barbadensis

Source: Native to Africa, this member of the lily family is grown in the southwestern United States and Mexico. The gel is obtained from the outer layer of the leaf. The inner leaf contains a yellow, bitter and drastic purgative.

Standardization: No specific standard, but should contain *manapol extract*.

Dosage: Available in the form of a gel or juice of varying concentrations. The gel or juice is used externally for skin problems or burns. Use internally according to directions, (begin with 1/4 cup daily of either gel or juice and increase gradually to 1–2 cups). The latex has a laxative effect but is known to cause undue cramping and spasms of the intestines.

Safety: The gel and juice may cause abdominal cramping and diarrhea when recommended doses are exceeded. Should not be used during pregnancy. The gel may decrease the body's need for insulin. Should not be taken by diabetics without professional advice.

American Ginseng—Panax quinquefolia

Source: American ginseng may be found growing wild in the damp woodlands of the northeastern United States. The tap root is a supreme adaptogen but is currently listed as a threatened species due to overharvesting. Milder and cooler in nature than Chinese ginseng.

Standardization: Standardized to 5–15% ginsenosides.

Dosage: Capsules: Start with low dose of 200 mg and work up to 600 mg daily. Do not take for more than 6 weeks without a break, or take in a cycle of 2 weeks on, 2 weeks off. Tincture: 1–4 ml, 3 times daily.

Safety: Not for individuals with estrogen-dependent conditions (e.g. breast cancer, uterine fibroids), high blood pressure, glaucoma. Can cause headache, insomnia, palpitations or high blood pressure.

Amla—Emblica officinalis

Source: Found in India, Amla, or Indian gooseberry, is considered one of the best tonifiers in Ayurvedic medicine. A highly absorbable source of Vitamin C and main ingredient of chyavanprash, a classic Ayurvedic longevity formula.

Standardization: None.

Dosage: Powdered herb: 6–15 g daily.

Safety: No known toxicity or contraindications.

Andrographis—Andrographis paniculata

Source: Originally from Southeast Asia and China, andrographis is a wonderful flu and cold remedy, usually combined with eleutherococcus and schisandra. The whole plant of this bitter herb is medicinal in nature. Its Chinese name translates to "thread-the-heart-lotus".

Standardization: Andrographolides 15%, 20%, and 30%.

Dosage: Capsules: 300 mg, up to 4 times daily.

Safety: A safe herb with very low toxicity and no known contraindications.

Angelica—Angelica archangelica

Source: This member of the carrot family is a remedy for respiratory and digestive ills and is the main flavoring agent in the liqueur Benedictine.

Standardization: None.

Dosage: Tincture: 1–5 ml, 3 times daily.

Safety: Avoid with bleeding disorders (e.g. hemophilia). Due to its uterine stimulating properties, do not take during pregnancy. There may be increased sensitivity of the skin to sunlight. Avoid prolonged sunbathing or sun exposure. Discontinue use if a rash develops.

Anise—Pimpinella anisum

Source: This member of the carrot family is a close relative to fennel and caraway. The seeds are a flavorful digestive aid and useful in colic type disorders.

Standardization: None.

Dosage: Tincture: 1/4 to 1 tsp, 3 times daily. Tea: 1–2 tsp of seeds in one cup water.

Safety: No known toxicity or untoward effects.

Arjuna—Terminalia arjuna

Source: Arjuna was used medicinally in Ayurveda for over 3,000 years. This evergreen tree grows in the foothills of the Himalayas, and its bark is used medicinally.

Standardization: None.

Dosage: Capsules: 1,500 mg daily.
Safety: Well tolerated at prescribed doses.

Arnica—Arnica montana

Source: A member of the daisy family and native to Europe, the flowering tops of this herb contain an essential oil that helps heal injured tissues.
Standardization: Use 15% arnica oil or 20–25% tincture.
Dosage: Creams or ointments: apply 3–4 times daily for pain and bruising.
Safety: For external use only in the form of creams or ointment. Internally, use only in homeopathic form.

Artichoke—Cynara scolymus

Source: Artichoke is a Mediterranean plant that is a member of the daisy family and has been used as a liver and digestive tonic since antiquity.
Standardization: 2.5–5% caffeylquinic acids, 15% chologenic acid, 2–5% cynarin.
Dosage: Capsules: 800–1,200 mg daily. Standardized extract: 250 mg, 3 times daily. Tincture: 10–40 drops, 4 times daily.
Safety: Quite safe, but those with blood-clotting disorders or taking anticoagulants should not use artichoke. Avoid if allergic to certain members of the daisy family (e.g. thistle, chrysanthemums, goldenrod).

Ashwaganda—Withania somnifera

Source: This shrub is in the nightshade family and a well-known Indian equivalent to ginseng. The leaves, root and fruit are harvested. Ashwaganda has been used for centuries and recent research studies have served to validate its many beneficial actions.
Standardization: 1.5–10% withanolides, alkaloids 1%.
Dosage: Capsules: 1–2g daily. Standardized extract: 450 mg, twice daily. Tincture: 30–60 drops, 3 times daily.
Safety: Contraindicated in pregnancy. Excellent for young people as a substitute for ginseng, which may be too stimulating.

Asian Ginseng—Panax ginseng

Source: The medicinal effects of this ancient Chinese tonic and adaptogen have been documented for over 4,000 years. The root of ginseng is harvested only after the plant has reached 5–7 years of age.
Standardization: Standardized to 5% ginsenosides.
Dosage: Start with low dose of 200 mg and work up to 600 mg daily. Do not take for more than 6 weeks without a break, or take in a cycle of 2 weeks on, 2 weeks off. Tincture: 30–60 drops, 3 times daily.
Safety: Not for individuals with high blood pressure, glaucoma or estrogen-dependent conditions (e.g. breast cancer, uterine fibroids). Can cause headache, insomnia, palpitations or high blood pressure.

Astragalus—Astragalus membranaceous

Source: A member of the pea family, used medicinally in its native China for over 4,000 years as an immune strengthener and general tonic.

Standardization: Minimum of 0.5% of specific complex isoflavones.

Dosage: Capsules: 500 mg, 3 times daily or up to 4,500 mg. Tincture: 30 drops, 3 times daily.

Safety: No known side effects or contraindications.

B

Balm of Gilead—Populus gileadensis

Source: The resinous leaf buds of the balsam poplar tree are collected during the winter months. Poplar trees are indigenous to North America and temperate regions of the globe. The closed leaf buds are used.

Standardization: None.

Dosage: Capsules: Take as directed. Tincture: 1–2 ml, 3 times daily.

Safety: Do not take if you are allergic to aspirin or other salicylates.

Balmony—Chelone glabra

Source: Balmony is a bitter herb found in the damp wetlands of northeastern United States and Canada. In Greek, chelone means tortoise, referring to the flowers striking resemblance to a turtle's head.

Standardization: None.

Dosage: Tincture: 10–20 drops in water 3–4 times daily for gallbladder or digestive complaints.

Safety: Safe for use in children. No known toxicity or contraindications.

Barberry—Berberis vulgaris

Source: Barberry shares many properties with its close relatives, goldenseal and oregon grape. A bitter herb originally from Europe, barberry is now cultivated in America as an ornamental and medicine.

Dosage: Capsules: 400–500 mg daily. Tincture: 2–4 ml, 3 times daily.

Safety: May inhibit beneficial gut flora. Supplement with probiotics during or after use. Contraindicated during pregnancy.

Bayberry—Myrica cerifera

Source: The root bark of this evergreen is native to the eastern part of North America and was listed in the U.S. National Formulary from 1916–1936 for its astringent properties.

Standardization: None.

Dosage: Capsules: 450 mg, up to 6 capsules daily. Tincture: 20–40 drops, 1–4 times daily. May be taken every 15 minutes to 1/2 hour acutely, not to exceed 360 drops in 24-hour period.

Safety: Do not take during pregnancy or nursing.

Bhringraja—Eclipta alba

Source: The whole plant is used in Asian, Indian and North American traditions. Eclipta is known as a hair tonic and general tonifying herb used to renew vitality. Also used as an astringent and hemostatic to stop bleeding anywhere in the body.

Standardization: None.

Dosage: Capsules: 6–15 g daily.

Safety: No known contraindications.

Bacopa—Bacopa monniera

Source: Known as "brahmi" or "water hyssop," this herb originates in tropical climates and southern Asia. Indian medicine utilizes bacopa for its mental and nervous system effects

Standardization: 20% barcoposides.

Dosage: Capsules: 100 mg twice daily. Tincture: 60 drops daily.

Safety: No known side effects.

Beet Leaf—Beta vulgaris

Source: The white and red variety of the beet root contain numerous medicinal nutritive substances and are grown worldwide as a food. White beet root served as the first source of sugar in 1760.

Standardization: None.

Dosage: Capsules: 605 mg, 2 capsules, 3 times daily.

Safety: No toxicity, even at high doses.

Beth Root—Trillium erectum or pendulatum

Source: A low-lying perennial member of the lily family. Beth root is also called "birth root," due to its powerful anti-hemorrhagic properties. Northern Native American's used the root and rhizome for reducing hemorrhaging after childbirth and difficult menstruation.

Standardization: None.

Dosage: Tincture: 1–4 ml, 3 times daily.

Safety: Due to its uterine-stimulating properties, avoid during pregnancy.

Bilberry—Vaccinium myrtallus

Source: A close relative to blueberry tree, this member of the heath family was known traditionally as a blood purifier and vision enhancer. Today bilberries are a recognized source of protective antioxidants highly concentrated in the pigmented skin of the fruit.

Standardization: 15–25% anthocyanidin content.

Dosage: Capsules: 80–160 mg, 3 times daily. Standardized extract: up to 450 mg daily. Consume the fresh berries on a regular basis.

Safety: No known side effects or interactions with conventional drugs. Quite safe, even in pregnancy. High doses may be mildly laxative.

Birch—Betula alba

Source: Birch is native to North America, Europe and parts of Russia where the bark and twigs are removed and dried for use. The medieval Saint Hildegard of Bingen was the first to extol the medicinal properties of betula.

Standardized: 3% flavonoids.

Dosage: 2–3 g drunk several times daily. Fluid intake should increase to at least 2 liters daily.

Safety: No known contraindications with therapeutic doses.

Bitter Melon—Momordica charantia

Source: The leaves, seeds, oils, ripe and unripe fruit of this Asian climber herb are harvested all year long for their medicinal properties.

Standardization: 3% bitters, 5.1% triterpenes.

Dosage: Capsules: 200 mg, 3 times daily. Standardized extract: 200mg, 3 times daily. Juice: 100 ml per day.

Safety: High doses can cause cramps and diarrhea. Contraindicated in children or hypoglycemia. Caution: May increase the effect of medical sugar-lowering drugs.

Bitter Orange—Citrus aurantium/Zhi Shi

Source: Native to the tropical regions of Asia, the fruit, leaves and flowers of this species of orange contain substances that act as a potent thermogenic agent—increasing metabolism and burning off fats. Bitter orange is the source of neroli and petigrain oils and its acidic nature promotes internal cleansing and weight loss.

Standardization: 6% Advantra Z.

Dosage: Standardized extract: 650 mg of Advantra Z before each meal. Tincture: 20–30 drops, 3 times daily.

Safety: Very safe at therapeutic doses. Does not have the unpleasant side effects associated with ephedra or yohimbe (e.g. palpitations, anxiety). Caution: Do not take the oil internally.

Black Cumin—Nigella sativa

Source: Native to western Asia and a member of the buttercup family, the seeds of black cumin are a popular culinary spice and medicinal herb throughout India and the Middle Eastern regions.

Standardization: None.

Dosage: Follow package directions.

Safety: Safe for use in children for colic and digestive complaints. No contraindications are known.

Black Cohosh—Cimicifuga Racemosa

Source: A member of the buttercup family and native to Canada and eastern United States. Different species of this dark root are utilized by Traditional Chinese Medicine for asthma and rheumatism, though in the West, it is known mainly as an herb for women.

Standardization: 1 mg triterpenes or 2.5% triterpenoid glycosides.

Dose: Capsules: 250 mg, 3 times daily. Standardized extract: 4 mg triterpenes daily for menopausal symptoms or up to 1,500 mg daily of the 0.2% triterpenes form. Tincture: 20–40 drops, 3 times daily.

Safety: Do not take during the first trimester of pregnancy. Since the herb is in such great demand, it may soon become endangered. Do not exceed the recommended dosage. If currently on estrogen therapy, seek professional advice before taking black cohosh.

Blue Cohosh—Caulophyllum thalictroides

Source: A Native American root used to facilitate childbirth by the Algonquin tribe, blue cohosh grows wild throughout the woodland regions of eastern North America.

Dosage: Tincture: 60–120 drops, 3 times daily.

Safety: Do not use prior to the ninth month of pregnancy due to the risk of miscarriage. Contains alkaloids and caulosaponin glycosides, which have the ability to constrict coronary blood vessels.

Blue Flag—Iris versicolor

Source: The rhizome of this lily family member is a cooling lymphatic cleanser and cholagogue. Especially useful when glandular tissues are swollen and spongy in nature.

Standardization: None.

Dosage: Tincture: 1–5 drops, 3 times daily.

Safety: Toxic in high doses. Use only under professional supervision. Overdoses cause gastroenteritis possibly resulting in death. Contraindicated during pregnancy.

Bladderwrack—Fucus versiculosus

Source: Bladderwrack or kelp is a common seaweed, which supplies trace minerals and iodine for rebalancing thyroid or metabolic disorders.

Standardization: None.

Dosage: Capsules: 600 mg, 1–3 times daily. Tincture: 1–2 ml, 3 times daily.

Safety: Contraindicated with high blood iodine levels, Hashimoto's thyroiditis, hyperthyroidism, pregnancy and nursing.

Black Radish—Raphanus sativus-niger

Source: Native to southern Asia. The radish was so valued through the ages that early Egyptian pyramid builders were thought to be paid in radish, onions and garlic. It is used as a stimulating digestive tonifier.

Standardization: None.

Dosage: 100–150 ml of fresh juice daily, taken for 4 days on, and 2 days off, repeating the cycle for several months.

Safety: Contraindicated with gallstones or obstructive gallbladder disease. May experience gastric upset in high doses.

Bloodroot—Sanguinaria canadensis

Source: Traditionally, Native Americans used this herb to treat fevers, vomiting and as a tool during divination ceremonies. So named for its dark earthy red root.

Standardization: None.

Dosage: Tincture: 2–4 ml daily. Mouth rinse: 1 tsp per cup of water, made as an infusion.

Safety: Contraindicated in pregnancy, breastfeeding, glaucoma. Excessive doses are toxic and will induce nausea and vomiting.

Bogbean—Menyanthes trifoliata

Source: Bogbean is an aquatic herb that prefers the damp swamplands of Asia, Europe and North America. Bogbean's fruit resembles a small bean, hence its name.

Standardization: None.

Dosage: Tincture: 1–2 ml, 2–3 times daily.

Safety: Because of bogbean's diuretic nature, drink plenty (6–8, 8 oz glasses) of water while taking this herb. Excessive doses may cause vomiting. Do not take with diarrhea or colitis conditions.

Boldo—Peumus boldus

Source: The lemon-scented leaves and bark of this Andean evergreen shrub are still utilized today by native people of Chile as a fruit and tonifying beverage. Include boldo in any gallstone formulation for increased effectiveness.

Standardization: None.

Dosage: Capsules: Up to 2.5 g daily. Tincture: 30–120 drops, 1–3 times daily.

Safety: Do not take during pregnancy.

Boneset—Eupatorium perfoliatum

Source: An eastern North American herb whose name originates from the ability of its leaves to relieve "bone breaking fevers" flus and rheumatism. Native Americans taught the European settlers of its many medicinal values, touting boneset as a "cure all" for many ills.

Standardization: None.

Dosage: Capsules: Take as directed. Tincture: 30–60 drops.

Safety: Toxic in high doses.

Boswellia—Boswellia serrata

Source: A relative of the frankincense, this Indian tree is tapped to acquire its anti-inflammatory resin. In Ayurveda, boswellia resin is known as

Sallai guggal.

Standardization: 37.5–65% boswellic acid.

Dosage: Capsules: 500–1,200 mg, 3 times daily, for 8–12 weeks duration.

Safety: Side effects are rare, but include diarrhea, skin rash and nausea.

Bromelain—Ananas comosus

Source: Bromelain's anti-inflammatory and wound-healing effects are actually due to protein-digesting enzymes found in the pineapple's stems.

Standardization: None.

Dosage: Capsules: 1,200 to 3,000 mcu, or 125–450 mg, 3 times daily.

Safety: No side effects or toxicity. Avoid with a known allergy to pineapples, with gastritis, stomach/duodenal ulcers or bleeding disorders.

Buchu—Barosma betulina

Source: This herb was originally used by the Khoikhoin people in South Africa as a stimulant and diuretic. During the 18th century, buchu was imported to Europe and was listed as a medicinal substance.

Standardization: None

Dosage: Capsules: 500 mg, twice daily. Tincture: 20–40 drops, 3 times daily.

Safety: Do not take during pregnancy.

Buckthorn—Rhamnus frangula/cathartica

Source: Buckthorn is a small tree native to the northeastern United States and Europe. The bark from four-year-old trees is harvested, dried and aged for one year prior to use. It is one of the cleansing herbs found in the Hoxsey cancer formula.

Standardization: None

Dosage: Tincture: 20–70 drops, 3 times daily. Milder laxative than senna leaves. Unlike most laxatives, buckthorn can be used on a long term basis, useful in cases of chronic constipation.

Safety: Do not use with colitis or other chronic gastrointestinal disorders. Use aged bark only. Berries may be toxic if eaten. The fresh bark is a violent purgative. If vomiting or severe gastrointestinal distress occurs, seek medical attention.

Bugleweed—Lycopus virginicus

Source: A North American herb that grows near water. The flowers, leaves and stems were valued since the 19th century for their sedative effects.

Standardization: None

Dosage: Tincture: 10–20 drops, 3 times daily.

Safety: Do not take in hypothyroidism, pregnancy or nursing. Use only under professional supervision. Seek medical attention if experiencing racing heartbeat or excessive nervous excitement.

Bupleurum—Bupleurum chinense

Source: Native to China, bupleurum root is a popular liver tonifier and protectant that has been recorded in Chinese medicinal formulations for over 2,000 years.

Standardization: None.

Dosage: Capsules: 500 mg, 3 times daily. Tincture: 30–90 drops, 1–3 times.

Safety: No known contraindications or toxicity.

Burdock—Arctium lappa

Source: This member of the daisy family is originally of Eurasian origin but has become a well-known weed in the northeastern United States. The root has been used medicinally for centuries as both a blood purifier and detoxifying agent.

Standardization: None.

Dosage: Capsules: 1–2 g daily. Tincture: 2–4 ml, 3 times daily.

Safety: Some caution may be required in psoriasis due to burdock's high inulin content. Discontinue if an increase in skin symptomology occurs. Generally, no other known side effects or safety issues.

Butcher's Broom—Ruscus aculeatus

Source: So named because butchers once used the bundled branches as brooms in Europe. Butcher's broom is a member of the lily family and native to northwestern European and Mediterranean regions.

Standardization: 10% of the saponin glycoside ruscogenin.

Dosage: Capsules: up to 2,400 mg of the encapsulated herb. Standardized extract: 50–100 mg, 1–3 times daily. Tincture: 10–60 drops daily.

Safety: Do not use if you have high blood pressure.

Butterbur—Petasites hybridus

Source: Of European origin, butterbur is now found in North America and Northern Asia. Historically used as a plague remedy, the leaves were once worn by country travelers in Europe as protection from pestilence.

Standardization: None.

Dosage: Capsules: 4.5–7 g daily.

Safety: Contains pyrrolizidine alkaloids. Daily dosages should not exceed 1 mg of the alkaloids due to possible liver toxicity. Contraindicated in pregnancy and nursing.

Butternut—Juglans cineraria

Source: Valued for its timber, the bark of this North American tree is a digestive aid, laxative and anti-parasitic that also decreases elevated cholesterol levels.

Standardization: None.

Dosage: Tincture: 10–30 drops, 3 times daily.

Safety: Do not take during pregnancy due to its laxative effects.

Calendula—Calendula officinalis

Source: A European native, calendula or marigold is one of the most popular garden herbs. A useful household remedy that is suitable for everyday applications. Soothes chapped skin, hastens healing time, reduces infection and quiets irritation. Its bright orange flowers contain the highest concentration of active compounds.

Standardization: None.

Dosage: Tincture: 5–20 drops, 3 times daily. External use: Place the flower and leaf directly on the affected area. Use the cream, infusion or ointment for topical skin conditions.

Safety: No known side effects or contraindications. If allergic to other daisy family plants, test on a small area of skin, watching for symptoms of redness or itching before applying or taking internally.

California Poppy—Eschscholzia californica

Source: This member of the poppy family is native to the sandy soil of California. The aerial parts were used by Native Americans for pain relief. A gentle and soothing remedy for children and the elderly.

Standardization: None.

Dosage: Tincture: 30–60 drops, 4 times daily for tension or bedwetting.

Safety: No adverse effects known. Use cautiously in pregnancy, as one animal study demonstrated uterine stimulant effects.

Caraway Seed—Carum carvi

Source: Of European origin, the seeds of the caraway plant are closely related to their carrot family cousins; anise and fennel. Thus they all share in their ability to relieve cramping in the entire digestive tract.

Standardization: None.

Dosage: Seeds: 1.5–6 gm daily in tea.

Safety: Caraway has very low toxicity, with no known drug interactions. The essential oil is for external use only.

Cardamon—Eletteria cardamomum

Source: One of the world's oldest medicinal spices. The seedpods contain fragrant antispasmodic volatile oils that relieve colic and digestive upsets. This member of the ginger family is native to India and Sri Lanka and flourishes at altitudes of up to 5,000 feet.

Standardization: None.

Dosage: Capsules: 1–5 gm daily. Tincture: 5–30 drops, 1–4 times daily.

Safety: Do not use cardamon with gallstones or gallbladder disease. May be associated with increased gallbladder pain.

Cardiospermum—Cardiospermum halicacabum

Source: Native to Bermuda, Florida and Texas, this herb is also named "heart seed" for the white heart that marks the seed's surface. The above-ground parts are used in a cream to treat eczema and dermatitis.

Standardization: None.

Dosage: Available in cream form. Apply externally as directed.

Safety: No adverse effects reported.

Carob—Certonis siliqua

Source: Carob pods have been appreciated since biblical times for their ability to ease diarrhea and digestive ailments. A member of the bean family, this now popular chocolate substitute is native to Arabia and Somalia.

Standardization: None.

Dosage: Powder: 15 g mixed with applesauce (for children) or 20 g daily for adults.

Safety: Carob is a very safe and well-tolerated herb with no known toxicity or side effects. Note that infants with severe diarrhea may require immediate care and should be evaluated by a health care practitioner.

Cascara—Cascara sagrada/Rhamnus purshiani

Source: The bark of this North American tree is aged at least one year, since the fresh bark causes vomiting and digestive toxicity.

Standardization: 25–30% hydroxyanthracene derivatives.

Dosage: Capsules:400–500 mg, up to 2 capsules as needed. Tincture: 1–5 ml daily. Children and elderly should take only 25–50 mg per dose.

Safety: Safe, but should not be used for prolonged periods (i.e. more than 10 days), as this may deplete the body of vital salts or cause dehydration. Avoid in pregnancy, serious ulceration or intestinal bleeding.

Castor Oil—Ricinus communis

Source: This African shrub in the evergreen family is harvested throughout the year for its medicinal seeds and oil. Used since Egyptian times as a bowel cleanser.

Standardization: 60–100% castor oil.

Dosage: Oil: 1–4 tsp orally per dose. Apply the oil topically in the form of a poultice to the abdomen, sore joints and swollen cysts.

Safety: Do not use internally with children, if pregnant (uterine stimulant) or for more than 1–2 days every 2–3 weeks. Caution: Do not eat the seeds or leaves as they contain lethal toxins, which are not found in the expressed, commercially available oil.

Catnip—Nepeta cateria

Source: This member of the mint family grows alongside roads and at altitudes up to 5,000 feet. Native to Europe and now grown in North America, the leaves and flowers are harvested during the spring and summer months.

Standardization: None.

Dosage: Tincture: 2–4 ml, 3 times daily.

Safety: Catnip is contraindicated in pregnancy and during nursing.

Cat's Claw—Uncaria tomentosa

Source: A member of the coffee family and related to quinine, this herb grows in the Peruvian rain forests of the Amazon. Its name comes from the claw-like thorns at the base of the plant's leaf. Known as the "sacred vine of the rainforest," the bark, root, stem and leaf are used in medicinal preparations.

Standardization: 10–15% phenolics, 4% alkaloids

Dosage: Capsules: 500–1,000 mg, 3 times daily. Standardized extract: 20–60 mg daily. Tincture: 1–2 ml, 3 times daily.

Safety: Though there is little inherent toxicity, avoid during pregnancy or if trying to conceive, as it can cause uterine contractions. Avoid if taking anti-ulcer medication or with organ transplants.

Cayenne—Capsicum fructescens

Source: Native to South America and a member of the nightshade family, this "red hot" pepper is the most widely used spice throughout the world. Benefits the digestion, increases circulation and relieves pain.

Standardization: 5–10% capsaicin or 150,000 Scoville heat units.

Dosage: Capsules: Up to 400 mg daily, in divided doses. Tincture: 1–10 drops in water, 3 times daily. External preparations: 0.25%-0.75% capsaicin creams.

Safety: Excess use can irritate the stomach and inflame the kidneys. May experience redness and irritation with topical use. Avoid eye contact. Do not exceed recommended dosages.

Celandine—Chelidonium majus

Source: A member of the poppy family, the latex (sap), flowers, leaves and stems possess medicinal properties. Native to Europe, western Asia and northern Africa, celandine flourishes in damp places and along roadsides across temperate North America.

Standardization: None.

Dosage: Tincture: 1–2 ml, 3 times daily. The juice applied to the skin must be surrounded by an oil or non-petroleum jelly to avoid irritation.

Safety: Do not use in pregnancy. Large doses will produce nausea, vomiting and watery diarrhea.

Chamomile—Matricaria recutita

Source: The flowers of both German chamomile (*Matricaria recutita*) and Roman chamomile (*Chamaemelum nobile*) have been taken for centuries as a digestive tonic. Chamomile grows wild in much of Europe and temperate regions.

Standardization: 1.2% Aperigenine,1.5 mg.

Dosage: Capsules: 2–3 g daily. Tincture: 1 tsp, 3 times a day.

Safety: Generally safe; toxicity is extremely rare, though occasionally those with severe hay fever have had allergic reactions to chamomile.

Chapparal—Larrea tridentata

Source: This bush may be found in the arid deserts of Mexico and the American southwest. Native Americans value the leaves and young twigs of this powerful herb as a cure-all for a variety of conditions.

Dosage: Capsules: 2–4 capsules daily. Tincture: 20–60 drops daily.

Safety: Cases of jaundice and hepatitis reported after using this herb; reports are inconclusive as to the cause. Use caution with liver disorders. Possibly toxic to the liver in high doses.

Chasteberry—Vitex agnus castus

Source: The berry of this Mediterranean tree is a member of the vervain family. So named for its anaphrodisiac properties, chaste trees were commonly found in monastery gardens during the Middle Ages.

Standardization: 0.8% agnuside and 0.6% aucubine.

Dosage: Capsules: 400 mg, 4–6 daily. Standardized extract: 200 mg daily. Tincture: 40 drops, 3 times daily. Used for at least 3 months; may require 18 months for optimal effects.

Safety: No serious toxicity or drug interactions are known; some people report an itchy rash with prolonged use. Vitex can cause headache or increased menstrual flow. Do not use during pregnancy. Also may interfere with other types of hormone therapies (e.g. the pill, estrogen therapy).

Chinese Rhubarb—Rheum palmatum

Source: Used for over 2,000 years in its native China and Tibet, the rhizome is gathered when the tree is ten years of age.

Standardization: None.

Dosage: Capsules: Follow manufacturer's directions. Tincture: 20 drops in water, twice daily.

Safety: Do not use if pregnant or breastfeeding, during menstruation or if prone to kidney stones. Gentle enough for children.

Chinese Skullcap—Scutellaria baicalensis

Source: The root of this perennial plant is native to Asia and grows in open fields up to 8,000 feet above sea level. Wooden tablets from 2nd century A.D. have recorded its value as a "bitter and cold" herb suitable for hot and damp conditions, such as diarrhea, fevers and inflammation. A member of the mint family, it is closely related to American skullcap.

Standardization: None.
Dosage: Capsules: 20–40 mg daily. Tincture: 30–40 drops in water, 3–4 times daily.
Safety: No known contraindications.

Chinese Wormwood—Artemesia annua
Source: Native to the grasslands of Asia and Russia, Chinese wormwood, or "qing hao" has been mentioned in Chinese medical texts since 168 B.C. for relief of heat conditions such as fever and diarrhea. This clearing herb has been verified as an effective anti-parasitic and anti-malarial remedy.
Standardization: None.
Dosage: Capsules: 300–600 mg daily. Tincture: 1–4 ml, 3 times daily. Should be taken as 500 mg, twice daily for 10 days. Recurrence of parasite infections are high, so the 10-day dosing cycle may need to be repeated.
Safety: No adverse effects are known.

Chickweed—Stellaria media
Source: Native to Asia and Europe, chickweed is regarded as a pleasant salad green and a beneficial herb for skin ailments.
Standardization: None.
Dosage: Tincture: 1–5 ml daily. Chickweed creams or compresses may be applied externally to relieve itching and soothe inflamed or irritated skin rashes.
Safety: Do not take during pregnancy or in high doses.

Cinnamon—Cinnamomum verum
Source: This evergreen tree is native to India and Sri Lanka. The inner bark has a long and well-documented history of use in Egyptian, Chinese and Indian traditions.
Standardization: None.
Dosage: Tincture: 20–30 drops, 3–4 times daily. Powder: 1/4 teaspoon, 2–3 times daily.
Safety: Do not use during pregnancy or in excessive doses. Do not take the essential oil internally.

Cleavers—Galium aparine
Source: This ground cover vine is found throughout most of the world. The leaves and stems have a history of being a lymphatic cleanser, coffee substitute and edible salad green.
Standardization: None.
Dosage: Capsules: 5–10 capsules daily. Tincture: 1/2–1 tsp, 3 times daily.
Safety: No known contraindications or side effects.

Clove—Syzygium aromaticum

Source: Native to the Molucca Islands and Phillipines, cloves were a much valued aromatic spice in trade routes around the world. This evergreen tree grows to about 50 feet in height and the unopened flower buds are used in medicinal and culinary practices.

Standardization: None.

Dosage: Capsules: Take as directed. Tincture: 20–40 drops, 3 times daily.

Safety: Do not use the essential oil internally, as it may cause irritation if applied directly to the skin.

Codonopsis—Codonopsis pilosula

Source: The adaptogenic and tonifying effects of this Chinese root are similar in nature to Chinese ginseng. It is usually preferred when ginseng's effects are too strong, yang, or hot-natured.

Standardization: None.

Dosage: Capsules: Take as directed. Tincture: 1/2–1 tsp, 3 times daily.

Safety: No contraindications or untoward side effects noted.

Coleus—Coleus forskohlii

Source: Coleus is a member of the mint family and flourishes along the dry hillsides of the Himalayan mountains. The roots and leaves are well respected in Ayurvedic medicine for their many beneficial effects.

Standardization: 10%–20%, 2.5–9 mg forskohlin.

Dosage: Capsules: 50 mg (18% forskohlin extract) 4 times daily or 250 mg (1% forskohlin extract) up to 3 times daily. Tincture: 2–4 ml, 3 times daily

Safety: No known side effects or contraindications. Monitor, or do not use if taking anti-asthmatic and anti-hypertensive drugs, as it may increase the medication's effects. Avoid in low blood pressure conditions and peptic ulcer disease.

Coltsfoot—Tussilago farfara

Source: An ancient European respiratory expectorant herb in the daisy family. The flowers and leaves were appreciated by Dioscorides and Pliny for their value in the treatment of coughs and lung ailments.

Standardization: None.

Dosage: Tincture: 10–15 drops, 3 times daily.

Safety: Should contain less than 1 ppm of PAs (pyrrolizidine alkaloids), which can cause liver damage with prolonged or excessive use. Use leaves, as the flowers contain a higher percentage of PAs. Not to be used by pregnant or nursing women or by children. Do not use for over one month.

Comfrey—Symphytum officinale

Source: A perennial herb from the borage family, comfrey's name alludes to its long history for mending broken bones, *confirma* means "to make firm," *symphytum* means "to make strong." The leaves and root are for external and internal use.

Standardization: None.

Dosage: Capsules: 250 mg, twice daily.

Safety: Comfrey root contains pyrrolizidine alkaloids, which can damage the liver. In most preparations, the alkaloids have been removed. Only the leaf and only American comfrey (not European or Russian) should be used. Prolonged use is contraindicated; it should not be taken by children or by pregnant or nursing women. External ointments should not be used for more than one month.

Coptis—Coptis chinensis

Source: A member of the buttercup family, coptis root contains bitter berberines, and is similar in nature to goldenseal and Oregon grape. Native to China, coptis is valuable in treating liver disorders and any condition characterized by excess heat and dampness, as defined in Traditional Chinese Medicine.

Standardization: None.

Dosage: Capsules: 40 mg daily. Tincture: 1–4 ml, 3 times daily.

Safety: Do not take during pregnancy. Berberines are uterine stimulants.

Cordyceps—Cordyceps sinensis

Source: Cordyceps is a black caterpillar fungus, which is a well-known tonifying herb in China to increase vitality and treat various lung and kidney ailments. It is a powerful immune stimulant and is used as an adjunct to mainstream cancer therapy for improving results and decreasing the side effects of medical treatments.

Standardization: 0.14% adenosine and 5% mannitol per dose.

Dosage: Standardized extract: 1–3.5 g daily. Tincture: 15–30 drops, 2 times daily.

Safety: Use caution when buying in bulk from Chinese distributors, as adulteration is common. Should be taken on an empty stomach. Do not use if there is active bleeding, bleeding disorders or if taking anticoagulant medication. Do not take along with MAO inhibitor drugs.

Corn Silk—Zea mays

Source: Native to North and South America, corn has been revered by many cultures for its practical, ceremonial and mythical value. *Zea* means "cause of life" and *mays* means "our mother." The inner silk of corn is utilized medicinally as a cooling anti-inflammatory.

Standardization: None.

Dosage: Capsules: 1–2 g daily. Tincture: 1–4 ml, 3 times daily.

Safety: No side effects or contraindications

Corydalis—Corydalis yanhusuo

Source: A member of the poppy family and native to China, Siberia and Japan, Corydalis has been used since the 8th century to relieve menstrual cramping. It is regarded today as an effective pain reliever.

Standardization: None.

Dosage: Capsules: 2,000 mg daily. Tincture: 1 tsp, 2–3 times daily.

Safety: Do not take during pregnancy.

Cowslip—Primula veris

Source: Cowslip may be found growing in chalky soil in Europe and Asia. Do not wildcraft, as it is becoming rare in its native land. The whole plant is used medicinally.

Standardization: None.

Dosage: Capsules: Take as directed. Tincture: 1–3 ml, 3 times daily.

Safety: Do not take during pregnancy, if allergic to salycilates, aspirin, or if taking anti-clotting medications.

Couchgrass—Agropyron repens

Source: A common weed found throughout much of the world, couchgrass has been used since the times of Dioscorides for urinary ailments.

Standardization: None.

Dosage: Capsules: 3,000–10,000 mg daily. Tincture: 1–4 ml, 3 times daily.

Safety: No ill effects or toxicity noted. Drink plenty of water (6–8, 8-ounce glasses) while taking this herb to flush out the urinary tract.

Crampbark—Viburnum prunifolia

Source: A popular anti-inflammatory herb that Native Americans used for strengthening and tonifying the uterus after childbirth.

Standardization: None.

Dosage: Capsules: 1,000 mg, 1–3 times daily. Tincture: 1–3 ml, 4 times daily.

Safety: No ill effects found at prescribed dosage.

Cranberry—Vaccinium macrocarpon

Source: The well-known cranberry is a member of the heather family and grows in boggy regions of North America and Europe.

Standardization: 75–80% cranberry solids in concentrate form.

Dosage: Capsules: 500–1,000 mg of extract. Juice: 300 mg of the pure unsweetened juice (one cup or 10 ounces). In one study, 16 ounces daily of sweetened cranberry juice showed beneficial effects in acute and recurrent urinary infections.

Safety: Avoid if taking diuretics or other kidney drugs, breastfeeding or during pregnancy.

Cranesbill—Geranium maculatum

Source: This rhizome grows in the shady forests of Europe and North America. Cranesbill is an astringent herb that helps to decrease bleeding in a variety of conditions.

Standardization: None.

Dosage: Tincture: 2–4 ml, 3 times daily. Powdered herb: 1–2 g daily. May also be used as a mouthwash for swollen or bleeding gums.

Safety: Due to the high tannin content it may cause gastric irritation. Combine with a soothing demulcent such as marshmallow or slippery elm to balance this effect.

Culver's Root—Leptandra virginica

Source: This North American root grows in meadows and woodlands. Culver's root was used by Native Americans and 19th century Physiomedicalists as a purgative and bile stimulant.

Standardization: None.

Dosage: Capsules: Take as directed. Tincture: 1–4 ml, 3 times daily.

Safety: The fresh root is toxic if taken internally. Do not use during pregnancy or nursing.

Curcumin—Turmeric/Curcuma longa

Source: A member of the ginger family and a native Indian spice, ginger has been revered as a panacea in Ayurvedic and Chinese medicine for several millennia.

Standardization: 95% curcuminoids or 97% curcumin

Dosage: Capsules: 250–600 mg, 3 times daily. Tincture: 1 tsp, 3 times daily. Turmeric powder: 8–60 g, 3 times daily.

Safety: Not for children. Older children and the elderly should begin with small doses. May cause heartburn or stomach upset in large doses. Do not use with anti-coagulants, in clotting disorders, gallbladder problems or immediately before surgery. Do not use if pregnant or trying to conceive, as one animal study showed decreased fertility.

D

Daisy—Bellis perennis

Source: The flowering plant is native to Europe and is now found throughout most of North America. Wild daisy is helpful for injuries and bruising.

Standardization: None.

Dosage: Tincture: 3 drops, 2–3 times daily.

Safety: Toxic in high doses do not take without professional advice.

Damiana—Turneria aphrodisiaca

Source: Native to Mexico, the southwestern United States and Central

America, the leaves and flowers of this herb have been used since ancient Mayan times as an aphrodisiac and nerve tonifier.

Dose: Capsules: 400 mg, up to 6 times daily. Tincture: 20–30 drops, 4 times daily. Take on an "as needed" basis rather than continually

Safety: Minor laxative effect at higher doses. High doses may cause euphoria, insomnia and headache.

Dandelion—Taraxacum officinalis

Source: A common weed in the daisy family, dandelion is a traditional European springtime liver tonic and cleansing diuretic. The plant is high in potassium, vitamins and minerals.

Standardization: 20% taraxisterol.

Dosage: Capsules: Root: 500 mg, 3 times daily. Leaf: 250–500 mg, 2–3 capsules daily. Tincture of the root or leaf: 5–10 ml, 3 times daily. Leaves are used in salads or juiced.

Safety: Avoid with gallbladder obstruction, gallstones, or stomach ulcers. Seek professional advice if taking diuretics for fluid retention.

Devil's Claw—Harpagophytum procumbens

Source: The root of this African plant possesses anti-inflammatory effects and has been used traditionally to treat a wide range of complaints.

Standardization: 1.5–5% harpagosides or 5 mg harpagosides per dose.

Dosage: Capsules: 400–500 mg, up to 6 times daily. Tincture: 15 ml daily.

Safety: Low toxicity. Due to its stimulating effect, should not be taken during pregnancy or with gastric or duodenal ulcers.

Devil's Club—Oplopanax horridus

Source: An herb in the ginseng family and native to the Pacific Northwestern United States, the root is indicated to strengthen the kidneys, adrenals and immune system.

Standardization: None.

Dosage: Capsules: 100–200 mg, twice daily. Tincture: 1–4 ml, 1–4 times daily.

Safety: No known contraindications or toxicity. May alter clotting time, so use caution in bleeding disorders.

Dong Quai—Angelica sinensis

Source: This herb is a member of the carrot family that is second only to ginseng in importance in Chinese herbal medicine.

Standardization: Standardized to 0.8–1% ligustilide.

Dosage: Capsules: 500–600 mg, 3–6 times daily. Take one month to one year for full effects.

Safety: Very low toxicity, but should not be used in those with stomach or intestinal ulcers (including ulcerative colitis). Avoid if taking blood thinners, if menstruating, or during pregnancy. May stimulate a menstrual period in higher doses. In general this is a tonifying herb with minimal or no side effects. May take months to see its regulatory effects.

Dulse—Rhodymenia palmata or Palmaria palmata

Source: Dulse is a good source of protein, iron, chlorophyll, enzymes and vitamins A and B. More total dietary fiber (33%) and soluble fiber (16%) than oat bran.

Standardization: None.

Dosage: Loose dulse: 1/3 of a cup or 1/4 oz or 7 g. Tincture: 4 drops daily, containing 225 mcg of iodine.

Safety: No known ill effects.

Dusty Miller—Cineraria maritima

Source: A member of the daisy family, this silver-white shrub is originally West Indian in origin, but has been naturalized to the Mediterranean and Europe. Its use has been limited solely to conditions of the eye.

Standardization: None.

Dosage: May also be taken internally, but most commonly used one drop in an eyewash, four or five times a day, for several months.

Safety: Contains pyrorrolizidine alkaloids, toxic to the liver when taken internally for more than a few weeks.

E

Echinacea—Echinacea angustifolia/purpurea/pallida

Source: Various species of this member of the daisy family (*Asteraceae*) possess immune modulating effects, mainly angustifolia, purpurea and pallidium. The root, leaves or whole plant may be used.

Standardization: 4% echinacosoides, (E. *angustifolia*), 4% sesquiterpene esters (E. *purpurea*) 10 mg echinacosides.

Dosage: Capsules: Up to 1,200 mg daily. Tincture: 4–5 ml daily. In acute infections dose frequently, 1/2–1 ml of tincture or 1–2 capsules every 1–2 hours. Reduce the dosage as symptoms begins to clear. May take preventively, continuing for at least 2 weeks, followed by 1 week off, then repeat cycle.

Safety: Acts to increase phagocytosis and as an immune modulator. No evidence exists to curtail use in AIDS, HIV, lupus, autoimmune diseases, multiple sclerosis and TB. Do not use in pregnancy. Some people may have an allergic reaction to plants in the daisy family.

Elderberry—Sambucus nigra

Source: The flowers, berries, leaves and bark of the American and European elderberry tree are renowned for their fever and flu fighting properties, and part of many traditional European cold formulas.

Standardization: 5–30% flavonoids

Dosage: Capsules: elderberries: 2,000 mg, up to 3 capsules daily; elderflowers: 500 mg, 3 times daily. Tincture: 10–60 drops, 3–4 times daily. Liquid or syrup: 15 ml, 2–3 times daily.

Safety: A popular children's herb that is safe at recommended doses. Note that the unripe berries, bark, leaves and root contain cyanide and are poisonous.

Elecampane—Inula helenium

Source: Southern Europe and Asia are home to this mucilaginous root which was known since the Roman times as both a food and herbal tonic for the lungs.

Standardization: None.

Dosage: Capsules: 1,000 mg, 3 times daily. Tincture: 1–4 ml, 3 times daily.

Safety: Do not take during pregnancy or breastfeeding.

European Snake Root—Asarum europaeum

Source: The root is indigenous to various parts of Europe and Siberia.

Standardization: None.

Dosage: Capsules: 30 mg of dry root extract. Tincture: 15 drops daily.

Safety: Do not take more than recommended dose. Older literature reports burning of the tongue, diarrhea, gastroenteritis symptoms and skin rashes with poisonings.

Eucalyptus—Eucalyptus globulus

Source: The eucalyptus tree is native to Australia where the Aboriginal people used the leaves as a treatment for wounds and fevers. Today Eucalyptol, the menthol-like compound from eucalyptus leaves, is an ingredient in many over-the-counter preparations.

Standardization: None.

Dosage: For external use only. Pour boiling water over the leaves and inhale for relief from congestion or place a handful of leaves in a bath.

Safety: Caution: Do not take internally; one teaspoon may prove fatal. Keep out of reach of children and away from pets.

Eyebright—Euphrasia officinalis

Source: Originally from Europe, this plant's use dates back to the Middle Ages where its aerial parts were used to treat eye inflammations.

Standardization: None.

Dosage: Capsules: 400–500 mg, up to 5 capsules daily. Tincture: 1–4 ml, 3 times daily. As a compress, place 1–2 tsp of dried herb with 1 pint of water. Boil for 10 minutes, cool and apply as needed or dilute 5–10 drops of the tincture in a glass of water and apply as an eye compress.

Safety: No known side effects or toxicity.

Evening Primrose—Oenethera biennis

Source: The leaves and seeds (oil) from the evening primrose are part of the Native American herbal tradition. The seeds are high in GLA, a precursor to many hormones.

Standardization: 8% gamma-linolenic-acid (GLA).

Dosage: Capsules: Up to 12 capsules or 500 mg of the oil daily. Or 6–8 g of oil for inflammatory conditions. Tincture: Up to 1/2 tsp. It may take three months before an effect is seen.

Safety: Safe for use in children and the elderly. Generally safe and without side effects. Do not combine with phenothiazine medications for schizophrenia; an increase in temporal lobe seizure activity may occur.

F

False Unicorn Root—Helonias dioica/Chamaelirium luteum

Source: Native to North America, false unicorn root (rhizome) was a favorite for uterine weakness and was listed in the U.S. National Formulary from 1916–1947 as a uterine tonic and diuretic herb.

Standardization: None.

Dosage: Tincture: 10–40 drops, 1–4 times daily. It may take a month or two before beneficial effects are seen.

Safety: Do not use during pregnancy or nursing. No other side effects or contraindications are noted.

Fennel—Eletteria cardamomum

Source: An herb similar in quality to anise and caraway, fennel originates in the Mediterranean region, but is naturalized to all parts of the world. The seeds are cultivated in the fall. In the Middle Ages, this plant was considered an antidote to witchcraft and snakebites.

Standardization: None.

Dosage: Capsules: 500 mg, up to 4 times daily. Tincture: 1–2 ml, 1–4 times daily.

Safety: No contraindications or side effects.

Fenugreek—Trigonella foenum-graecum

Source: A member of the bean family and native to the eastern Mediterranean area, fenugreek possesses a sweet maple-like flavor and has a balancing effect on blood sugar levels.

Standardization: None, though general isoflavone content may be cited.

Dosage: Capsules: 1–6 g daily. Tincture: 1–2 ml, 3 times daily. Studies using 25g/day, 100g/day and 15 g/day all showed a lowering of blood sugar levels.

Safety: Safe, though over 100 g daily can cause nausea and diarrhea.

Feverfew—Tanacetum parthenium

Source: Feverfew is a member of the daisy family, native to Europe and grown throughout Australia and North America.

Standardization: 0.1–0.2% parthenolide, 0.7% parthenolide

Dosage: Capsule: 400 mg, 3 times daily. Standardized extract: 125–370 mg feverfew or 240–600 mcg parthenolide. The freeze-dried herb is known to be very effective.

Safety: Eating the fresh leaves can cause mouth ulcers. May take weeks before anti-inflammatory effects are seen.

Figwort—Scrophularia nodosa

Source: Figwort is similar in appearance to the snapdragon plant, which originated from Europe, Asia and North America. The flowering parts are gathered during the summertime. Figwort was well known for its ability to treat swollen lymph node conditions.

Standardization: None.

Dosage: Capsules: Take as directed. Tincture: 30 drops, 3 times daily.

Safety: Do not take during pregnancy.

Flaxseed—Linum usitatissimum

Source: Archeologists have traced the use of flax back to 10,000 years ago. Flax's many uses are as a fiber for linen clothing, as linseed oil in paints and varnishes, waxes and feed for animals. The seeds, oil and fiber are used medicinally. Flax is a source of essential oil, highest in omega 3.

Standardization: 58% alpha linolenic acid.

Dosage: 1–2 tbsp of flax oil, 3 times daily. Buy only in a glass container, as the oil will break down the plastic bottle. The seeds can be soaked in water overnight for a gelatinous mixture to relieve constipation, or may be ground in a coffee grinder and sprinkled over food. Topically, use 30–50 g of flax as a hot, moist compress.

Safety: Drink plenty of water or other liquids while taking flaxseeds. Do not use in bowel obstructive diseases. Flaxseeds promote healthy bowel movements; if diarrhea occurs, decrease dose.

Fleabane—Erigeron canadensis

Source: Originating in dry wastelands of North America, the aerial parts of fleabane are its medicinal parts.

Standardization: None.

Dosage: Tincture: 1–2 tsp daily.

Safety: No recorded adverse effects.

Fo-Ti—Polygonum multiflorum

Source: An herb in the buckwheat family, fo-ti root is best known in Chinese medicine as "ho-shou-wu" and is used for deficient kidney and liver "yin." In Traditional Chinese Medicine, fo-ti is one of the most widely prescribed tonifying herbs for debility and weakness.

Standardization: None.
Dosage: Capsules: 500–1,000 mg daily. Tincture: 1–4 ml, 2–3 times daily.
Safety: Contraindicated with diarrhea. Rarely, gastric upset may occur, or loose stool may result at high doses.

Fringetree—Chionanthus virginicus
Source: The root of this olive family tree is native to the United States and Eastern Asia. Native Americans and herbalists treated bruises, wounds and liver derangements with this cooling and bitter herb.
Standardization: None.
Dosage: Capsules: Take as directed. Tincture: 10–30 drops, 3 times daily.
Safety: No contraindications or side effects noted.

G

Galangal—Alpinia officinarum
Source: The rhizome of this Chinese herb in the ginger family is used for treating colds and flus. Hildegarde of Bingen employed it as a heart tonic during the Middle Ages.
Standardization: None.
Dosage: Capsules: 3,000–6,000 g daily. Tincture: 1–2 ml, 3 times daily.
Safety: No known side effects or toxicity known.

Garcinia—Garcinia gambogia
Source: An Asian tree whose extract, hydroxycitric acid (HCA), is derived from the fruit's rind. It is both an appetite suppressant and energy enhancer, promoting weight loss.
Standardization: 50% hydroxycitric acid.
Dosage: Capsule: 1–1.3 g daily.
Safety: Up to 4 g daily produces no adverse effects. It is proposed that over 10 g could prevent mineral absorption or cause gastric irritation.

Garlic—Allium sativa
Source: A member of the lily family and native to Asia, garlic is the world's largest-selling herb. Apart from its culinary qualities, it has powerful antibiotic and heart-protective properties.
Standardization: Various standards are used, including allicin, sulfur, alliin and s-allyl cysteine. Usually 1.3% alliin.
Dosage: Capsules: 500–7,000 mg daily or as directed. There are a wide variety of preparations. Fresh garlic: One or two cloves per day.
Safety: Very safe; large doses may cause irritation, gas or indigestion. Do not use therapeutic doses just before surgery or if on anticoagulants. Do not combine with other blood thinners like aspirin.

Gentian—Gentiana lutea

Source: Native to Eurasia, this bitter root has been used since Egyptian times to treat problems related to a weakened digestive system.

Standardization: None.

Dosage: Tincture: 5–15 drops before meals. To be effective, gentian should be held in the mouth to increase and strengthen digestive secretions.

Safety: Avoid with gastric ulcers.

Ginger—Zingiber officinale

Source: The well-known Asian spice is made from the underground rhizome and has been revered as a medical panacea for 5,000 years.

Standardization: 20% of the pungent compounds, gingerols and shagols or 5% zingiberene.

Dosage: Capsules: 500–2,000 mg, 2–4 times daily. Ground root: 1/2–1 tsp daily. Fresh ginger:1/4 inch slice daily or as desired. Tincture:10–30 drops 3 times daily. Ginger syrup: 1–2 tbsp daily. For motion sickness, begin taking 500 mg ginger capsules several days before trips.

Safety: May irritate the digestive system at high doses. Do not use excessively during pregnancy or for prolonged periods (i.e. usually not more than two capsules daily). Do not use at all with a high-risk pregnancy. Do not use if on anticoagulant drugs.

Ginkgo—Ginkgo biloba

Source: Ginkgo is one of the oldest surviving species of trees and has been the subject of over 300 scientific studies. It is the number one prescription for poor circulation and memory loss in Europe and the third best selling herb in the United States.

Standardization: 24% ginkgosides, 6–7% triterpenes.

Dosage: Capsules: 120–240 mg daily. Standardized dose: 40 mg, 3 times daily. Tincture: 10–15 drops, 1–3 times daily.

Safety: No serious side effects. Can cause mild headache or mild stomach upset. No contraindications during pregnancy or lactation. Avoid if on anticoagulants or blood-thinning medications such as warfarin.

Ginseng—Panax ginseng

Source: Chinese and Korean ginseng should be harvested from six-year-old roots. Only purchase from a reputable manufacturer. Red ginseng is subjected to steaming and is considered stronger and "hotter" than white ginseng.

Standardization: 4–7% ginsenosides.

Dosage: Capsules: 1–2.5 g of the root daily. Standardized extract: 100 mg-300 mg, 1–2 times daily. Tincture: 30 drops, 3 times daily. Should be taken for some time for immune and adaptogen benefits. Take one month on, two months off.

Safety: Generally safe at normal dosages. Occasionally gastric upset, breast tenderness, nervousness, insomnia, headache and menstrual disturbances have been reported. Avoid during pregnancy, with fever, asthma, emphysema, bronchitis, kidney failure, high blood pressure or an irregular heart beat (arrhythmias). Use with phenelzine may increase manic symptoms. Avoid with anticoagulants or blood-thinning medications. Seek professional advice if also taking blood sugar or antidepressant medications.

Goldenrod—Solidago virgaurea

Source: Originally a European member of the daisy family, this herb now grows wild across the United States. Since the 13th century it has been used to treat urinary symptoms and conditions of the upper respiratory tract.

Standardization: None.

Dosage: Capsules: 6–12 g dried herb daily. Tincture: 2–4 ml, 3 times daily.

Safety: Contraindicated in heart or kidney disease-related edema. Drink at least two liters of water daily while taking this herb. There is a possibility of allergic sensitization if allergic to other daisy family members.

Goat's Rue—Galega officinalis

Source: Originally from Europe and Asia this perennial herb has a long history of protecting against the plague and increasing the quantity of breast milk in nursing mothers.

Standardization: None.

Dosage: Capsules: Take as directed. Tincture: 1–3 ml, 3 times daily.

Safety: Use caution if on insulin or diabetic drug treatment, as it may lower blood sugar. Monitor glucose levels closely.

Goldenseal—Hydrastis canadensis

Source: Native to the woodlands of eastern North America, this herb was prized by Native American medicine traditions. It is now rare in the wild due to overharvesting. Barberry or oregon grape may used as substitutes.

Standardization: 10% alkaloids, berberine; 5% hydrastine, canadine.

Dosage: Capsules: 500–1,000 mg, 3 times daily. Standardized extract: 250–500 mg, 3 times daily. Tincture: 2–4 ml, 3 times daily.

Safety: Not recommended in pregnancy or breastfeeding. Generally for acute disorders requiring an antibacterial herb.

Gotu Kola—Centella asiatica

Source: A member of the carrot family, gotu kola grows by riverbanks and marshy places in Madagascar, India and Sri Lanka. It was traditionally used for leprosy, wound healing, as a nervous system and memory stimulant. It was purported to increase longevity because elephants would be seen chewing the herb. Leaves and stem are used.

Standardization: 20–25% mg total triterpenic acids, 10–30% asiaticosides, 2–4% tripterpenes.

Dosage: Capsules: 400–500 mg, up to 8 times daily. Standardized extract: 250 mg, 3 times daily. Tincture: 30 drops, 3 times daily.

Safety: Well tolerated; rarely, contact dermatitis may occur if applied topically. No hazards if therapeutic dosage is followed.

Grapefruit Seed Extract—Citrus paradisi

Source: A concentrated source of antimicrobial compounds derived from the grapefruit seed.

Standardization: 40% citricidal.

Dosage: Capsules: 125 mg, up to 3 capsules, 3 times daily. Tincture: 8–12 drops mixed well in 5 oz or more of juice, tea or water, 3 times daily, may be taken before, during or after meals.

Safety: No known contraindications. Do not take the concentrated drops directly, as it will irritate mucus membranes.

Grape Seed Extract—Vitis vinifera

Source: The grape has a long history of health benefits. Wine making dates at least to the Egyptian times. Though all parts of the grape plant have been used medicinally in one form or another, the seeds have only recently been researched for their proanthocyanidin (antioxidant) content.

Standardization: 95% oligomeric proanthocyanidins (PCOs).

Dosage: Capsules: 150 mg of proanthocyanidin daily.

Safety: No side effects or contraindications noted.

Gravel Root—Eupatorium purpureum

Source: This perennial root is native to the eastern United States and is a member of the daisy family. "Joe pye weed" is another name for this herb widely used by the Native Americans to treat typhus and ailments of the genitourinary tract.

Standardization: None.

Dosage: Tincture: 5–30 drops daily.

Safety: No contraindications or side effects known.

Green Tea—Camellia sinensis

Source: Tea is the world's most popular drink—after water—with over 5,000 years of usage. Green tea is prepared by light steaming, while black tea is fermented and oxidized, losing much of its therapeutic benefit.

Standardization: 90% polyphenols, 55% epigallocatechin gallates (EGCG).

Dosage: Capsules: 250–500 mg daily. Standardized extract: 1–3 capsules daily (1 capsule = 2 cups of tea). For tea, use 1 ounce of leaves to 1 pint of water; add leaves after water boils and steep for 5–20 minutes.

Safety: No adverse effects. Caffeine sensitivity may necessitate obtaining commercially available decaffeinated green tea products. Adding milk to the tea decreases the antioxidant effects.

Grindelia—Gum Plant/Grindelia robusta

Source: This daisy family member grows in the arid soil of the American southwest and Mexico. The leaves and tops contain substances that benefit the lungs in respiratory ailments.

Standardization: None.

Dosage: Capsules: 3–6 g daily. Tincture: 1.5–3 ml daily.

Safety: Grindelia can be toxic in high doses and should be avoided in those with advanced kidney or heart disease. Avoid if allergic to other daisy family members.

Ground Ivy—Glechoma hederacea

Source: This European member of the mint family is a traditional plant for promoting sweating and reducing fevers. It is also an astringent for sinusitis and bronchitis.

Standardization: None.

Dosage: Tincture: 1–4 ml daily.

Safety: No known toxicity.

Guaiacum—Guaiacum officinale

Source: The resin of the heartwood from this South American evergreen tree relieves the pain and inflammation associated with rheumatism. Its greenish-brown wood is heavier than water and its shavings turn green upon exposure to the air.

Standardization: None.

Dosage: Capsules: 4–5 g daily. Tincture: 20–40 drops, 2–3 times daily.

Safety: No interactions or adverse effects are known to occur.

Guggul—Commiphora mukul

Source: The resin of this thorny tree is native to Arabia and India and has been used for over 2,600 years in Ayurvedic medicine to treat obesity, lipid disorders and rheumatoid arthritis

Standardization: 2.5%–10% guggulosterones E and Z.

Dosage: Capsules: 500 mg, containing 25 mg guggulosterones, 3 times daily. Tincture: 20–40 drops, 3 times daily. May take 3–4 weeks to notice cholesterol-lowering effects; generally used for 12–24 weeks.

Safety: Guggul is non-toxic and well tolerated, though long-term use may be associated with mild stomach upset. It may stimulate the thyroid and the uterus so best avoid in hyperthyroidism and pregnancy.

Gymnema—Gymnema sylvestre

Source: Used since the 6th century B.C., in India it is known as "gurmur," the destroyer of sugar, due to its ability to interfere with or block the perception of sweet and bitter tastes for up to three hours.

Standardization: 25%–85% gymnemic acids.

Dosage: Capsules: 300–400 mg daily. Tincture: 5–60 drops, 3 times daily. Use for 18–24 months for optimal effects.

Safety: Use under medical supervision and monitor closely, as one may require less insulin or a decrease in the dosage of diabetic drugs such as glipizide. Effects during pregnancy and lactation are not known.

H-J

Hawthorn—Crataegus oxycantha

Source: The berry of the hawthorn, a member of the rose family, was a symbol of hope in the Middle Ages and was hung over doorways to prevent the passage of evil spirits. Today, it is recognized as the world's most safe and effective heart tonic.

Standardization: 1.8–3.2% vitexin-2'-rhamnoside, or 10–18.75% proanthocyanidins.

Dosage: Capsules: Up to 5 g daily. Standardized extract: 100–250 mg daily. Tincture: 10–60 drops, 4 times daily. Standardized fluid extract: 5 ml per day.

Safety: There are no known interactions with mainstream cardiac drugs, but hawthorn may strengthen the effect of cardiac glycosides (i.e. digitalis). Hawthorn is similar to rose hips and of minimal toxicity. Excess can produce fatigue, sweating, nausea and rashes on the hands.

Holy Basil—Ocimum sanctum

Source: Holy basil is a warm and aromatic member of the mint family and native to the Indian subcontinent. An important Ayurvedic herb, its leaves can be eaten raw in salads; its stems have been used to make into rosary beads.

Standardization: None.

Dosage: Capsules: Take as directed. Tincture: 1–2 ml, 1–4 times daily. Apply leaves directly to skin to relieve insect bites or take the tincture internally for respiratory or nervous conditions.

Safety: Due to basil's ability to lower blood sugar, use with caution in diabetic or hypoglycemic disorders. May alter insulin's effects.

Hops—Humulus lupulus

Source: Hops have been enjoyed for centuries as an ingredient of ale and beer by many societies. The flowers, known as strobiles, possess estrogenic and sedative qualities.

Standardization: 5.2% bitter acids, 4% flavonoids.

Dose: Capsules: 500–1,000 mg daily. Tincture: 1–4 ml, 3 times daily.
Safety: Hops are generally safe and without adverse effects or toxicity. May be anaphrodisic in effect.

Horehound—Marrubium vulgare
Source: Horehound is indigenous to the Mediterranean region and central Asia. The velvety gray-green leaves, flowers and stems are harvested for their medicinal value. Unlike many fragrant plants in the mint family, horehound has a bitter taste and no appreciable aroma.
Standardization: None.
Dosage: Capsules: 1–2 g, 3 times daily. Tincture: 10–30 drops, 3 times daily for acute respiratory or digestive ailments.
Safety: Horehound should not be used during pregnancy or nursing.

Horse Chestnut—Aesculus hippocastanum
Source: Horse chestnut, a large North American shade tree, is native to Asia and was introduced to Europe in 1576. Preparations are made from the young bark, fruit seeds and leaves.
Standardization: 20% aescin.
Dosage: Capsules: 250 mg, twice daily. Standardized extract: 30–150 mg, 1–2 times daily. Tincture: 1–4 ml, 3 times daily.
Safety: No interactions or contraindications are known. Rarely side effects such as gastric upset or nausea may occur.

Horsemint—Monarda punctata
Source: Horsemint is a perennial herb in the mint family, similar in fragrance to thyme and grows in eastern and central United States.
Standardization: None.
Dosage: Tincture: 1–3 ml, 2–3 times daily.
Safety: Contraindicated in pregnancy and nursing.

Horseradish—Amoracia rusticana
Source: This deep taproot is native to Europe and western Asia. Horseradish has been used as a popular spice, diuretic and decongestant since earliest recorded history.
Standardization: None.
Dosage: Capsules: Take as directed. Tincture: 1–2 ml, 4 times daily. The fresh root may also be taken as desired for respiratory complaints.
Safety: Do not use if thyroid is underactive. Large doses can irritate the stomach and intestines.

Horsetail—Equisetum arvense
Source: Also called shavegrass, this flowerless herb is a relative of prehistoric trees from 270 million years ago. High in silica, horsetail's ability to reduce bleeding in wounds was known from the Grecian times.

Standardization: 10% silicic acid, 7% silica

Dosage: Capsules: 400–500 mg, up to 6 times daily. Tincture: 20–40 drops, 2–5 times daily.

Safety: Do not use in children, pregnancy or nursing, heart disease, kidney disease.

Hydrangea—Seven Barks/Hydrangea arborescens

Source: Hydrangea is a ten-foot shrub native to eastern North America, found in damp woodlands and along streams. The root (rhizome), was used by Native Americans and early herbalists for kidney problems.

Standardization: None.

Dosage: Capsules: 400–800 mg daily. Tincture: 1–3 ml, 2–3 times daily.

Safety: Generally safe. No side effects or toxicity known.

Huperzine A—Hyperzia serrata

Source: A rare type of club moss growing in the cool mountainous lands of China, known as "qian ceng ta." This herb is quickly becoming well known for its ability to improve various kinds of memory defects, particularly Alzheimer's and related dementias.

Standardization: 98% Huperzine A.

Dose: Capsules: 50–100 mcg twice daily.

Safety: Contraindicated in pregnancy, hypertension and diseases that have increased bronchial mucus secretion. Only the purified extract has been studied; the crude herb is thought to be toxic in nature.

Hyssop—Hyssopus officinalis

Source: Hyssop's budding leaves and clusters of purple-blue flowers are of European origin but common to many American gardens. The volatile oil is a flavoring in such liqueurs as Chartreuse and Benedictine.

Standardization: None.

Dosage: Capsules: 500 mg–1,000 mg, 3 times daily. Tincture: 1–4 ml, 2–3 times daily. May also be used as a gargle or compress for bruises. Use in combination with horehound for respiratory disorders.

Safety: Keep out of reach of children. Do not give to children under 2 years of age. In elderly or children 2–12 years of age, use a very low dose or avoid. Contraindicated in pregnancy or nursing.

Irish Moss—Chondrus crispus

Source: This fan-shaped seaweed, found on the coasts of the Europe and North America, is collected at low tide and is high in minerals and trace elements.

Standardization: None.

Dosage: Capsules: Take as directed.

Safety: Do not use if taking anticoagulants or with bleeding disorders.

Jamaican Dogwood—Piscidia erythrina

Source: A small tree native to the southern United States, Caribbean and Central and South America, dogwood is used as lumber for boats, but its root bark has long been used in folk medicine as an effective pain reliever.

Standardization: None.

Dosage: Capsules: 500–1,000 mg every 4–6 hours as needed for pain. Tincture: 2–3 ml, up to 15 ml daily.

Safety: Do not use during pregnancy or with heart disease. Avoid if taking any other pain medication or with alcohol as it may increase drowsiness and sedation. Can be toxic in high doses; decrease dose according to vitality or age. Use cautiously or not at all in children or the aged.

Jiaogulan—Gynostemma pentaphyllum

Source: This member of the cucumber family is also known as the "herb of immortality" in Southern China. Its antioxidant and adaptogenic qualities promote vitality, endurance and virility.

Standardization: 10% total gypenosides.

Dosage: Capsule: 20–60 mg, 2–3 times daily. Standardized extract: 1–20 mg, 3 times daily. Standardized liquid: Sold in 10 mg per dose vials.

Safety: No known toxicity.

Juniper—Juniperus communis

Source: A North American shrub in the pine family, juniper's fresh or dried berries (cones) are used in kidney and digestive disorders.

Standardization: None.

Dosage: Capsules: 400–500 mg, up to 6 daily. Tincture: 15–30 drops, 3 times daily. Berries: 1–5 daily not to exceed 2 weeks.

Safety: Do not use for longer than 4 weeks. Contraindicated in pregnancy and inflammatory kidney diseases. People with diabetes may wish to avoid this herb as it may cause an increase in blood sugar levels.

Kava Kava—Piper methysticum

Source: Kava is a South Pacific member of the pepper family, where it has been used for centuries as a pain reliever and aphrodisiac. In ceremonial practice, the root was chewed to induce euphoria and visions.

Standardization: 30–70% kavalactones.

Dosage: Capsules: 200–1,000 mg, 3 times daily. Standardized extract: 120–240 mg of kavalactones daily. Tincture: 1–4 ml, 3 times daily.

Safety: Do not take with alcohol or other pharmaceutical tranquilizers. Excess use can lead to a temporary scaly rash. Use for only 3 months at a time. Should not be taken by those with Parkinson's disease.

Kelp—Bladderwrack/Fucus vesiculosis/Ascophyllum nodosum

Source: Growing on the shores of both the north Atlantic and western Mediterranean, this brown seaweed has been used as an edible vegetable, fuel, cattle feed and goiter treatment since antiquity.

Standardization: None.

Dosage: Capsules: 500 mg, 1–2 times daily.

Safety: Use this herb only under medical supervision with thyroid disease, since iodine may worsen some thyroid conditions. Avoid if pregnant or breastfeeding.

Khella—Ammi visnaga

Source: A member of the parsley family, khella is native to Middle Eastern and Egyptian countries. The active compounds are found in khella's seeds and fruit.

Standardization: 12% khellin.

Dosage: Capsules: 200–300 mg of standardized khellin daily. Tincture: 20–60 drops, 1–4 times daily as needed.

Safety: Contraindicated in pregnancy due to its ability to induce menstruation. Decreases the toxicity of the cardiovascular drug, Digitoxin.

Kudzu—Pueraria lobata

Source: Kudzu's root may grow to be larger than a human in size. In Asia, kudzu was once a staple food of the people. Mentioned as early as 600 A.D. in Japan for its medicinal properties, this fast-growing vine is used today for angina and to reduce alcohol cravings.

Standardization: 1.5% daizen 0.95% daidzen.

Dosage: Capsules: 150 mg, up to 6 times daily. Tincture: 20–60 drops, 4–5 times daily.

Safety: No toxicity or side effects are known for this herb.

Lady's Mantle—Alchemilla vulgaris

Source: Native to Europe, the leaves and stems are used medicinally. Rich in history, alchemilla refers to the word "alchemy" because of the miraculous cures purported to have occurred through this herb's use.

Standardization: None.

Dosage: Capsule: Take as directed. Tincture: 2–4 ml, 3 times daily

Safety: Do not use during pregnancy or breastfeeding.

Lady's Slipper—Cypripedium pubescens

Source: This plant is a member of the orchid family and grows in the forests of North America and Europe, where it is considered endangered. Do not wildcraft this herb.

Standardization: None.
Dosage: Capsule: 2–4 g daily. Tincture: 2–4 ml, 3 times daily.
Safety: Do not use if pregnant or breastfeeding.

Larch—Larix decidua/europea

Source: The inner bark and resin is the source of the arabinogalactan extract. Originally from Europe, the Alps and Carpathian mountains region, it was introduced into Britain in 1639.
Standardization: None.
Dosage: Powder: For acute symptoms, 2 tbsp, dissolved in water or juice, 3 times daily. For prevention, 1/2 tablespoon daily. Tincture: 30–60 drops, 3 times daily.
Safety: No known toxicity or side effects.

Lavender—Lavandula officinalis/angustifolia

Source: Lavender is a member of the mint family and native to the Mediterranean. This popular ornamental is an essential part of perfumes, potpourri and sachets, as well as being an ancient Greco-Roman medicine.
Standardization: None.
Dosage: Capsules: 800 mg daily. Tincture: 10–30 drops, 3–4 times daily. May be applied directly to the skin or diluted; 20 drops of essential oil in 20 drops of a carrier oil. Lavender oil is an external antiseptic and pain reliever. The tincture is used internally as a relaxant and antidepressant.
Safety: Do not use internally during pregnancy due to its emmenagogue effects.

Lemon Balm—Melissa officinalis

Source: This lemon-scented member of the mint family was used for over 2,000 years to soothe nervousness and treat insomnia. Lemon balm was originally from the Mediterranean regions, Asia and Africa.
Standardization: None.
Dosage: Capsules: 300–400 mg, up to 9 daily. Tincture: 10–60 drops, 1–6 times daily. A cream has been shown in research studies to decrease the time it takes herpes simplex lesions to heal. Apply at first signs of an outbreak.
Safety: Unlike sedative drugs, lemon balm does not interfere with one's ability to drive or perform other duties. No adverse effects or toxicity is noted. Safe for children.

Licorice—Glycyrrhiza glabra

Source: The root of this member of the bean family is native to Eurasia and has been used in Chinese and Grecian medicine for over 2,000 years.

Standardized: 5% glycyrrhetinic acid, less than 2% glycyrrhizin.

Dosage: Capsules: 400 mg, 3–4 times daily. Tincture: 1–4 ml, 3 times daily. Use for only 4–6 weeks at a time. DGL: 250 mg, 3 times daily of 2% glycyrrhizin before meals. Ointment or cream form with glycyrrhietinic or glycyrrhizic acid available for topical use.

Safety: High doses can cause diarrhea. Do not exceed 5 g daily. Can raise blood pressure and cause water retention and potassium loss. Not for those with hypertension or during pregnancy. Do not use with diuretics, heart medications or corticosteroid drugs. Available in a deglycyrrhizinated form (DGL), which eliminates these potential side effects.

Linden—Tilia europaea

Source: Growing over 100 feet high, the lime tree has white flowers, which are used for heart and nervous conditions. Linden may be found growing in temperate regions around the world.

Standardization: None.

Dosage: Capsules: 800 mg daily. Tincture: 20–40 drops, 1–4 times daily.

Safety: No health hazards have been recorded with therapeutic use.

Lobelia—Lobelia inflata

Source: Lobelia is native to North America, where it has a long history of medical use by Native Americans and "Thompsonian" herbalists.

Dosage: Capsules: 400 mg, 1–3 times daily. Tincture: 15–30 drops daily. Usually used in combination with other synergistic herbs.

Standardization: None.

Safety: Toxic levels cause nausea and vomiting; lethal doses are rare, as an overdose causes vomiting and little absorption occurs.

Lomatium—Lomatium dissectum

Source: A member of the carrot family and native to the United States where Native American healers used this root to treat all kinds of respiratory infections including tuberculosis.

Standardization: None.

Dosage: Tincture: 20–60 drops, 3 times daily. Isolate tincture: 5–10 drops, twice daily.

Safety: Contains coumarins and may increase clotting time. A skin rash may occur in some individuals with the fresh plant. Discontinue use if this occurs. Using the isolate avoids these possible skin effects.

Lungwort—Sticta pulmonaria

Source: Part of the lichen family, lungwort may be found growing along the base of oak or beech trees and is common to many parts of Europe. The aerial parts are used medicinally.

Standardization: None.

Dosage: Tincture: 10–40 drops, 1–4 times daily.

Safety: No contraindications are known.

Lungwort—Pulmonaria officinalis

Source: A member of the borage family, this native of Europe and Russia flourishes in moist pastures and mountainous areas.

Standardization: None.

Dosage: Tincture: 1–4 ml, 3 times daily.

Safety: Do not use if pregnant, breastfeeding or with bleeding disorders.

M

Maca—Lepedium meyenii

Source: This root, nicknamed "Peruvian ginseng," was used by Incan warriors before battle. Maca is a superb adaptogenic herb that increases stamina and vitality in a variety of conditions.

Standardization: 0.6% macamides and macacenes.

Dose: Powdered herb: 3–5 g daily. Standardized extract: 1–2 g daily.

Safety: No contraindications or toxicity known.

Ma Huang—Ephedra sinica

Source: The Chinese have used ma huang for over 5,000 years for colds flus and lung afflictions. This evergreen shrub with a pine-like odor can be found throughout the desert regions of China. Ephedra's active parts are its dried green stems and seeds. American ephedra does not appear to contain the same active components as the Asian species.

Standardization: 6–8% total ephedrine alkaloids.

Dosage: Capsules: 500–1,000 mg, 2–3 times daily. Standardized extracts: 12–25 mg total alkaloids, 1–3 times daily. Tincture: 10–30 drops, 3 times daily.

Safety: Do not use in high blood pressure, diabetes, thyroid disorders, heart disease, while taking MAO inhibitors, during pregnancy or lactation. Side effects of overdose include high blood pressure, anxiety, insomnia and palpitations. In Traditional Chinese Medicine, ephedra was never used alone, but in combination with balancing herbs. Individuals may react differently to the stimulant effects of ephedra so begin with low dosages and gradually increase if necessary.

Maidenhair Fern—Adiantum pedatum

Source: Native to southern Europe and the North Atlantic coast, the dried leaves are used as an expectorant and hair tonic.

Standardization: None.

Dosage: Tincture: 15–60 drops, 1–3 times daily.

Safety: Do not take during pregnancy.

Maitake—Grifola frondosa

Source: This Chinese mushroom was a common medicinal food for over 3,000 years. It has been revered for its ability to maintain health and longevity; as an immune stimulator and for its tumor-inhibiting properties. It is now a recognized cancer treatment in Japan.

Standardization: D-fraction form.

Dose: Capsule: 3–7 g daily. Tincture: 12–20 drops of D-fraction extract, 3 times daily.

Safety: No toxicity even at high doses.

Marshmallow—Althea officinalis

Source: Althea is a Greek word for "associated with healing." Found throughout Europe and in North America, marshmallow is a soothing mucilage for the digestive, urinary and respiratory tracts.

Standardization: None.

Dosage: Capsules: 400–500 mg, up to 6 times daily. Tincture: 1–2 ml, 3–4 times daily.

Safety: No side effects are known. May interfere with the absorption of other drugs due to its mucilin content.

May Apple—Podophyllum peltatum

Source: May apple grows in the northeastern United States region and exudes an acrid odor. Its singular white flowers bear yellow fruit that resemble swollen rosehips.

Standardization: Tincture: a 5%–25% solution in alcohol or tincture of benzoin is available.

Dosage: Tincture: 1–10 drops, 1–2 times daily.

Safety: Avoid in diabetes, with prescription steroids, pregnancy or nursing. Do not use in children. The whole plant is poisonous except for the ripe fruit. In excessive doses may cause diarrhea and nervous system effects, dizziness and coma. Largely restricted to medical use.

Meadowsweet—Filipendula ulmaria

Source: This member of the rose family can be found growing by rivers and meadows in Europe. Meadowsweet's small white flowers and upper parts are a wonderful remedy for flus and rheumatic pains due to its aspirin-like compounds.

Standardization: None.

Dosage: Capsules: Up to 2,400 mg daily. Tincture: 10–60 drops, 1–4 times daily.

Safety: Avoid if allergic to aspirin. No other contraindications are known.

Milk Thistle—Silybum marianum

Source: A member of the daisy family and found throughout Europe, milk thistle's use as a liver herb dates back over 2,000 years.

Standardization: 80% silymarin. Must be alcohol extracted.

Dosage: Capsules: 200 mg, 3 times daily. Standardized extract: 100–600 mg daily. Tincture: 1–2 ml, 1–4 times daily.

Safety: Loose stools may occur in the first few days of use. If troublesome, reduce the dose accordingly and build up gradually. Avoid if allergic to other daisy family members. No other contraindications are noted.

Motherwort—Leonarus cardiaca

Source: The aerial parts of this member of the mint family are collected during the flowering season. It is indigenous to Europe and Scandinavia and is used for nervous heart conditions.

Standardization: None.

Dosage: Tincture or extract: 10–40 drops, 1–4 times daily.

Safety: Avoid in pregnancy; uterine-stimulating effects in animal studies.

Muira Puama—Ptychopetalum olacoides

Source: Known as potency wood, the wood or bark of this Brazilian plant is known for its powerful aphrodisiac, tonifying and stimulating effects.

Standardization: None.

Dosage: Capsules: 300–1,000 mg daily. Tincture: 10–60 drops, 1–3 times daily.

Safety: No known contraindications.

Mullein—Verbascum thapsus

Source: A member of the snapdragon family and of European and Asian origin, mullein's soft leaves were smoked by Native Americans for relief of coughs. The herb is a soothing demulcent for respiratory ailments.

Standardization: None.

Dosage: Capsules: 500 mg, twice daily. Tincture: 1–3 ml, 1–4 times daily.

Safety: No known contraindications.

Myrrh—Commiphora myrrha

Source: Native to the Middle East and Africa, the resinous extract from this desert shrub boasts a recorded history of use spanning thousands of years. It is an effective antiseptic, astringent and vulnerary.

Standardization: None.

Dosage: Capsules: 1,000 mg, 3 times daily. Tincture: 1–4 ml, 1–4 times daily. As a gargle, use 30–60 drops in water a few times daily. Dental powder comes as a 10% formula of powdered resin extract.

Safety: Contraindicated in pregnancy.

N

Neem—Azadirachta indica

Source: A member of the mahogany family, the neem tree is known in Asia as "free tree" for its ability to free up nutrients from dry soil. Renowned in India for centuries, all parts of this tree are medicinal in nature, treating everything from malaria to gum disease.

Standardization: None.

Dosage: Capsules: 400–500 mg, up to 6 daily. Tincture: 1–4 ml daily.

Safety: Neem oil should not be ingested. Use as directed.

Nettles—Urtica dioica

Source: The stinging nettle plant is closely related to the hemp family and has been used medically since antiquity in both Western and Eastern medicine. Its formic acid content causes a blistering skin irritation, but this is lost in the dried plant. The root is used for the prostate, while freeze-dried nettle leaf provides relief of allergy symptoms and inflammation.

Standardization: 1.2% plant silica.

Dosage: Capsules: 500–1,000 mg, 3–4 times daily. Tincture: 2–4 ml, 3 times daily.

Safety: No known contraindications.

O

Oats—Avena sativa

Source: Oats are grown worldwide in temperate regions as a food crop. Medicinal products are made from the seed, ripe dried fruit, leaf and stem of the husk. The most effective nervines are from the milky seed.

Standardization: None.

Dosage: Capsules: 500 mg, up to 8 times daily. Tincture: 3–5 ml, 3 times daily. For external relief of itch associated with eczema or other skin conditions, use 1 lb of oat straw in a bath or apply a paste directly to skin.

Safety: No side effects or toxicity are known, but if there is allergy to gluten, one may wish to avoid oats as well.

Olive Leaf—Olea europaea

Source: Olive trees have been cultivated for millennia in the Mediterranean and are now a worldwide crop in warmer climates. The fresh or dried leaves are used medicinally.

Standardized: 6–15% oleuropein.

Dosage: Capsules: 250 mg, 2–4 times daily. Tincture: 1–2 ml, 1–3 times daily.

Safety: Avoid olive leaf in gallbladder disease, as it may cause cramps.

Oregano Oil—Origanum vulgare

Source: This widely used spice is a member of the mint family and a close relative of marjoram. Oregano was once a ritual herb in wedding and funeral ceremonies. The oil is now used as a powerful fungicide and antimicrobial.

Standardization: 5% thymol.

Dosage: Capsules: 450 mg, twice daily with meals. Powder: 0.5–1 tsp with food. Standardized extract: 260 mg daily dose, containing 13 mg thymol. Oregano oil 90 mg daily, containing 18 mg thymol. Also use as a gargle or compress.

Safety: No associated side effects or contraindications are known.

Oregon Grape—Berberis aquifolia

Source: A member of the barberry family, oregon grape or mahonia is native to the Rockies, Colorado and the Pacific Northwest. The bark and root of this holly-like plant is used similarly to goldenseal.

Standardization: None.

Dosage: Capsules: 500–600 mg, up to 6 times daily. Tincture: 2–4 ml, 3 times daily.

Safety: May decrease the effectiveness of tetracycline and doxycycline. Contraindicated in pregnancy.

P

Papaya—Carica papaya

Source: Originally from Mexico and Central America, papaya's sap, seeds and fruit are utilized as medicine. The enzymes papain and chymopapain have digestion-enhancing and anti-inflammatory effects.

Standardization: Papain/chymopapain.

Dosage: Capsules and chewable tablets: 5–25 mg, 4 times daily. For anti-inflammatory effects take one hour before or one to two hours after meals.

Safety: Generally safe, but papaya has been reported to induce delayed menses so do not take in capsule or tablet form if pregnant. The fruit is fine to eat in moderation.

Parsley—Petroselinum crispum

Source: A wild herb in the carrot family and found originally in the Mediterranean region, parsley boasts a long history of culinary, medicinal and ritual use. A known diuretic and nutritive herb, parsley is a fine addition to any meal.

Standardization: None.

Dosage: Capsules: 400–500 mg, up to 6 times daily. Tincture: 30–60 drops, 3 times daily.

Safety: Parsley seed is a known abortifacient. Avoid excessive use (2 or more cups daily) of fresh parsley or its juice during pregnancy. Use caution in inflammatory kidney disease or in clotting disorders as it possesses blood-thinning properties.

Partridge Berry—Mitchella repens

Source: An evergreen herb in the coffee family that was widely used by Native Americans in preparation in childbirth. Partridge berry can be found flourishing around the bottom of trees throughout woodland areas of eastern and central North America.

Standardization: None.

Dosage: Capsules: 2–4 g daily. Tincture: 30–60 drops, twice daily.

Safety: Do not use in the first six months of pregnancy or with liver disease.

Passionflower—Passiflora incarnata

Source: Passionflower grows from Southeastern America to Brazil and has been used in South American and Native American medicine for centuries. It is not named for aphrodisiac properties, but for its purple and white flowers representing the crucifixion (i.e. purity and heaven).

Standardization: 3.5–4% isovitexin or flavonoids.

Dosage: Capsules: 200 mg of the standardized capsule daily. One or two capsules half hour before bedtime encourage sleep. Tincture: 20–40 drops, 4 times daily.

Safety: There are no reported side effects, but toxicity is not well researched. Thus it is not recommended in pregnancy or for children under two. May increase the sedative effects of barbiturates.

Patchouli—Pogostemon cablin

Source: This plant may be found in the tropical regions of the world and is native to Malaysia and the Phillipines. Apart from its well-known fragrance, the young shoots and leaves are used medicinally in Chinese preparations.

Standardization: None.

Dosage: Powdered herb: 3–9 g in a decoction daily.

Safety: Do not take the essential oil internally.

Pau D'Arco—Lapacho/Tabebuia avellanedae

Source: This flowering evergreen tree in the bignonia family is native to

Florida, Central and South America. In Portuguese pau d'arco means "bow stick," as it is used to make bows for hunting. The inner bark is utilized for its medicinal effects.

Standardization: 3% naphthoquinones.

Dosage: Capsules: 500 mg, 1–2 capsules, 3 times daily. Tincture: 1–3 ml, 1–4 times daily.

Safety: No contraindications or toxicity known.

Pellitory of the Wall—Parietaria judaica

Source: Native to Europe, the plant may be found climbing on walls, as its name suggests. It has been used for over 2,000 years for kidney complaints.

Standardization: None.

Dosage: Tincture: 1–3 ml, 3 times daily.

Safety: No side effects have been reported.

Peony—Paeonia lactiflora

Source: A famed woman's herb, with over 1,500 years of documented medical use, white peony is indigenous to northern China and Mongolia. After 4–5 years the root is harvested in the spring and summer months.

Standardization: None.

Dosage: Capsules: Take as directed. Tincture: 1–30 drops, 4 times daily.

Safety: No known contraindications.

Peppermint—Mentha piperita

Source: Peppermint is the most popular member of the mint family, enjoying a rich history of folklore and medicinal attributes. Peppermint was originally from Africa, but is now native to most of Europe and cultivated in North America. Today mint is an ingredient in many "mentholated" medicinal preparations such as cough drops. The leaves and flowering tops are used.

Standardization: None.

Dosage: Capsules: 400 mg, up to six times daily, preferably, between meals. A coated capsule is recommended. Tincture: 10–20 drops in water. Essential oil may be diluted in a carrier oil and applied to skin for pain or itching.

Safety: Avoid with gallbladder disease, bile duct obstruction, esophageal reflux and during pregnancy. Do not use oil on broken skin.

Periwinkle—Vinca minor

Source: Indigenous to Spain and naturalized to Europe, the plant is cultivated for its purple flowers in gardens around the world. Lesser periwinkle can be found growing by roadsides, in orchards, wooded areas and bordering hedges. The leaves are used medicinally.

Standardization: Vinpocetine (5 mg), vinblastine, vincristine.

Dosage: Capsule: 5–30 mg daily. Tincture: 1–2 ml, 3 times daily.
Safety: Avoid in pregnancy. Can increase pressure in the brain. Avoid with brain tumor or head injury.

Pipsissewa—Chimaphila umbellata
Source: Pipsissewa is a creeping perennial and member of the heath family. Originally from Eurasia and North America, its arial parts or leaves are used for their effects on the bladder and prostate.
Standardization: None.
Dosage: Capsules: Take as directed. Tincture: 1–3 ml, 3 times daily.
Safety: Wildcrafting is discouraged. Use in pregnancy is generally contraindicated due to the arbutin content.

Plantain—Plantago lanceolata
Source: Native to Europe and Asia, wild plantain is widespread throughout most of the temperate regions of the globe. In Gaelic Ireland, plantain was called "the healing plant" for its properties of relieving bruises and wounds of all kinds.
Standardization: None.
Dosage: Capsule: 400 mg, 3 capsules, 4 times daily. Tincture: 1–2 ml, 3 times daily. As a poultice mix the bruised leaf with water to form a gelatinous paste and apply to affected areas, cover and leave on for two hours.
Safety: No known contraindications or toxicity.

Poke Root—Phytolacca decandra
Source: Poke root is a perennial weed-like shrub indigenous to North America and is now common to the Mediterranean area. It grows best in damp woody climates. This herb was widely valued by Native Americans and English settlers for its lymphagogue properties.
Standardization: None.
Dosage: Tincture: 1–20 drops daily. The oil can be applied topically to swollen glands; use 1/4 to 1 tsp per application.
Safety: Berries are toxic and prolonged contact may induce a dermatitis rash. May induce vomiting and diarrhea in high doses.

Pomegranate—Punica granatum
Source: Pomegranate is a tropical shrub originating in northwestern India whose growth has spread to many tropical regions. It has been associated with fertility rites and with the myth of Persephone and Hades. The bark of the root is most effective against parasites and worms. The fruit is used in Ayurveda as a cooling agent and blood tonic. The peel has astringent properties.
Standardization: None.
Dosage: Tincture: 5–45 drops at bedtime, followed by a morning laxative.

Safety: Contraindicated during pregnancy or breastfeeding. Due to the alkaloid content of this herb, over 80 g of the root or stem have induced poisoning symptoms of vomiting, dizziness and eventual death through respiratory failure.

Prickly Ash—Xanthoxylum americanum

Source: A tree found throughout the United States and a member of the rue or citrus family. Prickly ash was once the most widely used herb in 19th century medicine, being coined the "toothache tree" by Native Americans for its ability to relieve tooth pain. Prickly ash bark also increases the flow of saliva and gastric secretions and is a fine anti-arthritic herb.

Standardization: None.

Dosage: Tincture: Up to 15 ml daily.

Safety: Its uterine-stimulant properties make it unsafe during pregnancy.

Psyllium Seed—Plantago ovata

Source: This species of plantain is native to Iran and India. In China and India this plant was valued for its ability to relieve symptoms of diarrhea, hemorrhoids, bladder problems, skin irritations and high blood pressure.

Standardized: None.

Dosage: 7.5 g of seeds or 5 g of the husk, mixed with water or juice, once or twice daily, or take as directed on individual products.

Safety: Some allergic reactions have occurred. Make sure to follow with an 8 oz glass of water. Do not use with abdominal pain or when nausea and vomiting are present. Do not take with meals or other supplements, as it will interfere with their absorption.

Pulsatilla—Pulsatilla pratense

Source: Pulsatilla, also known as "windflower," is a member of the buttercup family. Its name is derived from the Greek god of the winds, *Anemos*, who sent this flower to announce his arrival during early spring. The French associate pasque flower with Easter. While known as a charm against diseases, in China it was considered the flower of death. The dried leaves, stems and flowers contain the active principles.

Standardization: None.

Dosage: Tincture: 0.5–3ml, 3 times daily.

Safety: Avoid handling the fresh plant, as it may cause skin and mucus membrane irritation. Do not use during pregnancy or nursing. Toxic doses cause kidney and urinary tract irritation, bloody urine, stomach upset and vomiting.

Pumpkin Seeds—Curcubita pepo

Source: For centuries, in all parts of the world, pumpkin seeds were a safe and gentle treatment for eliminating intestinal worms. The ripe dried or fresh seeds are used.

Standardization: None. (Seeds contain the amino acids cucurbitin 0.18–0.66% as well as L-tryptophan and alpha linolenic acid).

Dosage: For worm removal, eat 1–3 oz or 10 g of whole or coarsely ground seeds. For prostate disorders, consume 10 g daily.

Safety: No known contraindications. Safe for use in pregnancy, debilitated conditions and children.

Pygeum—Pygeum africanum

Source: Native to Africa, the bark of pygeum has been well researched in Europe since the 1960s for prostate disorders.

Standardization: 13% phytosterols or triterpenes and 0.5% n-docosanol.

Dosage: Standardized lipophilic extract: 200 mg daily. Tincture: 1–3 ml, 1–3 times daily.

Safety: Excess use may cause stomach irritation.

Q

Quassia—Picrasma excelsa

Source: A tropical tree named after the Surinam healer "Quassi." Quassia was introduced to Germany and Europe in the mid 1700s. A bitter digestive tonic, its bark was prized for its ability to reduce the craving for alcohol.

Standardization: None.

Dosage: Tincture: 10–30 drops, 2–3 times daily.

Safety: Safe, though has occasionally caused dizziness, headache and uterine pain. Excess may cause gastric irritation and vomiting.

Quebracho—Aspidosperma quebracho

Source: A South American tree that may reach heights of over 100 feet. The thick bark is a respiratory stimulant and one of the most bitter-tasting herbs known.

Standardization: None.

Dosage: Tincture: 5–60 drops daily.

Safety: No ill effects have been recorded with prescribed dosage; however, some side effects may occur such as sweating, dizziness, salivation and headache. In higher doses, toxicity may occur. Symptoms of overdose include queasiness and vomiting.

R

Red Clover—Trifolium pratense

Source: A member of the bean family and native to Eurasia, the flowers of several species of clover are used for their hormone-like isoflavone content. Traditionally the plant is a blood purifier and detoxifier.

Standardization: Standardized extracts should contain all four known isoflavones (formononetin, daidzein, biochanin and genistein).

Dosage: Capsules: 500 mg, 2 capsules, 3 times daily. Tincture: 2–6 ml, or 1–3 ml of fluid extract, 3 times daily. It may take at least 3 weeks for hormone-balancing effects to be seen.

Safety: Due to estrogen effects, should not be taken by pregnant or lactating women, children under two or during hormone therapy.

Red Raspberry—Rubus idaeus

Source: A member of the rose family and native to North America. Raspberry leaves and berries have been used medicinally for some 2,000 years to heal wounds and as a pregnancy tonic. Women traditionally drink raspberry tea throughout their pregnancy to relieve morning sickness and to strengthen the womb for childbirth.

Standardization: None.

Dosage: Capsules: 400 mg, up to 6 capsules daily. Tincture: 4–8 ml, 3 times daily.

Safety: Some texts recommend avoiding raspberry during the first three months of pregnancy except under a practitioner's supervision. Do not take with a history of rapid labor. Loose stools may occur in maximum dosages.

Red Root—Ceanothus americanus

Source: This member of the buckthorn family was introduced to English settlers by Native Americans as a spleen and lymphagogue remedy. As the name implies, the ochre-colored root is used.

Standardization: None.

Dosage: Capsules: Take as directed. Tincture: 1–4 ml, 3 times daily.

Safety: No contraindications or side effects.

Red Sage—Dan Shen/Salvia miltiorrhiza

Source: This Chinese root is a member of the mint family. Its value for heart and circulatory ailments has recently been "validated" by Western scientific research. Red sage is similar to hawthorn in safety and popularity in circulatory formulations.

Standardization: None.

Dosage: Capsules: 5–10 g after meals. Tincture 1–4 ml, 3–4 times daily.
Safety: No known contraindications or side effects.

Rehmannia—Rehmannia glutinosa

Source: The root of this Chinese herb is used for kidney and adrenal disorders. It strengthens the adrenal glands, benefiting the effects of overwork, stress or sexual excess, while improving insomnia, palpitations and vertigo. One of ingredients in the Chinese tonic "four things soup."
Standardization: 1% glutannic acid.
Dosage: Capsules: 250 mg, 1–3 times daily. Tincture: 2–3 ml, 4 times daily.
Safety: No side effects or contraindications known at prescribed dosages.

Reishi—Ganoderma lucidum

Source: This mushroom is still picked wild in its native China, where it has been used medicinally for 4,000 years. Renowned by Taoists for increasing both awareness and longevity, its traditional name is ling zhi, the herb of spiritual potency.
Standardization: 4–12.5% polysaccharides and 10% triterpenes.
Dosage: Capsules: 250 mg, totaling 6,000 mg daily. Tincture: 30 drops, 3 times daily. In severe illness, up to 31,000 mg daily has been used.
Safety: Avoid during pregnancy or nursing. May increase bleeding time. Stop using if dizziness, sore bones, itchy skin, increased body movements, pimple-like eruptions, or digestive upset occur.

Rhubarb—Rheum officinale

Source: Since ancient times, rhubarb root has been used in China to treat dysentery and constipation, in small doses it is a anti-diarrheal, and in larger doses, a laxative. The stems are used to make rhubarb pie.
Standardization: None.
Dosage: Capsules: Take as directed. Tincture: For diarrhea, 1/4 teaspoon daily. For constipation, 1/2–1 tsp daily.
Safety: The leaves are poisonous. Do not use with colitis or other intestinal conditions or while pregnant, as rhubarb may stimulate uterine contractions. Use for less than two weeks. Rhubarb may alter the urine's color.

Rosemary—Rosmarinus officinalis

Source: This aromatic shrub of the mint family is native to the Mediterranean basin. The leaves are a traditional culinary spice and cosmetic additive. Various herbalists throughout history have remarked upon rosemary's memory-enhancing and mood-elevating qualities.
Standardization: Europeans extract the antioxidant carnosol.
Dosage: Capsules: 800 mg, 1–3 daily. Tincture: 1–4 ml, 3 times daily.
Safety: Rosemary has no contraindications or adverse side effects when used as a spice or medicinal herb.

S

Sage—Salvia officinalis

Source: A well-known garden ornamental and spice, sage originated in the Mediterranean and Baltic regions. Now widely cultivated in Europe and North America, this mint family member has been used internally and externally for over 2,000 years.

Standardization: None.

Dosage: Tincture: 1–4 ml, 3 times daily. Apply fresh leaves to inflamed joints or sprains. Gargle with 1–4 g of the leaf in a tea.

Safety: Contraindicated in pregnancy due to its emmenagogue effects and during nursing because of its ability to reduce the flow of milk. Prolonged use is not recommended.

St. John's Wort—Hypericum perforatum

Source: This herb is a European and North American native. The red marks that appear on its leaves in mid-summer were associated with the blood of St. John. Long used as a magical herb and vulnerary, it has reached enormous popularity for its anti-depressant and antiviral effects.

Standardization: 0.3% hypericin or 3–5% hyperforin.

Dosage: Capsules of the extract: 300 mg, 1–3 times daily. Standardized extract: 900 mg daily. Tincture: 1/2 tsp, 3 times daily. Needs to be taken for 4–6 weeks before properly assessing effectiveness.

Safety: Hypericum causes photosensitivity of skin in animals, but this is rarely seen in people. Avoid tyrosine-containing foods: red wine, aged cheese, yeast, pickled herring. Do not use if taking prescription anti-depressants and avoid during pregnancy or lactation. For HIV/AIDS patients, do not take while using Indinavir.

Sarsaparilla—Smilax officinalis

Source: This member of the lily order is a tropical plant native to Mexico, South America and the Caribbean. Sarsaparilla was one of the famous beverages in the 18th and 19th centuries and was considered a cure for syphilis. Today the root is prescribed for its steroidal hormone-like effects.

Standardization: None.

Dosage: Capsules: 800 mg daily. Tincture: 10–40 drops, 3 times daily.

Safety: Do not take with prescription medications, as it may enhance their absorption rate. May rarely cause gastric or kidney inflammation. Avoid during pregnancy or breastfeeding due to its steroid-like components. Avoid inhaling the dust from the root as it may induce asthma in susceptible individuals.

Saw Palmetto—Seronoa repens

Source: Native to the American Southwest, the berry of this palm tree has been extensively researched and is the most widely used prostate herb.

Standardization: 85%–95% liposterolic acids.

Dosage: Capsules: 160 mg, 2 times daily. Standardized extract: 300 mg daily. Tincture: 10–60 drops, 4 times daily. Improvement may occur in 4–6 weeks, but a full year is required for maximum prostate or hair effects. Can be taken indefinitely, on and off.

Safety: Rarely, large amounts can cause stomach irritation. Due to a slightly estrogenic effect, it has been known to increase breast size.

Schisandra—Schisandra chinensis

Source: A woody vine native to Southeast Asia, it is known as "five flavored herb" or "wu wei zi" in Chinese medicine. Used as an astringent tonic for thousands of years, it is now a lung, kidney and adrenal adaptogen.

Standardization: 1.0% schisantherins, A &B; 9% schisandrins (18 mg).

Dosage: Capsules: 500 mg, up to 6 times daily. Tincture: 30–60 drops, 3 times daily.

Safety: No contraindications are known. Can be used for long periods. Higher doses may cause insomnia and restlessness.

Senega Snakeroot—Polygala senega

Source: The dried root has a history in Native American lore as a heart remedy and insect sting neutralizer. A member of the milkweed family.

Standardization: None.

Dosage: Tincture: 2.5–5 ml, 3 times daily.

Safety: Not for use during pregnancy. Gastric irritation may occur with prolonged use. Signs of overdose may include nausea, diarrhea, queasiness and gastric complaints.

Senna—Cassia senna

Source: Native to India, China and Pakistan, senna is a popular component of over-the-counter laxatives worldwide. The leaves and seed pods of this member of the bean family are responsible for its medicinal effects.

Standardization: 5% sennosids.

Dosage: Capsules: Children 6–12 years, 1 capsule twice daily for a maximum of 4 tablets daily. Adults and children over 12 years of age may take two 187 mg tablets at bedtime for a maximum dose of 8 tablets daily. Tincture: 2–7 ml, 3 times daily. Drink 1–2 8-ounce glasses of water per dose.

Safety: Contraindicated in intestinal obstruction, appendicitis or acute inflammatory diseases of the colon. Do not use in children under two years old. Abdominal cramping may occur as a side effect. Chronic use (more than 3 times weekly for more than one year) may lead to dependence, electrolyte imbalances and subsequent irregular heart activity.

Shativari—Asparagus racemosus

Source: An Indian root that was used for centuries in Ayurvedic traditions as a female tonic, reproductive strengthener and adaptogen.

Standardization: None.

Dosage: Capsules: 500 mg, twice daily.

Safety: Do not use for cold or damp conditions (i.e. mucus or phlegm, diarrhea, cold limbs, low energy).

Shepherd's Purse—Thlapsi bursa pastoris

Source: This member of the mustard family originated in southern Europe and western Asia. Shepherd's purse is a tender weed-like plant with heart-shaped pods and can be found growing in all non-tropical regions of the world.

Standardization: None.

Dosage: Tincture: 15–30 drops, 3 times daily.

Safety: Do not use in pregnancy or nursing due to the uterine-stimulating effects of this herb. No other contraindications or side effects are noted.

Shiitake—Lentinus edodes

Source: Japan's top agricultural export, Shiitake mushroom is a delicacy in Korea, Japan and China and has been a medicinal and culinary mushroom since the times of the Sung Dynasty, over 1,000 years ago.

Standardization: 3.2% KS-2 polysaccharides (peptidomannan).

Dosage: Capsules: 800 mg, 3 times daily. Standardized extract: 1–3 g daily. Whole dried mushroom: 6–16 g daily. Tincture: 1–4 ml, 3 times daily.

Safety: Shiitake has no contraindications. In high doses, it may induce bloating or diarrhea.

Siberian Ginseng—Eleutherococcus senticosus

Source: This member of the ginseng family grows in Russia (Siberia), Korea, China and northern Japan, where the root or bark is utilized to make dried powder, capsules, tablets or tinctures.

Standardization: Eleutherosides B, D, E or total eleutherosides. Some preparations include: 0.3% eleutheroside B or 0.5% eleutheroside E.

Dosage: Capsule: 400–500 mg, up to 9 capsules daily. Tincture: 2–12 ml daily. Standardized extract: 100–200 mg, 3 times daily.

Safety: Excess can cause anxiety, depression, insomnia, irritability, diarrhea or skin rashes. Do not use while taking antibiotics, digitalis or hexobarbitol. May slightly raise blood pressure.

Skullcap—Scutellaria lateriflora

Source: Eastern North America is home to this nourishing nervine of the mint family. It was used by Native Americans and early settlers as it is today: an effective herb for anxiety and the effects of stress.

Standardization: None.

Dosage: Capsules: 400 mg, up to 6 times daily. Tincture: 1–2 ml, 3 times daily.

Safety: No side effects are known to occur with the recommended dosage. No information exists for pregnancy or nursing safety.

Slippery Elm—Ulmus fulva

Source: Slippery elm was revered by Native Americans and early English settlers for its versatility as both a source of lumber and medicine. The inner bark is harvested from ten-year-old North American trees.

Standardized: None.

Dosage: Capsules: 1,500 mg, 3 times daily. Tincture: 10–30 drops, 3 times daily. For a nutritious food in debilitated conditions (in the elderly, infants or to sooth irritated membranes), mix 1 tablespoon of slippery elm powder with enough boiling water to make a porridge-like consistency. Consume 1–3 times daily or as desired. May also be prepared in this way as a compress for external skin conditions.

Safety: A very safe herb, with no known side effects or contraindications.

Spikenard—Aralia racemosa

Source: This North American root in the ginseng family is a strengthening tonic used by Native Americans. It was included in the U.S. National Formulary from 1916 to 1965.

Standardization: None.

Dosage: Capsule: Take as directed. Tincture: 1–4 ml, 3 times daily.

Safety: Do not use during pregnancy.

Spilanthes—Spilanthes oleracea

Source: A member of the daisy family, spilanthes is native to the Amazon. The flower buds are chewed and create a tingling sensation that dulls toothaches. This is a strong herb with lovely yellow flowers.

Standardization: None.

Dosage: Capsules: Take as directed. Tincture: 1–4 ml, 3 times daily.

Safety: No side effects known.

Stevia—Stevia rebaudiana

Source: The leaves and flowers of the South American shrub provide a natural sweetener enjoyed for hundreds of years in Latin countries.

Dosage: Dried leaves, powdered extract and liquid extract are used according to taste. Approximately 1–3 drops extracted to 1 cup liquid is appropriate. Its taste is not affected by heat.

Safety: There is an ongoing FDA resistance to allowing stevia to be marketed as a sweetener in spite of widespread use in Japan for thirty years—based on the economics of the sugar industry. No known human toxicity.

Stone Root—Collinsonia canadensis

Source: This aromatic and bitter rhizome in the mint family is native to the northern United States and central European regions.

Standardization: None.

Dosage: Tincture: 20–60 drops, 3 times daily.

Safety: No contraindications or side effects.

Suma—Pfaffia paniculata

Source: Suma is a South American adaptogenic herb known as the "Brazilian ginseng" for its rejuvenating qualities. Though it bears no botanical relationship to ginseng, suma's attributes are similar in nature.

Standardization: 5% beta-ecdysterones.

Dosage: Capsules: 500 mg, 2–4 times daily.

Safety: No known contraindications.

T

Tea Tree Oil—Melaleuca alternifolia

Source: An Australian tree traditionally used for a wide variety of ills by native Aboriginals, tea tree has been researched since the 1920s for its antiseptic qualities. The leaves and twigs are the source of the oil.

Standardization: 10–65% terpinen-4-ol, cineol. Topical oil is 5–15% strength.

Dosage: Externally, tea tree oil can be used full strength or diluted for application to nails or in acne, while 2–4 drops may be used in a vaginal douche. Foot soaks may require 20 drops of oil in warm water.

Safety: Do not take oil internally. Do not apply to broken or open skin, as burning may occur. Full strength doses can be an irritant.

Tribulus—Tribulus terrestris

Source: Tribulus is also known as "burra googeroo" in its East Indian homeland. Its seeds are touted for their male energizing and aphrodisiac properties.

Standardization: 20–30% total saponins.

Dosage: Capsules: 500 mg, 3 times daily. Tincture: 10–30 drops.

Safety: No known side effects.

Triphala

Source: An age-old Indian combination of three herbs that serves to cleanse and regulate the digestive and elimination processes in the body. Amla fruit (*Emblica officinalis*), behada fruit (*Terminalia belerica*) and harada fruit (*Terminalia chebula*) are the three herbs that make up triphala.

Standardization: None.

Dosage: Capsules: 300 mg, 2–3 times daily. Increase dose for a more laxative effect.

Safety: No known contraindications.

True Unicorn Root—Aletris farinosa

Source: Native to swamps and damp woodlands of eastern North America, the root of this lily-related plant is a traditional ingredient in native medicines to initiate menses, promote digestion and relieve colic.

Standardization: None.

Dosage: Tincture: 1–2 ml, 3 times daily.

Safety: The fresh or dried root is toxic in overdose, causing diarrhea and vomiting.

UVW

Usnea—Usnea barbata

Source: Also known as "old man's beard" for it mossy, beard-like appearance, this lichen grows on trees in cool damp environments. Usnea has the ability to inhibit gram-positive bacteria and is good for upper respiratory infections and urinary tract disorders.

Standardization: None.

Dosage: Capsules: 600 mg daily. Tincture: 60–70 drops, 3–4 times daily.

Safety: In large quantities, usnea is safe as an antibiotic and diuretic herb.

Uva ursi—Arctostaphylos uva ursi

Source: Uva ursi is a Central European native, where the leaves have been used since the Greek and Roman times for treating urinary tract symptoms.

Standardization: 20% arbutin.

Dosage: Capsules: 400 mg, up to 9 capsules daily. Tincture: 1–4 ml, 3 times daily.

Safety: Contraindicated in pregnant and breastfeeding women and children under the age of twelve.

Valerian—Valeriana officinalis

Source: A European herb that has been used for over 2,000 years to calm and sooth the nervous system. In the first century A.D., the Roman naturalist Dioscorides named the plant "phu" to reflect its distinct odor.

Standardization: 0.2–1% valerenic acids.

Dose: Capsules: 300 to 600 mg, 1–2 capsules at bedtime. Tincture: 1/2 to 1 tsp, forty-five minutes before bed or as needed. The tincture seems to be the most effective form. May be taken during the day for anxiety in similar doses.

Safety: Valerian causes no morning hangover, impaired mental or physical performance or other side effects associated with most sedatives. Long-term use may cause depression, headache, anxiety or palpitations. Should not be used for prolonged periods. May increase the effects of barbiturates and alcohol. No adverse effects cited during pregnancy or nursing. Not advised for children under two.

Vervain—Verbena officinalis

Source: Native to the Mediterranean region, this plant has been revered by the Druids as one of the most sacred herbs, next to mistletoe.

Standardization: None.

Dosage: Capsules: 350 mg at bedtime or 1–2 capsules, 3 times daily. Tincture: 1–4 ml, 3 times daily.

Safety: Do not use if taking blood thinners, as it may delay clotting time.

Walnut—Juglans nigra

Source: According to folklore, the gods lived on walnuts when they walked the earth. The hulls and inner bark of the black walnut tree were listed in the U.S. Pharmacopoeia as a laxative and a treatment for liver disorders. A popular Revolutionary War remedy, walnut was hailed for its beneficial digestive effects.

Standardization: None.

Dosage: Capsules: Take as directed. Tincture: 1–10 drops, 1–3 times daily.

Safety: Do not use in pregnancy or for long periods of time. In large doses it may sedate the heart functioning and circulatory system.

White Ash—Fraxinus excelsior

Source: A large deciduous European tree which has been venerated in Celtic folklore. Medicinally, its tender flowering tops are useful as a gentle laxative and for rheumatic disorders.

Standardization: None.

Dosage: Follow package directions.

Safety: No adverse effects have been noted with prescribed dosages.

White Cedar—Thuja occidentalis

Source: Arbor vitae, or the "tree of life," is native to northeastern North America. The active constituents are found in its needles and young twigs. Thuja is useful as a respiratory mucus expectorant and an external remedy for warts and growths.

Standardization: None.

Dosage: Tincture: 1 ml, 3 times a day for expectorant effects. Externally: Apply to warty growths or fungal infections.

Safety: Contraindicated during pregnancy, nursing, epilepsy or gastritis. Thuja contains the volatile oil, thujone, which is toxic and found mainly in the fresh twigs and needles. Avoid tea made from fresh twigs. Symptoms of toxicity include queasiness, vomiting, painful diarrhea and bleeding from mucus membranes. Deaths have been reported when thuja is used as an abortifacient. Keep the essential oil away from children and pets as it may prove fatal if ingested.

White Oak—Quercus alba

Source: The young bark of the oak was an important remedy in European and Native American medicine and the most sacred tree of the Celtic Druids. Oak's astringent and antiseptic properties help combat many conditions. If gathering it from the wild, take care never to remove a full ring of bark from an oak trunk, as this will kill the entire tree.

Standardization: None.

Dosage: Capsules: 500 mg, 1–3 times daily. Tincture: 1–2 ml, 2 times daily. Externally: For compresses or gargles, use 20 g to 1 liter of water. For baths, add hot water to 5 g of bark and then add into bath water.

Safety: Do not use externally on large areas of exposed skin, such as in eczema or psoriasis. Baths containing oak bark are contraindicated in advanced cardiac disease or with high fevers of an infectious nature.

White Pine—Pinus sylvestris

Source: A tree indigenous to North America, the pine needle shoots are used for skin conditions and respiratory disorders.

Standardization: None.

Dosage: Capsules: 2–3 g of the herb several times a day. Externally: Use a 20–50% strength ointment rubbed on affected areas, 2–3 times daily.

Safety: No known contraindications. Do not add pine preparations to a bath with extensive skin damage, cardiac insufficiency, or high fever.

Wild Cherry—Prunus virginiana

Source: Related to the rose family, the dried bark of this North American tree is used as a component in many cough syrups for various bronchial complaints. It was a favorite of 19th-century physicians.

Standardization: None.

Dosage: Capsules: 1–2 g of the dried bark daily. Tincture: 1–2 ml, 1–4 times daily.

Safety: The bark is safe in prescribed dosages. Do not use if pregnant or nursing. All parts of wild cherry (except the fruit) contain varying amounts of the poison hydrogen cyanide. Symptoms of cyanide overdose include difficulty breathing or speaking, spasms, stupor and coma leading to death. Milder signs include nausea, vomiting, headache, muscle weakness and irregular heartbeat.

Wild Indigo—Baptisia tinctoria

Source: An antiseptic herb in the bean family, wild indigo is a Native American herb used for chronic, deep-seated infections. The leaves and roots are used medicinally.

Standardization: None.
Dosage: Tincture: 10–20 drops, 3 times daily.
Safety: Excess causes nausea and vomiting. Very high doses are extremely toxic or even fatal. Use caution. Do not take if pregnant or nursing.

Wild Lettuce—Latuca virosa
Source: The dried leaves of wild lettuce contain trace or minute amounts of opium-like substances. As far back as Egyptian times, this herb was used for insomnia, mild sedation and pain. The latex or juice was used as a substitute for morphine and codeine during World War I.
Standardization: None.
Dosage: Tincture: 1–3 ml. Dried latex: 0.3–1.0 g. Dried leaves: 0.5–3.0 g. All forms can be taken up to 3 times daily.
Safety: Excessive use should be avoided due to its sedative effects. No clear data for pregnancy or nursing has been established. Wild lettuce is generally safe. No documented side effects or toxicity have occurred.

Wild Pansy—Viola tricolor
Source: Native to Europe, Asia and Africa. This herb is able to flourish in a wide variety of climates, including North and South America. Gentle enough for use in children.The aerial parts are used medicinally.
Standardization: None.
Dosage: Capsules: Take as directed. Tincture: 1–4 ml daily.
Safety: No side effects or contraindications are known.

Wild Thyme—Thymus serpyllum
Source: A Mediterranean native, which was touted by Pliny and the ancient Romans for its ability to cleanse the bites of snakes and scorpions. Wild thyme's leaves contain powerful oils, possessing a more stimulating nature than the common garden variety (*Thymus vulgaris*).
Standardization: None.
Dosage: Capsules: 400 mg, 1–3 times daily. Tincture: 2–4 ml, 3 times daily.
Safety: Do not use during pregnancy or nursing. Do not ingest the essential oil; a few drops have been fatal in children. Keep out of reach of children and away from pet areas.

Wild Yam—Dioscorea villosa
Source: Wild Yam is a vine that may reach up to 20 feet and grows in the damp woodlands of North and Central America. The root is used for its hormonal precursor, diosgenin, but does not supply estrogen, progesterone or DHEA directly.
Standardization: 10% diosgenins.
Dosage: Capsules: 400 mg, 1–3 times daily. Tincture: 1–10 ml, 1–2 times daily for hormonal balancing.
Safety: Some people experience oily skin, acne or nausea on wild yam. If

this occurs, the dosage should be decreased until symptoms subside, and resumed at a lower level.

Willow Bark—Salix spp.

Source: Willow, native to Europe (white willow) and America (black willow), was traditionally used to treat fevers and was one of the first herbs investigated scientifically. In 1899, acetylsalicylic acid or aspirin was synthetically produced based upon this tree's active constituent.

Standardization: 7–15% salicin.

Dosage: Capsules: 250–500 mg (with 30 mg salicin per capsule), up to 4 times daily. Tincture: 1–3 ml, 2–3 times daily.

Safety: Avoid if pregnant or nursing, if allergic to aspirin, with gastric ulcer disease, or bleeding disorders. Do not use if currently on blood-thinning medications such as Coumadin.

Witch Hazel—Hamamelis virginiana

Source: The bark, twigs, branches and leaves of the witch hazel shrub contain medicinal constituents. A native to North America, it has been popular commercially for over 150 years for its astringent and pain-relieving qualities.

Standardization: None.

Dosage: Tincture: 2–4 ml in water or applied directly a few times daily. Externally: Apply as a compress or use as a gargle.

Safety: Due to the high tannin content of this herb, use internally only under supervision of a licensed practitioner. No adverse effects are noted in the literature with external use. The store-bought brands have little or no tannins, thus, they are less drying but not as effective as the tincture or infusion.

Wood Betony—Stachys officinalis

Source: This mint family member was once valued as a protective amulet during the Middle Ages. The above ground parts are used as a soothing nervine and sedative.

Standardization: None.

Dosage: Capsules: 400 mg, 1–3 times daily. Tincture: 1–6 ml, 1–3 times daily.

Safety: Do not take during pregnancy, as this herb is a uterine stimulant.

Wood Sage—Cat Thyme/Teucrium scorodonia

Source: A member of the mint family that may be found growing throughout most of the Mediterranean region. The leaves of wood sage possess vermifuge properties and exude a leek-like fragrance when cut.

Standardization: None.

Dosage: Capsules: Take as directed.

Safety: No adverse effects or contraindications with therapeutic dose.

XYZ

Yarrow—Achillia millefolium

Source: Derived from Achilles—the Greek hero who used the herb to treat wounds in the Trojan war—it has been a major wound remedy throughout history. In folklore yarrow was called "nosebleed" for its ability to stop bleeding. The flowers and leaves are utilized.

Standardization: 0.2% volatile oils and .02% alchillicin (a proazulene).

Dosage: Capsules: 600 mg, 3 times daily. Tincture: 15–30 drops, 3 times daily or every 1–2 hours for fever. In sitz baths: 100 g yarrow to 5 gallons of warm water. For wounds: Apply poultice topically.

Safety: Do not take if pregnant. Allergic reactions may occur if sensitive to other members of the daisy family.

Yellow Dock—Rumex crispus

Source: The iron-rich root of yellow dock was originally from Europe and is valued in the Americas and Asia as a blood purifier and mild laxative.

Standardization: None.

Dosage: Capsules: 500 mg, 1–4 daily. Tincture: 1–4 ml, 3 times daily.

Safety: Contains oxalic acid and is toxic in large quantities. Avoid this herb with any diseases of the kidney.

Yerba Mansa—Anemopsis californica

Source: An herb similar in action to goldenseal, it is an astringent and may be applied topically to fungal infections.

Standardization: None.

Dosage: Tincture: 10–40 drops daily.

Safety: May increase the action of sedative medications. Excessive use may irritate the kidneys.

Yerba Santa—Eriodictyon californicum

Source: An evergreen shrub found growing in the mountains of California and Mexico, this herb is one of the most valued herbs in northern California. It was quickly adopted by Spanish missionaries for treating respiratory disorders and also shows promise as a cancer therapy.

Standardization: None.

Dosage: Tincture: 1–2 ml, 3–4 times daily.

Safety: No known contraindications.

Yucca Root—Yucca spp.

Source: The yucca is in the agave family, found in the desert Southwest and a relative to the tequila agave. It was valued by the Cherokee Nation as a skin and hair cleanser. It is now used for diabetes, arthritis and digestive ailments.

Standardization: None.

Dosage: Capsules: 500 mg, 1–4 times daily. Tincture: 1–2 ml, 3 times daily.

Safety: Safety in pregnancy and lactation has not been established.

Yohimbe—Pausinystalia yohimbe

Source: The inner bark of this African tree was traditionally used as an aphrodisiac and mild hallucinogen by the Bantu tribe. It is now both a prescription drug for impotency and a freely available herb.

Standardization: 6% indole alkaloids.

Dosage: Capsules: 15–30 mg daily. Tincture: 5–10 drops daily. Prescription drug: For male impotency, 2.7 mg to 5.4 mg, twice daily or as directed.

Safety: A short-term MAO inhibitor, standard doses can cause indigestion, nausea, dizziness, headaches, tremors, irregular heart rhythms, hypertension, sweating and anxiety. Not to be used with liver or kidney diseases, peptic ulcer, glaucoma, in pregnancy or during lactation. Avoid tyramine-containing foods (cheese, chocolate, beer, aged meats, nuts), non-prescription stimulants, such as caffeine, cold medications containing phenylephedrine or phenylpropanolamine, and antidepressants. Also available by prescription,

Part 5

Herbal Resources

HERBAL PRACTITIONERS

American Association Naturopathic Physicians
601 Valley Street, Suite 105
Seattle, WA 98109
(703) 610-9037

American Botanical Council
PO Box 144345
Austin, TX 78714
(512) 926-4900
www.herbalgram.org

American Herb Association
PO Box 1673
Nevada City, CA 95959
(916) 265-9552

American Herbal Products Association
8484 Georgia Avenue, Suite 370
Silver Springs, MD 20910
(301) 588-1171
AHPA@ix.netcom.com

American Herbalists Guild
PO Box 70
Roosevelt, UT 84066
(435) 722-8434
www.healthy.net/herbalists

American Holistic Health Association
PO Box I 7400
Anaheim, CA 92817
email: ahha@healthy.net

Ayurvedic Institute
PO Box 23445
Albuquerque, NM 87192-1445
(505) 291-9698

Herb Research Foundation
1007 Pearl Street, Suite 200
Boulder, CO 80302
www.berbs.org

HERBAL PRODUCTS

AYURVEDIC HERBS

Sushakti
1840 Iron Street, Suite C
Bellingham, WA 98225
(360) 752-0575
www.ayurveda-sushakti.com

CHINESE HERBS

Crane Herb Company
745 Falmouth Road
Mashpee, MA 02649
(800) 227-4118

Kan Herb Company
6001 Butler Lane
Scotts Valley, CA 95066
(800) 543-5233
www.kanherb.com

Mayway Corporation
1338 Mandela Parkway
Oakland, CA 94607
(800) 262-9929

Tashymin Tong Herbs
5221 Central Avenue, Suite 105
Oakland, CA 94804
(800) 538-1333

Western Herbs

Avena Botanicals
219 Mill Street
Rockport, ME 04856
(207) 594-0694

Aroma Vera
5901 Rodeo Road
Los Angeles, CA 90016-4312

Cheryl's Herbs
836 Hanley Industrial Court
St. Louis, MO 63144

Eclectic Institute Inc.
14385 Southeast Lusted Road
Sandy, OR 97055-9549

Frontier Herb
PO Box 299
Norway, IA 532218
(800) 669-3275

Gaia Herbs
108 Island Ford Road
Brevard, NC 28712

Green Terrestrial
328 Lake Avenue
Greenwich, CT 06830

Herb Pharm
PO Box 116
Williams, OR 97544

Herbalist and Alchemist
PO Box 553
Broadway, NJ 08808

Horizon Herbs
PO Box 69
Williams, OR 97544

Jean's Greens
119 Sulphur Spring Road
Newport, NY 13416
(888) 845-8327

Longherb Health Products
307 E. Washington Avenue
Fairfield, IA 52556-3148

Mountain Rose School
20818 High Street North
North San Juan, CA 95960
(800) 879-3337

Pacific Botanicals
4350 Fish Hatchery Road
Grants Pass, OR 97527

Rainbow Light
207 McPherson
Santa Cruz, CA 95060
(800) 635-1233

Reevis Mountain School of Survival
321 E. Northern
Phoenix, AZ 85020

Simpler's Botanicals
PO Box 2534
Sebastopol, CA 95473
(800) 652-7646

Terra Firma Botanicals
28653 Sutherfin Lane
Eugene, OR 97405
(503) 485-7726

Way of Life
1210 41st Avenue
Capitola, CA 95010

Wise Women Herbal
PO Box 279
Creswell, OR 97426
(800) 532-5219

Vitality Works
134 Quincy Street
Albuquerque, NM 87108

Zand Herbals
1722 14th Street, Suite 230
Boulder, CO 80302
www.zand.com

Herbal Training

Blazing Star Herbal School
PO Box 6
Shelbourne Falls, MA 01370
(413) 625-6875

California School of Herbal Studies
PO Box 39
Forestville, CA 95436

Dry Creek Herb Farm
13935 Dry Creek Road
Auburn, CA 95602
(530) 878-2441

Pacific NW Herbal Symposium
PO Box 279
Creswell, OR 97426
(800) 476-6518

Pacific Institute of Aromatherapy
PO Box 6723
San Rafael, CA 94903

Pacific School of Herbal Medicine
PO Box 3151
Oakland, CA 94609
(510) 845-4028

Rocky Mountain Center for Botanical Studies
2639 Spruce Street
Boulder, CO 80302
(303) 442-6861

Sage Mountain
PO Box 420
E. Barre, VT 05649
(802) 479-9825

Wild Rose College of Natural Healing
#400, 1228 Kensington Road NW
Calgary, Alberta, CAN T2N 4P9
(403) 270-0936

Herbal Magazines

American Herb Association Newsletter
PO Box 1673
Nevada City, CA 95959

Herbs for Health
Herb Companion Press, LLC
201 East Fourth Street
Loveland, CO 80537-5655
www.interweave.com

Herbalgram
PO Box 144345
Austin, TX 78714-4345
(800) 373-7105
www.herbalgram.org
custserv@herbgram.org

Medical Herbalism
PO Box 20512
Boulder, CO 80308

Medical Herbalist Magazine
PO Box 20512
Boulder, CO 80308
www.medherb.com

Meno Times
1108 Irwin Street
San Rafael, CA 94901

Mothering
PO Box 1690
Santa Fe, NM 87504
www.mothering.com
mother@ni.net

HERBAL READING LIST

The bibliography below lists the majority of texts and journals used in the writting of this book. It also has a built-in grading system that allows it to be a reference to further herbal reading and knowledge. The grading system is based on its value to the comsumer and professional alike. This evaluation is based on several criteria, including accuracy and depth of information, completeness, style, accessibility of information and format. The idea is to distinguish books that are truly useful, practical and easy to use and ultimately worth purchasing and owning. Another important criteria is the balance between taking a "scientific" approach to herbs and a traditional one. Some texts do not give credibility to any information whatsoever, unless it has been subjected to scientific investigation. Because of the great margin of error and poor design of such studies, it is a mistake to rely on this data exclusively and ignore all traditional knowledge. Likewise, those books that are just "folksy" provide no real understanding of the power and effectiveness of herbal treatment. The grading system is simple:

- *** *Excellent*. Reserved for a small number of extremely worthwhile texts.
- ** *Good*. Many books have an average value and contain reasonable amounts of useful information. This grading also applies to some good books, but that have a narrow focus or are merely outdated.
- * *Fair*. Such books are either inaccurate, quickly put together for commercial purposes, or are extremely limited in approach.
- ° *Poor*. Zero ratings are reserved for only a few books. Some may even be popular or heavily marketed, but contain superficial, erroneous or misleading information. Some are well-meaning, but poorly written, while others are designed to sell books, not profer herbal wisdom.

Medicinal Plants

Bartram, Thomas. *Encyclopedia of Herbal Medicine.*** Christchurch: Grace Publishers, 1995.

Bellamy, David and Pfister, Andrea. *World Medicine: Plants Patients & People.** Oxford: Blackwell, 1992.

Bezanger-Beuquesne. *Plantes Medicinale des Regions Temperees.*** 2nd Edition, Maloine, 1990.

Blumenthal, M. *The Complete German Commisssion E Monographs.*** Austin: American Botanical Council, 1998.

_______________. *Herbal Medicine: Expanded Commission E Monographs.**** Austin: American Botanical Council, 2000.

Blumert M and Liu Jialiu. *Jiaogulan: China'a Immortality Herb.** Badger: Torchlight Publishing, Inc. 1999.

Boyle, Wade. *Official Herbs: Botanical Substances in the U.S Pharmacopoeias, 1820-1890.*** East Palestine. Buckeye Naturopathic Press, 1991.

Brown, Deni. *Encylopedia of Herbs and Their Uses*.*** New York: Dorling Kindersley, 1995.

Buhner, Stephen. H. *Herbal Antibiotics*.** Pownal: Storey Books, 1999.

_______________. *Herbs for Hepatitis C and the Liver*.*** Pownal: Storey Books, 2000.

Bunny, Sarah, editor. *The Illustrated Encyclopedia of Herbs*.** London: Chancellor Press, 1992.

Castleman, Michael. *The Healing Herbs; the Ultimate Guide*.***New York: Bantam Books, 1995.

Chevallier, Andrew. *The Encyclopedia of Medicinal Plants*.*** London: Dorling Kindersley, 1996.

Chmelik, Stefan. *Chinese Herbal Secrets*.* Garden City Press: Avery Publishing, 1999.

Coon, Nelson. *Using Plants for Healing*.* Emmaus: Rodale Press, 1979.

Culbreth, David. A. *Manual of Materia Medica and Pharmacology*.** Philadelphia: Lea & Febiger, 1927.

Dobels, Inge, editor. *Magic and Medicine of Plants*.** New York: Reader's Digest Books, 1986.

Dodge, Bertha. *Plants That Changed the World*.* Boston: Little Brown & Company, 1959.

Duke, James. *The Green Pharmacy*.* Emmaus: Rodale Press, 1997.

Elias, J., Masline, S.R., *The A to Z Guide to Healing Herb Remedies*.* New York: Dell Publishing, 1995

Felter, Harvey Wickes, *The Eclectic Materia Medica and Pharmacology and Therapeutics*.** Cinncincinnati: John K. Scudder, 1922.

Fetrow, C.W., Avila J.R. *The Complete Guide to Medicinal Herbs*.* Springhouse: Springhouse Corporation, 2000.

Foster, Steven. *Herbs for Your Health*.** Loveland: Interweave Press, 1966.

__________. *101 Medicinal Herbs*.** Loveland: Interweave Press, Inc., 1998.

Foster and Duke, *Field Guide to Medicinal Plants*.***Boston: Houghton Mifflin, 1990.

George, Stephen, editor. *The Doctor's Book of Herbal Home Remedies*.* Emmaus: Rodale Press, 2000.

Grieve, Mrs. M. *Modern Herbal*.*** London: Johathan Cape Ltd, 1931.

Grime, William Ed. *Ethnobotany of the Black Americans*.** Algonac: Reference Publishing, 1979.

Gruenwald, Brendler, Jaenicke, editors. PDR *for Herbal Medicine*.* Montvale: Medical Economics Company, 2000.

Harris, Ben Charles. *The Compleat Herbal*.* New York: Bell Publishing, 1985.

Heinerman, John. *Heinerman's Encyclopedia of Healing Herbs and Spices*.** Prentice Hall, Englewood Cliffs, 1996.

Hobb, Christopher. *Herbal Remedies for Dummies*.° Foster City: IDG Books, 1998.

Hoffmann, David. *The Complete Illustrated Holistic Herbal*.*** New York: Barnes and Noble Books, 1996.

__________________ .*Healthy Bones & Joints*.** Pownal: Storey Books, 2000.

__________________ .*Healthy Heart*.** Pownal: Storey Books, 2000.

Kay, Margarita. *Healing with Plants in the American and Mexican West*.** Tucson: University of Arizona Press, 1996.

Kenner, Dan and Rquena, Yves. *Botanical Medicine: A European Professional Perspective*.** Brookline: Paradigm Publications, 1996.

Keville, Kathi. *The Illustrated Herb Encyclopedia*.** London: Grange Books, 1991.

Kurch, Joseph Wood. *Herbal*.* Boston: David R. Goodine, 1976.

Lesley Bremness. *Herbs*.* London: Dorling Kindersley, 1994.

Lewis and Elvin-Lewis. *Medical Botany*.**New York: John Wiley & Sons, 1977.

Llloyd, J. U and Lloyd, C. G. *Ranunculaceae (Drugs and Medicines of North America)*.** Cincinnati: Robert Clarke & Co., 1885.

Lust, John. *The Herb Book*.** New York: Bantum Books, 1974.

McCleb, Robert, Leigh, Evelyn and Morgan, Krista. *The Encyclopedia of Popular Herbs*.*** Roseville: Primat Health, 2000.

Manniche L. *An Ancient Egyptian Herbal*. ** Austin: University of Texas Press, 1999.

Millspaugh, Charles F. *American Medicinal Plants*.** New York: Dover Publications, 1892 (reprint 1974).

Mitchell, William A. *Plant Medicine: Applications of the Botanical Remedies in the Practice of Naturopathic Medicine*.*** Seatle: William A Mitchell Press, 2000.

Moore, Michael: *Los Remedios: Traditional Herbal Remedies of the Southwest*. ** Santa Fe: Red Crane Books, 1990.

______________. *Medicinal Plants of the Pacific West*.** Sante Fe: Red Crane Books, 1993.

______________. *Medicinal Plants of the Desret and Canyon West*.** Santa Fe: Museum of New Mexico Press, 1989.

______________. *Medicinal Plants of the Mountain West*.** Santa Fe: Museum of New Mexico Press, 1979.

Moss, Ralph W. *Herbs Against Cancer: History and Controversy*.** Brooklyn: Equinox Press, Inc., 1998.

Mowry, Daniel B. *The Scientific Validation of Herbal Medicine**. New Canaan: Keats Publishing, 1998.

Murry, Michael T. *The Healing Power of Herbs*.*** Rocklin: Peima Publishing, 1995.

______________. *Natural Alternatives to Over-the-Counter and Prescription Drugs*. *** New York: William Morrow and Company, 1994.

Newall, Carol, Anderson, Linda, Phillipson, David. *Herbal Medicines: A Guide for Professionals**. London: Pharmaceutical Press, 1996.

Ody, Penelope. *The Complete Medicinal Herbal*.* London: Key Porter Books, 1993.

Patnaik, Naveen. *The Garden of Life: An Introduction to the Healing Plants of India*.* New York: Doubleday, 1996.

Polunin and Robbins. *The Natural Pharmacy.*** London: Dorling Kindersley, 1992.

Schulick Paul. *Ginger: Common Spice and Wonder Drug.* Brattleboro: Herbal Free Press Ltd, 1996.

Schulick, P, Newark, T. *Beyond Aspirin.*** Prescott: Hohm Press, 2000.

Schilcher, Heinz. *Phytotherapy in Paediatrics.** Stuttgart: Medpharm Scientific Publishers, 1997.

Schmidt, Micheal. *Childhood Ear Infections.**** Berkeley: North Atlantic Press, 1997.

Sherman, John A. *The Complete Botanical Prescriber.** John A. Sherman Press, 1993.

Stary, Frantisek. *The Natural Guide to Medicinal Herbs and Plants.** Prague: Aventinum, 1991.

Svoboda Robert. *Ayurveda for woman.* Devon: David and Charles, 1999.

Taylor L. Herbal *Secrets of the Rainforest.*** Rocklin: Prima Health, 1998.

Tierra, Michael. *Planetary Herbology.**** Twin Lakes: Lotus Press, 1992.

_______________.*The Way of Herbs.**** New York: Pocket Books, 1998.

Tobyn G. *Culpeper's Medicine: The Practice of Western Holistic Medicine.*** Rockport: Element Books, Inc., 1997.

Tyler, Varro. *Herbs of Choice.** Pharmaceutical Products Press, New York, 1994.

_____________. *The Honest Herbal.** Pharmaceutical Products Press, New York, 1994.

Vaughan, J. G., Geissler, C. and Nicholson B. E. *The New Oxford Book of Food Plants.*** Oxford: Oxford University Press, 1997.

Vermeulen N. *Encyclopedia of Herbs.*** Netherlands: Revo Productions, 1999.

Watt M. and Sellar W. *Frankincense and Myrrh.*** Esseex: CW Daniel Company Limited, 1996.

Weiner, Micheal and Janet. *Herbs That Heal.*** Mill Valley: Quantum Books, 1994.

Weiner, Michael. *Man's Useful Plants.** New York: Macmillan, 1976.

Weiss, Rudulph Fritz, *Herbal Medicine*, 6th edition.** Beaconsfield, England: Beaconsfield Publishers,

White L.B. and Foster S. *The Herbal Drugstore.** Emmaus: Rodale Press, 2000.

Willard, Terry. *Textbook of Advanced Herbology.*** Calary: Wild Rose College of Natural Healing, 1992.

Wood, Matthew. *The Book of Herbal Wisdom.**** Berkeley: North Atlantic Books, 1997.

_____________. *Vitalism: The History of Herbalism, Homeopathy and Flower Essences***. Berkeley: North Atlantic Books, 1992.

Yance, Donald R. *Herbal Medicine, Healing and Cancer.*** Chicago: Keats Publishing, 1999.

INDEX

A

C

D

E

F

J

K

L

M

N

O

P

Q

R

S

T

U

V

W

X

Y

Z

NOTES